MOSQUITOPIA

This edited volume brings together natural scientists, social scientists and humanists to assess if (or how) we may begin to coexist harmoniously with the mosquito. The mosquito is humanity's deadliest animal, killing over a million people each year by transmitting malaria, yellow fever, Zika and several other diseases. Yet of the 3,500 species of mosquito on Earth, only a few dozen of them are really dangerous—so that the question arises as to whether humans and their mosquito foe can learn to live peacefully with one another.

Chapters assess polarizing arguments for conserving and preserving mosquitoes, as well as for controlling and killing them, elaborating on possible consequences of both strategies. This book provides informed answers to the dual question: could we eliminate mosquitoes, and should we? Offering insights spanning the technical to the philosophical, this is the "go to" book for exploring humanity's many relationships with the mosquito—which becomes a journey to finding better ways to inhabit the natural world.

Mosquitopia will be of interest to anyone wanting to explore dependencies between human health and natural systems, while offering novel perspectives to health planners, medical experts, environmentalists and animal rights advocates.

Marcus Hall is an environmental historian and professor at the University of Zurich. In exploring changing human relationships with the natural world, Hall has turned to such subjects as restoring, rewilding, invasive species, warfare, earth art, chronobiology, malaria, and parasites. His books include *Earth Repair*, *Restoration and History*, *Crossing Mountains*, and (with Marco Armiero) *Nature and History in Modern Italy*.

Dan Tamïr is environmental historian and research associate at the University of Zurich. His research examines the global circulation and the local adaptations of ideologies, species and resources. His current research focuses on the global political cooperation in targeting mosquito-borne diseases during the past century.

The *Routledge Environmental Humanities* series is an original and inspiring venture recognising that today's world agricultural and water crises, ocean pollution and resource depletion, global warming from greenhouse gases, urban sprawl, over-population, food insecurity and environmental justice are all *crises of culture*.

The reality of understanding and finding adaptive solutions to our present and future environmental challenges has shifted the epicenter of environmental studies away from an exclusively scientific and technological framework to one that depends on the human-focused disciplines and ideas of the humanities and allied social sciences.

We thus welcome book proposals from all humanities and social sciences disciplines for an inclusive and interdisciplinary series. We favour manuscripts aimed at an international readership and written in a lively and accessible style. The readership comprises scholars and students from the humanities and social sciences and thoughtful readers concerned about the human dimensions of environmental change.

For more information about this series, please visit: www.routledge.com/Ro utledge-Environmental-Humanities/book-series/REH

MOSQUITOPIA

The Place of Pests in a Healthy World

Edited by
Marcus Hall and Dan Tamïr

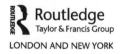
LONDON AND NEW YORK

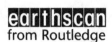
from Routledge

First published 2022
by Routledge
2 Park Square, Milton Park, Abingdon, Oxon OX14 4RN

and by Routledge
605 Third Avenue, New York, NY 10158

Routledge is an imprint of the Taylor & Francis Group, an informa business

British Library Cataloguing-in-Publication Data
A catalogue record for this book is available from the British Library

Library of Congress Cataloging-in-Publication Data
Names: Hall, Marcus, 1959–editor. | Tamïr, Dan, editor.
Title: Mosquitopia: the place of pests in a healthy world / edited by Marcus Hall and Dan Tamïr.
Description: Milton Park, Abingdon, Oxon; New York, NY: Routledge, 2022. | Series: Routledge environmental humanities | Includes bibliographical references and index.
Identifiers: LCCN 2021011825 (print) | LCCN 2021011826 (ebook)
Subjects: LCSH: Mosquitoes. | Mosquitoes–Control–Environmental aspects. | Mosquitoes as carriers of disease.
Classification: LCC QL536 .M696 2022 (print) | LCC QL536 (ebook) | DDC 595.77/2–dc23
LC record available at https://lccn.loc.gov/2021011825
LC ebook record available at https://lccn.loc.gov/2021011826

ISBN: 978-0-367-52011-3 (hbk)
ISBN: 978-0-367-52005-2 (pbk)
ISBN: 978-1-003-05603-4 (ebk)

Typeset in Bembo
by Deanta Global Publishing Services, Chennai, India

CONTENTS

FIGURES

CONTRIBUTORS

Tim Acott is a Reader in Human Geography at the University of Greenwich. His work focuses on understanding the social and cultural importance of natural resources including small-scale fisheries, wetlands and coastal environments. Tim specializes in thinking about the sense of place (with a particular emphasis on art and photography), cultural ecosystem services, social well-being, responsible tourism and co-constructionism.

Uli Beisel is Professor of Human Geography at the Free University of Berlin. She has worked on "mosquito–parasite–human entanglements" in malaria control in Ghana and Sierra Leone, and continues to be fascinated by practices of demarcation between human and non-human organisms, and the possibilities for their coexistence.

Sarah Chaney is an entomologist and mosquito enthusiast who does her bug-hunting and writing about public health, insects and vector-borne diseases from Quito, Ecuador. She has lived, worked and chased insects in the United States, Kenya, China and Argentina and is always striving to learn more about the intersection between human and insect behaviour.

Peter Coates is an environmental historian at the University of Bristol, UK, who has written books on subjects such as the Trans-Alaska Pipeline, attitudes to nature in the Western world, the salmon, invasive species, and rivers. Current interests include eels and the exploits of species from North America in Britain.

Isabelle Dusfour is research entomologist at the Institut Pasteur. She has worked on mosquito vectors in Southeast Asia and across the American continent. For ten years, she has addressed questions about vector control and insecticide resistance in

French Guiana (South America), developing an interest in the human components of these questions.

Adriana Ford is Centre Manager of the Leverhulme Centre for Wildfires, Environment and Society, at Imperial College London and King's College London. Her expertise lies in relationships between society and the environment, including attitudes and values, well-being, and sustainable development. Her research topics have included wildfires, wetlands, fisheries and coastal communities, invasive species, ecosystem services and community-based wildlife management.

Mary Gearey is a Senior Lecturer in Human Geography at the University of Brighton. A social scientist, she has worked globally with diverse communities and stakeholders in support of the integrity and sustainability of local water resources. Her research includes: community activism in response to changing water environments; renaturing cities through blue-green infrastructure; articulations of human and more-than-human relationships within wetland environments.

Marcus Hall is an environmental historian and professor at the University of Zurich. In exploring changing human relationships with the natural world, Hall has turned to such subjects as restoring, rewilding, invasive species, warfare, earth art, chronobiology, malaria and parasites. His books include *Earth Repair, Restoration and History, Crossing Mountains,* and (with Marco Armiero) *Nature and History in Modern Italy.*

Frances Hawkes is a Senior Research Fellow at the Natural Resources Institute, University of Greenwich. Incorporating laboratory and field-based studies on mosquito behaviour and ecology, her research spans temperate and tropical species, identifying traits that can be exploited in supporting vector control. Her work developing new mosquito surveillance techniques was recognized in a 2019 Queen's Anniversary Prize for smart and sustainable pest management.

Richard Hopkins is Professor of Behavioural Entomology at the Natural Resources Institute, University of Greenwich. His research involves the study of the searching behaviour of crop pests and vectors of diseases in temperate and tropical regions. A particular interest in piecing together the different aspects of how mosquitoes locate breeding and resting sites reflects the importance of understanding the ecology of vectors in the wider sense, and contributed to the award of the 2019 Queen's Anniversary Prize for smart and sustainable pest management to NRI.

Ashwani Kumar is Director of the ICMR-Vector Control Research Centre, Puducherry, India and adjunct Professor of Georgetown University, USA. Dr Kumar has over 33 years of experience in the field of vector-borne diseases, publishing some 127 articles and four books, including the WHO handbook *Vector Surveillance and Control at Points of Entry.* He is advisor to the WHO's "Vector Control Advisory

Group" and President of the World Mosquito Control Association and Society for Vector Ecology (Indian region).

Helmut Lemke is a sound artist. Through creative, deep engagement with more-than-human elements of environments he explores and uncovers connections. Thus Lemke aims to communicate alternative strategies of experience and acceptance.

Kerry Morrison is an independent artist, researcher and creative producer. Merging social art practice with ecology and embedded, responsive processes that build relationships and collaborative working, Kerry nurtures into existence art and co-creations that address environmental issues and discourse.

Clifford Mutero is an entomologist based at the International Centre of Insect Physiology and Ecology, Nairobi. He currently coordinates research on integrated vector management for malaria control while also serving as an Extraordinary Professor with the School of Health Systems and Public Health, University of Pretoria, South Africa. He has authored an autobiography entitled *Mosquito Hunter: Chronicles of an African Insect Scientist.*

Alex Nading is Associate Professor of Anthropology at Cornell University. He is the author of *Mosquito Trails: Ecology, Health, and the Politics of Entanglement* (University of California Press, 2014), and he is the editor of the journal *Medical Anthropology Quarterly.*

Ramya M. Rajagopalan is a research scientist at the Institute of Practical Ethics, University of California, San Diego. She uses ethnographic and archival methods to examine the social impacts of genome technologies and big data in biomedicine. Her current projects investigate ethical issues in genome editing and gene drive, and the impact of emerging tools in precision medicine understandings of race and health care practices.

Jean Segata is a social anthropologist. He is an Associate Professor in the Department of Anthropology at the Federal University of Rio Grande do Sul (Brazil) where he is the director of the NEAAT – Centre for Animal, Environmental and Technology Studies, and the COVID-19 Humanities MCTI Network. His teaching and researching experiences intersect multi-species and environmental health and anthropology of science and technology.

Frederic Simard is an expert in vector biology and control at the Institut de Recherche pour le Développement (IRD) in Montpellier, France. He has spent 15 years in tropical Africa exploring the population biology, ecology and genetics of major mosquito disease vectors. Bridging field and lab studies, medical entomology and evolution, he has explored issues related to mosquito adaptation to their environment, speciation and disease transmission.

Nancy Leys Stepan is Professor Emerita of History at Columbia University, New York. Previously she was Senior Research Fellow at the Wellcome Unit for the History of Medicine at the University of Oxford. Her books include *The Hour of Eugenics: Race, Gender, and Nation in Latin America*, and *Eradication: Ridding the World of Diseases Forever?*

Willem Takken is a medical entomologist and Professor Emeritus at Wageningen University & Research, Wageningen, the Netherlands. He has worked on alternative strategies for malaria control, with emphasis on behavioural manipulation of malaria vectors. Much of his work was conducted in endemic malaria settings. As advisor to the WHO, he participated in the development of the Global Vector Control Response.

Dan Tamïr is environmental historian and a research associate at the University of Zurich. His research examines the global circulation and the local adaptations of ideologies, species and resources. His current research focuses on the global political cooperation in targeting mosquito-borne diseases during the past century.

Indra Vythilingam is a Professor at the Department of Parasitology, University of Malaya. Her work involves the bionomics of mosquitoes of medical importance. Her early works were on vectors of human malaria but of late she has switched to studying mosquitoes biting both humans and macaques. With respect to dengue, she and her team work on proactive measures to inform the public before cases occur.

James L.A. Webb, Jr. is Professor Emeritus of History at Colby College. His research is in the field of the historical epidemiology of contemporary disease challenges. His recent books include *The Long Struggle Against Malaria in Tropical Africa* (Cambridge, 2014) and *The Guts of the Matter: A Global History of Human Waste and Infectious Intestinal Disease* (Cambridge, 2020).

Carsten Wergin is Associate Professor of Anthropology at Ruprecht-Karls-University Heidelberg. His research is located at the intersections of heritage, culture and ecology with regional foci in the Mascarene Archipelago, Northwest Australia, and the wider Indian Ocean World.

Anna Wienhues is a postdoctoral researcher at the Department of Philosophy and affiliated with the University Research Priority Programme Global Change and Biodiversity of the University of Zurich, Switzerland. Her work focuses on environmental ethics and green political theory. She is the author of *Ecological Justice and the Extinction Crisis: Giving Living Beings their Due* (Bristol University Press, 2020).

Urmi Engineer Willoughby is an Assistant Professor of History at Pitzer College. She was the 2019–2020 Molina Fellow in the History of Medicine and Allied Sciences at the Huntington Library. Her first book, *Yellow Fever, Race, and Ecology in Nineteenth-Century New Orleans* (Louisiana State University Press, 2017) was awarded the 2017 Williams Prize for the best book in Louisiana history.

FOREWORD

Clifford Mutero

Imagine a world without mosquitoes. They have all died. Everywhere. It would be an easy thing to envision, because most people consider them too dangerous for health, and a great nuisance due to their irritating whine. Now imagine there were no lions, not even in the zoo. This starts to sound sad and scary, doesn't it—as though human beings will be next on the list? But why does one feel that way about lions but not mosquitoes? After all, both are dangerous animals. Both view people as food.

I borrow the poetic opening to this foreword from John Lennon's 1971 iconic song "Imagine." Songs are powerful in giving us words with which to express thoughts about issues that may initially appear simple but which are, upon closer scrutiny, complex and could benefit from an external dose of inspiration. The songs that work for me are from the 1960s and 1970s eras, the kind you can whistle during your morning shower. That very song, "Imagine," provided the backdrop to my thoughts as I grappled with the scenario of the world being inhabited peacefully by mosquitoes and people when the editors of *Mosquitopia* approached me to write a foreword for this book. From the initial description of the multi-author chapters envisaged here, it was clear that there were no easy answers to the mosquito question. As one who has spent more than half of his life conducting research into mosquito-related issues, my informed position is that it is all about setting boundaries: dealing with mosquitoes is no different than how we address other human—wildlife conflicts, assuming that one can even imagine mosquitoes to be an integral part of wildlife!

Coming from Nairobi, I should know something about human—wildlife conflict; ours is the only city in the world to have a real national park within the city boundaries. Occasionally a stray lion escapes and will be spotted outside the confines of the park fence. The sighting sends equal ripples of excitement and panic through the adjacent residential area and across the city, until our well-trained game rangers spring into action and manage to divert the beast back into the park, with or without a little help from a tranquillizer dart. And just like that, the drama is over. All is quiet again, until the next big escape, which occasionally ends in the dispatching of the feline to the next world, thanks to a fatal shot from the rifle of an overzealous rookie ranger. From prehistoric times, people have proactively attempted and learned to manage the lion and keep it in its place. As Keith Somerville explains eloquently in his *Humans and Lions* (2019), another volume in the Routledge Environmental Humanities Series, proper lion management helps to keep the peace. And therein lies the explanation about why we would feel sad if all the lions were to die, while no such emotion manifests itself when we contemplate mosquitoes disappearing for good, overnight.

In contrast to the case of lions and other big game, researchers and society at large have failed to engage proactive approaches to keeping mosquitoes at bay via simple management methods. Lions for their part are kept away from humans by respecting and allocating them their space, delineated with the occasional length of electric fencing where necessary. In the case of mosquitoes, people have access to various means with which they could fence *themselves* in. Bed nets, mosquito-proof screens on house eaves and windows and doors, or the occasional topical repellent are all available at no significant cost. In settled areas considered no-go zones for mosquitoes, people could also push mosquitoes back to the jungle, to cohabit with lions and other wildlife by denying them breeding grounds around human habitations. No-go zones could be accomplished by ensuring that stagnant water habitats are unavailable for egg-laying. A range of insecticide-free tactics such as drainage, tight-fitting lids for domestic water containers, or the introduction of predators such as fish in open ponds can be employed. The list of possibilities certainly does not end there, for one might rely on any of several forms of environmental management or manipulation. Suffice it to say, the knowledge has been gathered over the decades, but decisive action is far below the threshold required to show mosquitoes their place. Researchers often resort to the argument that mosquitoes have co-evolved to live with humans for millennia; it would be difficult to change this narrative. Furthermore, we typically prefer to take the easy way out when we hear that irritating whining sound: grabbing a can of insecticidal spray and aiming short bursts at the tiny vampires as they flit about. I would not be surprised to hear that someone even sprayed a bit of insecticidal killer while reading Rachel Carson's *Silent Spring* (1962), the landmark book about people's fatal attraction to insecticides and the consequent scenario of a world without birdsong—if that knee-jerk trend for eliminating mosquitoes prevailed.

The pitch of my plot so far is that people and wildlife *can* coexist peacefully, and in a mutually beneficial way. Among the local communities where I come from, the term wildlife often connotes the big game animals capable of eating human beings alive or trampling them to death in a matter of seconds. Along with lions, leopards and hyenas rank high in the man-eating category while elephants, rhinos and buffalo are viewed as the big tramplers. Hippos are capable of both; their enormous bite often kills, and they are pretty good at stomping, too. Snakes are in a special category all of their own, feared by both humans and beasts. Ironically, as noted above, mosquitoes are hardly ever featured as wildlife, until one comes across a popular graphical representation from a 2014 blog by Bill Gates depicting the mosquito as "The deadliest animal in the world."

Even one and a quarter centuries after mosquitoes were discovered as the spreaders of several of the most deadly diseases known to humans, such as malaria, managing mosquitoes using the most basic and safe approaches has been largely all talk, some action and very little learned in terms of how to sustain momentum. It is as though the research community and society at large resist the truism that mosquitoes can be effectively managed with incredibly simple and commonplace approaches.

Intentional forestalling of potential conflict has come to be accepted as the best practice for human-wildlife co-existence, with expected mutual benefits for people and environmental conservation. Virtually all people on the planet are aware of the various benefits human beings derive from the natural environment, be they in relation to food, water, building materials and the entire range of other resources and ecosystem services that contribute to people's health and well-being. But visceral fear and phobias are also commonplace among people with regard to the many potential dangers lurking in the wild, especially in the form of large carnivores and snakes. Consequently, peaceful and fulfilled coexistence is difficult to imagine without a red line being deliberately drawn by human beings to separate humans from wildlife. The delineation is also made by the natural environment itself, when the feeling of "trespassers will be eaten" hits a crescendo of goosebumps as we venture to explore the wild side. Failure to respect such red lines can only lead to dire consequences for the human race.

A key take-home point from the foregoing is that mosquitoes belong to wildlife. Period. For this reason alone, there ought to be that red line limiting their flirtation with people. Assuming this argument holds water, our mindsets then need to change, to be able to view mosquitoes as wildlife, with a right to exist, just as do lions, seal pups, pandas and polar bears. Should mosquitoes breach the protective barriers we set for ourselves, we could for a time allow these beautiful creatures with highly sophisticated mouthparts to draw the small amount of blood they need to develop a batch of eggs; at least until we ramp up environmental management measures that can drive these critters back to the wild. If mosquitoes are denied access to human habitations, they will over time learn to spend the rest of their lives in the wild, participating in the food web shenanigans that characterize all of nature's biodiverse fauna and flora. The human-mosquito relationship could be that of live and let live, achievable through an ecosystem management approach that ensures both human health and well-being, and the health of our ecosystems.

Way back in 1976, I somehow figured we should not be too quick to reach for the insecticide spray can when mosquitoes come calling after listening to the late Professor Thomas Odhiambo, a renowned Kenyan entomologist and environmentalist, who delivered an exhilarating lecture about "anophelism without malaria." As an undergraduate student and budding entomologist, I had keenly hung on Prof Odhiambo's every word since he was the founder and Director of the International Centre of Insect Physiology and Ecology (ICIPE) in Nairobi. The lecture focused on the nascent scientific revelations about the existence of *An. maculipennis* as a species complex. Before there was knowledge about the occurrence of sibling species and their attendant vectorial capacities, it was a mystery why malaria was absent in parts of Europe where the mosquito species complex existed. Of course, we are now aware that malaria's scarcity arose because certain sibling species found in such areas were inefficient vectors of the disease. Odhiambo's lecture opened my eyes to the reality that we do not need to kill every mosquito in sight, and certainly not with insecticides that are potentially harmful to human health and to non-target organisms. His follow-up lecture dwelt at length on the insecticidal horrors highlighted in Carson's *Silent Spring*. Many years later, I came to appreciate Odhiambo's and Carson's views even more while conducting malaria research in a rice-irrigation scheme in central Kenya. In this setting, malaria habitually affected people on a seasonal basis up to about 2006. After this, malaria declined to non-detectable levels, suggesting local elimination of the disease. And the population of *Anopheles arabiensis*, a well-known vector of malaria in most of Africa, never declined in the rice-irrigation scheme. This mosquito continues to thrive to this day and hundreds of them can still be collected as they rest during the day inside a single unprotected house, having either fed on people indoors or outdoors, or on cattle. Yet locally transmitted malaria cases are a thing of the past, at least as of the last time I checked in 2018.

The question therefore is, would it still be necessary to eliminate mosquitoes in settings where there is no current evidence of mosquito-borne diseases and no strong predicters for the emergence or re-emergence of these maladies? I am more inclined to think that unless a situation is forecast to lead to a definite outbreak of disease, anti-mosquito activities should be strictly ecologically friendly and aimed mainly at minimising—not eradicating—the biting nuisance in situations where mosquitoes are attacking people near human habitations and during social gatherings. Deviations and exemptions to this rule should be for short periods only. Mosquito control products should be re-evaluated regularly for their effectiveness and assessed for unintended or known negative impacts on the health of people and their environments, including those products that eliminate Chironomid larvae, thereby denying food to many fish species. Entomological surveillance should nonetheless continue to be an essential means of determining whether parasites and viruses are circulating in a residual mosquito population, a practice that will promote environmentally benign mosquito control efforts in a time-bound and cost-effective manner.

A preoccupation with eliminating mosquitoes with expensive frontier technology in settings devoid of evidence of the diseases they transmit may be a luxury—and an unjustified way of spending limited resources which could be more meaningfully diverted to stocking health facilities with medications for emergency cases, or helping strengthen health systems in general. Pre-emptive strikes could be analogous to game rangers, accompanied by community members, invading the national park to kill the lions and green mambas just in case they escaped their confines and harmed innocent people. True, mosquitoes may be different because some of them have become used to living in domestic habitats and won't leave people alone without a bite, not to mention their high nuisance value certainly linked to their annoying buzz! But these bothers are not strong enough reasons to pander to people's whims by running mosquitoes out of town at whatever cost.

I believe many of these views are articulated in clearer and more detailed ways in the chapters of this volume. If the reader has misgivings, I recommend reading *Mosquitopia* alongside my own *Mosquito Hunter* (2017). Both are insightful and informative in their own ways, not only about mosquitoes but also about the much wider natural world of which we are all a part of. Learning to live with our pests and with our enemies is the only way the world will truly be as one.

Bibliography

Carson, Rachel. 1962. *Silent Spring*. Boston: Houghton Mifflin.

Gates, Bill. 2014. The deadliest animal in the world. *GatesNotes: The Blog of Bill Gates*, 25 April at https://www.gatesnotes.com/health/most-lethal-animal-mosquito-week on 15.02.2021.

Mutero, Clifford. 2017. *Mosquito Hunter: Chronicles of an African Insect Scientist*. Bloomington: AuthorHouse.

Somerville, Keith. 2019. *Humans and Lions: Conflict, Conservation and Coexistence*. London: Routledge Series in Environmental Humanities.

PART I

Could we (should we) eliminate mosquitoes?

1

KILLING MOSQUITOES

Think before you swat

Marcus Hall and Dan Tamïr

> Am I not mosquito enough to out-mosquito you?
> —D.H. Lawrence, "The Mosquito" (1920)

Global warming is ushering us into a new mosquito epoch. Ready or not, mosquitoes are coming faster than before, both indigenous and non-, human-biting and not, disease-carrying and sometimes–disease-carrying. What are we to do with these buzzing creatures, and what has been done with them so far? Usually perceived as a pest or at least as a nuisance, their mere presence often prompts us to take action. Are we able to control, or locally exterminate them, and with what side effects? Or is it more realistic to admit that the three most threatening mosquito genera—the disease carrying *Aedes*, *Anopheles* and *Culex*—are really controlling us? In recent years, yellow fever has kept spreading even as malaria has been retreating, but over half of the world's population is still exposed to these and other dangerous mosquito-carried diseases which also include dengue, West Nile, chikungunya and Zika. Control them we should; we must do, if we are to avoid the next pandemic and survive our mosquito-borne Anthropocene. COVID-19 has been humanity's latest collective horror, but across deep time, and likely into the foreseeable future, mosquitoes will be responsible for inflicting incalculably greater degrees of suffering and anguish.

But there are important reasons to protect mosquitoes, and not just because these creatures are amazing products of millions of years of evolution—since protecting them may in some instances assist us in the battle against various human diseases. Most obviously, we may want to save some mosquitoes for the simple reason that one needs to preserve a few of them in order to figure out how to kill the rest of them—with other practical reasons detailed below. Yet more subtle justifications for saving mosquitoes centre, for instance, on food web dynamics, whereby in our efforts to poison these creatures, or disrupt their

DOI: 10.4324/9781003056034-1

habitat, or rearrange their DNA, we may, through ecological loops, actually cause damage to other biological entities, such as mosquito predators, and end up *increasing* a mosquito's fitness and its ability to multiply and spread across the earth. Perhaps the sciences of mosquito control, or certain sectors of them, have not yet advanced to a stage that we can trust.

Some years ago, *Nature* journalist Janet Fang posed the simple but powerful question about what the ecological consequences might be of eradicating mosquitoes (Fang 2010). A concerted campaign across the twentieth and twenty-first centuries, after all, has been dedicated to this very goal. In sifting through the evidence, Fang's final answer is that in the case of this blood-sucking insect, humanity and even ecosystems could probably get along just fine without it. She reports on the views of one ecologist who feels that mosquitoes could readily be replaced in the food web, with many mosquito predators eventually able to switch to moths or houseflies or other sources of food. Although she outlines a host of possible disruptions stemming from the disappearance of mosquitoes, such as the loss of their pollination activities and other ecosystem services, she concludes by quoting entomologist Joe Conlon who believes that ecosystems "will hiccup and then get on with life. Something better or worse would take over." Or as Conlon elaborates in his own blog, "I would rather eat raw onions and celery for the rest of my life if I could do away with the little bastards" (Conlon 2011).

In these introductory pages we highlight some of the main arguments for saving mosquitoes, before reminding ourselves of vital reasons for setting out to control and eradicate them. Ours is not a comprehensive list, and our main goal here is to stimulate readers to begin thinking about the many reasons for saving or else exterminating these creatures, while outlining some pressing points that will be taken up in subsequent chapters. Confronting this question of how far we can, or should, pursue the goal of mosquito elimination is our central purpose of this book, seeing if there may be a kind of peaceful coexistence that we can achieve with these creatures. In the end, rather than pushing an ultimatum that it must be us or them, can humanity promote and practice a kind of "Mosquitopia" with these little humming creatures, humanity's most dangerous companions? Could we develop a relationship with this insect that will allow healthy cohabitation?

The project of searching for and identifying a possible harmonious coexistence involving humans and mosquitoes has implications for the lives and lifestyles of many millions of people affected by mosquito-borne pathogens. But it also becomes a crucial test case for identifying the proper place of people in the natural world. Although mosquitoes are amongst the most intimate of animals accompanying humanity across millennia, similar questions may be asked about scores of other species, including such charismatic ones as bears, dolphins, rhinos and orangutans, whose prospects are shaky, to say the least. The majority of human–animal interactions, as well as the greater part of the sixth species extinction crisis we are experiencing, involve many smaller jewels in the treasure box of creation. The mosquito then becomes one example, and an emblematic one to start with.

Some reasons for saving mosquitoes

The first reason for making our truce with mosquitoes is *strategic*. We must remind ourselves that we are ultimately battling diseases, not mosquitoes, and that there may be more effective, more economical, and more ethical ways to do this than killing that little, ubiquitous insect. Malaria, for instance, once emanated from swamps and the bad air they produced, although with more evidence it became clear that mosquitoes, rather than effluvia, were the vectors (or transmitters) of the malaria parasite. Should we be putting greater efforts into battling this microscopic *Plasmodium* rather than the carriers of them, as by developing more effective malaria drugs? Or should we be focusing at still-smaller levels, as by managing the chemical reactions set in motion by the *Plasmodium*, or else by treating the resulting symptoms, to let the body take care of itself? Two generations ago, zoologist Marston Bates considered the use of the powerful insecticide, DDT, to be the "sledge hammer approach to mosquito control" since this chemical caused so much collateral damage to other living things, from birds and fish to desirable insects such as bees (Bates 1953). An early anti-malarial medication such as Atabrine was itself a sledge hammer approach in the human bloodstream, since people often felt quite nauseous after taking it. With the ecological knowledge accumulated and the microbiological techniques developed since then, isn't it more realistic to see all population-level control techniques, whether applied to wetlands or to human bodies, as sledge hammers? And as our understanding of mosquito-borne diseases becomes more precise and accurate, the surgical response of today may seem like a sledge hammer tomorrow.

Eradicating any of the mosquito-borne diseases may therefore necessitate the extermination not of mosquitoes, but of the pathogens themselves. The malariologists' phrase of "anophelism without malaria" (or, the presence of anopheles mosquitoes without malaria) is known in many countries where the disease practically disappeared decades ago. Notwithstanding the differences in ecologies of other vectors and their transmission mechanisms, can we aim at parallel situations of "aedeism without dengue" or "culexism without West Nile"? The distancing of a pathogen from a human population—and even its total elimination—may be less challenging and less problematic than insect eradication. Because there are pros and cons to every health remedy, we need to return to ecological principles as well as cost–benefit analyses, before marching forward with any one strategy for disease control.

A second justification for preserving mosquitoes centres on *medical* reasoning. Modern epidemiological research reveals that there may be important benefits to maintaining discrete, residual levels of pathogens in a population so as to maintain immunological signals that our bodies can react to and maintain resistance against. Madagascar provides a telling example: when malaria was largely eradicated from parts of that large island between 1960 and 1980, it returned there several years later with more deadly virulence. Maintaining some mosquitoes there, and with them the diseases they transmit, means that human physiologies would not become naively adapted to an environment only temporarily free of this or that disease (Carter and Mendis 2002). A related issue is that certain kinds of less dangerous malaria can provide a degree of protection from more dangerous forms of it: a person infected by *Plasmodium vivax* is often given some resistance against being infected by the more lethal *Plasmodium falciparum* (Snounou and White 2004). In this case, a normal, mosquito-transmitted *vivax* malaria can be the lesser evil of contracting *falciparum* malaria.

There are also important *ecological* reasons for keeping mosquitoes buzzing, based on arguments pointing to the special role of these arthropods in ecosystems. Metric tons of flying biomass certainly alter natural processes, whether as foodstuff for other organisms or as modifiers of animal behaviour, as in the case of caribou and *Homo sapiens* who move or migrate to avoid them. Enormous numbers of friendly insects fall victim to the many projects of mosquito control (Török et al. 2020). Mosquitoes carry parasites and pathogens, not only to humans, but also to many other mammals, birds and reptiles. Microbes transmitted by mosquitoes to bats help control the numbers of the latter, thereby controlling the human diseases spread by these winged mammals. Moreover, it is only female mosquitoes that transmit pathogens by feeding on blood while their male counterparts generally subsist innocuously on plant nectars. Some mosquitoes even control other species of mosquitoes, since certain adult species feed on larvae of other species (Roux and Robert 2019). These mosquito-borne benefits are a sampling of reasons for maintaining at least some mosquitoes in ecosystems, or else bringing many of them back if drastically reduced.

Yet another rationale for saving mosquitoes is the *evolutionary* one. As an example, parasites and hosts coevolve, sometimes with beneficial results for both, since both members in such relationships generally become more tolerant of the other through time. Or at least this is the argument of Nobel laureate Joshua Lederberg for why the virulence of parasites can diminish over decades and centuries (Méthot 2012). Cautious hands-off approaches to vector control therefore allow nature to take its course, with harmful results balanced increasingly by beneficial ones over the longer run. There appear to be indispensable long-term roles for many of our bodily symbionts, and human acts of interference in their transmission may, over the short or long term, cause more harm than good.

From a more cognitive perspective, we may identify *ethical* reasons for leaving mosquitoes alone. Do humans have the right to kill or exterminate other creatures—or the right to transform or disrupt whole ecosystems? Is it justifiable to exterminate when we are still quite unsure how the many parts of an ecosystem fit together? If we are placing humans at the top of the pyramid of creation, what does that tell us about ourselves and our place in the future? To date, we have never been able to rid islands or continents of mosquitoes despite dogged efforts to do so—or at least not for very long: what makes us believe we can exterminate them now? More often than not, hubris has been the rule, not the exception, in describing humanity's attitude towards managing the non-human world. The question of eliminating mosquitoes should not be undertaken while being detached from wider global and environmental contexts. Our current and ongoing sixth mass extinction episode is gathering force, already eliminating thousands of species, while impoverishing the biosphere and annihilating millions of years of evolution. Such dramatic changes carry with them exceptional uncertainty, notably as potential adverse repercussions, be they ecological, political and/or economic. A key general guideline is the precautionary principle which may be phrased: "in case of doubt, stop." Such precautions may be more applicable to biodiversity preservation than to almost any other environmental problem (Myers 1993).

The scope of the extinction crisis may contribute to a notion of helplessness, by assuming that the saving of a few species of insects is a marginal concern that would not change much. Yet the severity of the crisis may pose a super-premium on applying the precautionary principle even more broadly: the burden of proof is on those aiming at eradication—call it deliberate extinction. As in so many other issues, a decent portion of modesty is a key strategy for making the right decision.

And yet—is it even thinkable that humans can propose a moral justification for *not* seeking every means possible to curtail or eliminate disease-spreading organisms? Is it ethically responsible to pay so much attention to insects and their needs when humans are made sick by them, and even die? Can it be advisable, or right, to rely on expert opinion, when the individuals directly affected by anti-mosquito treatments hold different viewpoints? Involving local communities in decisions about the tactics and timing of mosquito control is a relatively new recommendation of pest-control agencies.

From an *economic* perspective, millions of Euros and thousands of researchers are now dedicated to finding more effective vector control. In terms of spending efficiency, should these limited resources be diverted to other measures, such as bed nets, tighter houses, better equipped hospitals, and health education? Mosquito control is one of many health measures, and may merit lesser priority depending on circumstance or period. Yet another economic issue focuses on the potential utility of mosquitoes to industry or science; for example, mosquitoes can detect minuscule quantities of carbon dioxide, and produce amazing anti-coagulants, with both traits suggesting entrepreneurial opportunities unless these are curtailed by exterminators.

Last but not least is the *aesthetic* dimension of mosquitoes. Insects in general, and mosquitoes in particular, are exquisitely engineered organisms, supremely adapted to their various roles, and elegantly effective in carrying them out. We cannot help but admire them, even paint them, sculpt them, and remark on their carefully tuned soundscapes. Mosquitoes manage to pair with each other by matching the frequencies of their beating wings, so that sound artists can amplify and project these harmonic vibrations to demonstrate this insect's underappreciated acoustic attributes (Borrell 2009, BBC News 2013). Even with all the harm these insects cause, they are also beautiful, inspiring creatures. Of course, beauty by itself cannot be a justification for sparing harbingers of disease; but it should certainly prompt us, at the very least, to ponder saving rather than squishing these little humming beasts.

Key reasons for killing mosquitoes

Of course, beyond the many motives and justifications for protecting mosquitoes, there are also urgent reasons for ridding ourselves and the planet of these creatures. The list here is shorter, but may be just as powerful. The first and obvious reason is *human health*. Despite reasons for saving mosquitoes some of the time, or at least saving certain mosquitoes under certain situations, there remains a dire need to eradicate the disease-carrying varieties, utilizing even extreme measures to accomplish this goal—since the mosquito may be humanity's deadliest foe (Spielman and D'Antonio 2001, Winegard 2019). A crucial reason why some mosquito-borne diseases are not more pervasive today than in past decades, at least in some regions, is that former mosquito controllers were reasonably successful in their missions, bringing mosquito numbers down long enough so that the pathogenic virus, bacteria and protozoa they carried dropped below dangerous threshold levels. Although the percentages of people contracting malaria around the world are lower today than ever before, outbreaks of dengue and yellow fever are more serious in many areas than they were a decade or two ago (Mosquito Reviews 2020, WHO 2014, Jones 2012). We must assume that pandemics of mosquito-borne diseases could be brought into better control by intensifying the many anti-mosquito campaigns being waged around the world.

A second and related reason for stepping up mosquito control centres on *practical* motives: the project of exterminating mosquitoes allows us to avoid other, undesirable health or economic side-effects of dealing with these diseases, such as ingesting nauseating medications or diverting resources away from other pressing social issues. A case in point is when malaria-exposed soldiers and civilians during World War II avoided taking their prophylactic quinine or Atabrine because of the sickening side effects of this drug (Hall 2010). Finding a magic bullet that removes mosquitoes from ecosystems may therefore have ulterior beneficial consequences beyond curtailing disease, including the ability to redirect healthcare to combat other illnesses. Systematic sterilization of mosquitoes might allow wetlands to remain wet, for example, since draining them would no longer be required to disrupt mosquito habitat.

The control of mosquitoes might also be justified through a consideration of striving for better *ecosystem management*. Our human-altered biosphere means that mosquito numbers and their distribution are no longer natural, no longer in balance, so that human action is required to bring those balances into better harmony.

After all, today's abundance of mosquitoes and their accompanying pathogens can be traced in part to human agency. Since irrigation projects, say, or water-filled containers and discarded car tyres have favoured mosquito breeding in many parts of the world, then we can be better justified in seeking ways to diminish mosquito numbers. Here, Stewart Brand's dictum that "We are as Gods, and may as well get used to it" holds true for mosquito management (Brand 1968).

In a related issue, it seems appropriate in the context of human–mosquito relations to mention the *Anthropocene*: the current geological era in which *Homo sapiens* is modifying the entire planet. No place on earth has been spared by our alteration of ecosystems and our movement of creatures, with mosquitoes being part of that trend. The long coexistence of humans and mosquitoes made it only natural that we bring our winged companions with us across oceans and continents, while setting the table for them and preparing comfortable breeding sites (Kennedy and Lucks 1999, Boomgard and 't Hart 2010). After Europeans settled in certain areas of coastal South Africa, for instance, mosquito swarms arose where they were once rare: one explanation is that newly erected metal roofs on houses concentrated rainfall into puddles, thereby multiplying mosquito habitat and so mosquito-borne disease. A rational human response would therefore aim at resetting environmental equilibria, seeking to shrink mosquito habitat there. Such an argument could be used for justifying efforts to exterminate invasive alien Asian Tiger mosquitoes (*Aedes albopictus*) that never used to buzz across the Americas and across Europe before being introduced there by humans, but are now propagating at least 20 threatening diseases in these continents (Bhaumik 2013). Altering stream ecology by introducing alien Gambusia fish for slurping up mosquito larvae, as has already been carried out in many areas of the world beyond their native North America, may be part of the necessary quest to re-engineer the earth.

In a different light, there are also strong justifications for killing mosquitoes from the perspective of *economic development*. Poverty levels tend to worsen in a malarial environment, for instance, but evidence is inconclusive about whether mosquito-borne diseases are causes or effects of this impoverishment. While some experts claim that malaria blocks a country's economic development to result in poverty (Gallup and Sachs 2001), others assert that it is the continuous and deep impoverishment in communities that fosters the spread of malaria (Packard 2007). The effects of disease on development may hinder globalization, polarize private and public sectors, and disrupt international trade. The project of killing mosquitoes can be a catalyst for escorting a nation out of dependency.

A last-but-not-least reason for exterminating mosquitoes is *human comfort*. Pesky and nuisance mosquitoes drive people inside or away from their favourite places. In areas where mosquito-borne diseases are not a threat, the act of removing these bloodthirsty insects would still seem a good reason to continue funding mosquito-control agencies. After all, clearing mosquito swarms allows other organisms easier access to their grounds, including humans. Coastal wetlands, as in New Jersey, were virtually uninhabitable until early-twentieth-century drainage measures decimated mosquito populations and brought up land values (Patterson 2009). There is also evidence predicting that mosquitoes that currently do not feed on people may, with climate change or other stressors, develop a preference for human blood to then transmit the pathogens they carry (Rose et al. 2020). So, yes, even when the level of nuisance is "bearable," the physical and mental well-being of humans cannot be ignored, especially if we want to mobilize fellow men and women to confront other environmental and health challenges.

The case for killing mosquitoes here, or conserving them there, therefore goes to the core of what it means to be human in the natural world. The above points offer just a sampling of reasons for supporting either side of the question about what should be done with these biting insects—and certainly there are many other reasons to be added. The following chapters take up these reasons, expanding them while suggesting still other areas that need to be addressed. How we interact with, show mercy for, declare war on, or learn to live with our most dangerous game becomes a parable of our future on this planet. "I do favor insect control in appropriate situations," the great naturalist Rachel Carson once declared, even if the question that obsessed her to the end of her days was "whether any civilization can wage relentless war on life without destroying itself, and without losing the right to be called civilized" (Carson 1962a, 1962b). Mosquitoes present us with a supreme case for identifying ways to simultaneously promote people and pests on the same earth. A "Mosquitopia" is therefore a balanced relationship between ourselves and our main insect adversary that can permit us to both survive and prosper into the next epoch. Acknowledging the benefits and rights of our pathogens, parasites and predators (large and small), and then adjusting our lives and lifestyles to make room for them, is the pathway to a better existence.

What is in this volume

The book you are holding includes five parts for exploring the general question of whether we could, or should, eliminate mosquitoes. A vast experience demonstrates that insect controllers have been able to eliminate some mosquitoes, in some places, some of the time, but they have never been able to eliminate them completely to finally achieve species eradication. To date, the eradication of a pest has been achieved for only two microbial creatures, these being the viruses that cause smallpox and rinderpest—and only a few laboratory samples of such viruses survive to this day. Yet in the case of mosquitoes, we need to ask whether we could ever manage to eradicate this creature, and just as importantly, whether we would want to see this creature disappear forever. Even if eradicators and controllers focus their efforts on just a handful of the deadliest of some 3,500 mosquito species, as several authors maintain in the following chapters, we still need to ask hard questions: are the resources dedicated to their elimination better diverted to other health projects; are the inevitable collateral damages of the battle worth the cost; and are we ever able to know what is best for the earth's ecosystems? Even the project of pest *control*, as the first step toward pest *eradication*, requires us to think hard about resource allocation, collateral harm and the limits of our human abilities.

The book's first part prepares the reader for subsequent chapters by including essential information about the mosquito, its habits and traits—especially those related to its often painful encounters with humans. Here the reader can ponder examples of the intricate and elaborate ways in which humans and mosquitoes interact and the manners in which their life paths are intertwined. Even entomologists and anthropologists will find new ideas here that will help them reflect on the rest of the book. The second part is historical in character, drawing attention to past case studies and experiences. These mosquito stories stretch from Africa to England, from North America to Malaysia, spanning zones tropical to temperate; from distant eons of prehistory to the twenty-first century. This is not an attempt at compiling a comprehensive social or environmental history of mosquitoes; rather, this retrospective part presents examples of evidence and experience for elucidating issues worth considering when thinking about and dealing with mosquitoes today.

The book's third part centres on what can be termed (not without some provocation) "the enemy" and our perception of it as such. Beyond the obvious view of the mosquito as humanity's clear and present danger, this part challenges that view. How deeply are we committed to mosquito-as-adversary, and what may be done to alter that perspective? This buzzing insect feeding on blood may be *anthropophilic* (human-loving), but it may never become *domestic* (human-obedient). The next, fourth part is focused on us, humans: how do we react to mosquitoes? How should we understand them and put them in context within our larger living planet? Mosquitoes present us with nuisance and pathogens, and one wonders to what extent we can expect to live out our lives without confronting hardship and disease. The fifth and concluding part presents recent techniques and practices used for coping with mosquitoes and mosquito-borne diseases, some of which involve genetic engineering (such as CRISPR-Cas9 technology) along with applied evolution. By reviewing conduct and experimentation in the laboratory and the field, these chapters show what is now being achieved, while putting the results in wider ecological and social contexts. Building successful new relationships with mosquitoes demands technological and scientific understanding to be carried out with social and political sensitivity.

The world is warming—and buzzing

Mosquitopia, as a project, emerged from *INFRAVEC2* (2017–2020), a European Union Horizon2020 research initiative aimed at understanding and controlling disease vectors, especially mosquitoes. Weighing mostly on the natural sciences, especially for identifying ways to repel or exterminate these creatures, a small part of *INFRAVEC2* was also dedicated to examining the human side of dealing with mosquitoes. Our mission as humanists and social scientists was to reflect on these creatures and suggest ways to better understand interactions between species, human and insect.

A first consideration of our collaborative project suggests that its mere existence is already a success, by providing more evidence of the necessity and feasibility of bridging the gap opened between the natural sciences on the one side, and the social sciences and humanities on the other. The separation of these "two cultures" has been one of the gaps of thinking throughout the twentieth century, precisely at a time when humans were conducting concerted campaigns against the mosquito (Snow 1959). Despite brilliant scientific innovations combined with enormous technological progress, such campaigns have hitherto not been crowned total successes. We may plausibly assume that strengthening the connections between natural and humanistic sides of our encounters with the mosquito will contribute to achieving more satisfactory results. Our multi-disciplinary collaboration might be considered an "environmental humanities of the mosquito," since the issues raised require environmental insights from many disparate fields (Hall et al. 2015). Mosquitoes evoke health questions, but also ecological, ethical, anthropological, historical and literary questions, with the theme of our book being that crucial answers to the mosquito question require the full range of human inquiry.

Here, we acknowledge with gratitude the financial and organizational contributions from *INFRAVEC2, EU Horizon2020* for helping develop this project, along with crucial support received for our initial symposium from the Rachel Carson Center for Environment and Society (Munich), as well as in our later publication stages from the University of Zurich, Department of Evolutionary Biology and Environmental Studies and the Swiss National Science Foundation. We also thank the many institutions that have supported our authors in developing their chapters, and Douglas Da Silva for developing the index and Jayanthi Chander for project management.

We close this brief introduction by reflecting on Italy's famous Sardinian Project (1946–1951), which in the annals of mosquito control stands out as perhaps the premier instance in which men, women and their machines, together with metric tons of insecticide, composed mostly of DDT, were unleashed in a concerted action against *Anopheles labranchiae*, this island's most notorious malaria mosquito vector. At the height of this five-year campaign, some 30,000 mosquito eradicators fanned out across the Mediterranean island, draining wetland habitat, straightening meandering rivers, introducing *Gambusia* mosquito fish, and spraying DDT—by hand and airplane, in liquid and powder form—in every open well, on every watery spring, inside almost every house and stall. The goal of the Sardinian Project was to eliminate across this large and rugged island every single *An. labranchiae*, whether in larva or adult form, so that this mosquito would never again fly here, and its future control would never again be necessary, finally extinguishing the age-old scourge of malaria from its shores. The campaign's final report explained that

> Eradication was regarded as an objective which could be attained only
> through a complete concentration of effort. The end result was to be either

success or failure, eradication or failure to eradicate, and any additional objectives would weaken the principal one.

(Logan 1953)

But in the end, following five seasons of dust and drudgery, spraying and respraying, and then scouting for surviving mosquitoes to spray again, it became clear that *An. labranchiae* had not been completely eliminated, and that these insects would continue to buzz into the foreseeable future. Meticulous field work demonstrated that Sardinia's eradicators had come very close to achieving their goal, calculating that 99.936% of this species of mosquito had been exterminated from the island. Yet by the standards of the Rockefeller Foundation that oversaw the campaign, the Sardinian Project was deemed a "failure" because eradication had not been achieved. Malaria had been expunged from the island, but a few *An. labranchiae* remained, with the survivors surely showing DDT resistance and passing this resistance to their offspring that would continue propagating across the land. Here there was failure to eradicate the mosquito, but success at controlling the main disease it carried (Brown 1998).

In our own more humble mosquito project that follows, we hope that any success of bringing together humanists, social scientists and natural scientists

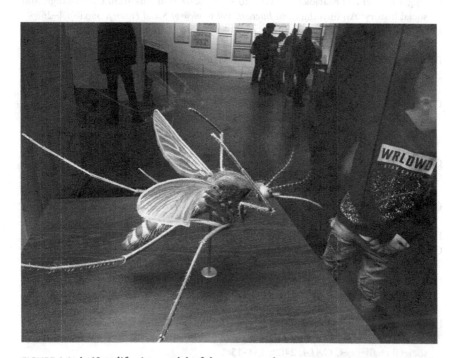

FIGURE 1.1 A 60 × life-size model of the common house mosquito (*Culex pipiens*), by Alfred Keller 1937. Museum für Naturkunde Berlin. Photograph by Marcus Hall.

will not be judged as narrowly as was the Sardinian Project. We believe that environmental humanities of the mosquito can show pathways to success, or at the very least, pathways that need to be taken to avoid failure in understanding the mosquito. The project of controlling and even eradicating mosquitoes must be scrutinized from many perspectives in order to judge whether it is technically feasible, ecologically compatible and ethically reasonable (Angelone et al. 2020). In the end, judging the success or failure of *Mosquitopia* will ultimately lie with the reader, and how the reader may build new relationships with the mosquito.

Bibliography

Angelone, Samer, Marcus Hall, and Dan Tamir. 2020. "Mosquitopia? Peaceful coexistence between humans and mosquitoes" (Video, 7 min.), https://www.youtube.com/watch?v=_-5BvgP78aI&t.

Bates, Marston. 1953. "Preface." In John Logan. *The Sardinian Project: An Experiment in the Eradication of an Indigenous Malarious Vector.* Baltimore: Johns Hopkins University Press.

BBC News. 2013. Can the buzz of mosquitoes be art? Nov. 1 at https://www.bbc.com/news/av/entertainment-arts-24766729 on 21.10.2020.

Bhaumik, Soumyadeep. 2013. Aggressive Asian tiger mosquito invades Europe. *Canadian Medical Association Journal*, 185(10): E464–4.

Boomgard, Peter and Marjolein 't Hart. 2010. Globalization, environmental change, and social history: An introduction. *International Review of Social History*, 55(s18): 1–26.

Borrell, Brendan. 2009. Mosquitoes mate in perfect harmony. *Nature.* doi:10.1038/news.2009.1167

Brand, Stewart. 1968. *Whole Earth Catalog 1* Menlo Park, CA: The Portola Institute, 2.

Brown, Peter. 1998. Failure-as-success: Multiple meanings of eradication in the Rockefeller Foundation Sardinia project, 1946–1951. *Parassitologia*, 40(1–2): 117–130.

Carson, Rachel. 1962a. Speech to the Women's National Press Club (Dec. 5). Quoted in Shirley A. Briggs, "Rachel Carson: Her Vision and Her Legacy." In G. Marco, R. Hollingworth, W. Durham, eds. 1987. *Silent Spring Revisited.* Wash., D.C.: American Chemical Society, 7.

Carson, Rachel. 1962b. *Silent Spring.* Boston: Houghton Mifflin, 99.

Carter, Richard and Kamini Mendis. 2002. Evolutionary and historical aspects of the Burden of Malaria. *Clinical Microbiology Reviews*, 15(4): 564–594.

Conlon, Joe. 2011. Mosquito genocide. *Nothing But Science* at https://nothingbutscience.wordpress.com/tag/joe-conlon/ on 28.5.19.

Fang, Janet. 2010. A world without mosquitoes. *Nature*, 466:432–434.

Gallup, John Luke and Jeffrey Sachs. 2001. The economic burden of malaria. *The American Journal of Tropical Medicine and Hygiene*, 64(1,2): 85–96.

Hall, Marcus. 2010. Environmental imperialism in Sardinia: Pesticides and politics in the struggle against malaria. In *Nature and History in Modern Italy*, Marco Armiero and Marcus Hall, eds. Athens: Ohio University Press, 70–86.

Hall, Marcus, Philippe Forêt, Christoph Kueffer, Alison Pouliot and Caroline Wiedmer. 2015. Seeing the environment through the humanities: A new window on grand societal challenges. *GAIA*, 24(2): 134–136.

Jones, Richard. 2012. *Mosquito.* London: Reaction Books.

Kennedy, Donald and Marjorie Lucks. 1999. Rubber, blight, and mosquitoes: Biogeography meets the global economy. *Environmental History*, 4(3): 369–383.

Logan, John. 1953. *The Sardinian Project: An Experiment in the Eradication of an Indigenous Malarious Vector.* Baltimore: Johns Hopkins University Press.

Méthot, Pierre-Olivier. 2012. Why do parasites harm their host? On the origin and legacy of Theobald Smith's 'law of declining virulence'. *History and Philosophy of the Life Sciences*, 34: 567.

Mosquito Reviews. 2020. *Statistics for Mosquito-Borne Diseases and Deaths* at https://mo squitoreviews.com/learn/disease-death-statistics/ on 21.10.2020.

Myers, Norman. 1993. Biodiversity and the precautionary principle. *Ambio*, 22(2/3): 74–79.

Packard, Randall M. 2007. *The Making of a Tropical Disease: A Short History of Malaria*. Baltimore: The Johns Hopkins University Press.

Patterson, Gordon. 2009. *The Mosquito Crusades: A History of the American Anti-Mosquito Movement*. New Brunswick: Rutgers University Press, 83.

Rose, Noah, et al. 2020. Climate and urbanization drive mosquito preference for humans. *Current Biology*, 30(18), https://doi.org/10.1016/j.cub.2020.06.092.

Roux, Olivier and Vincent Robert. 2019. Larval predation in malaria vectors and its potential implication in malaria transmission: An overlooked ecosystem service? *Parasites & Vectors*, 12: 217.

Snounou, Georges and Nicolas White. 2004. The co-existence of plasmodium: Sidelights from *falciparum* and *vivax* malaria in Thailand. *Trends in Parasitology*, 20(7): 333–339.

Snow, Charles Percy. 1959. *The Two Cultures and the Scientific Revolution*. New York: Cambridge University Press.

Spielman, Andrew and Michael D'Antonio. 2001. *Mosquito: The Story of Man's Deadliest Foe*. New York: Hyperion.

Török, Edina, et al. 2020. Unmeasured side effects of mosquito control on biodiversity. *European Journal of Ecology*, 6.1: 71–76.

Winegard, Timothy C. 2019. *Mosquito: A Human History of Our Deadliest Predator*. New York: Hutton.

World Health Organization. 2014. Yellow fever global annual reported cases and YFV coverage, 1980–2014 at http://158.232.12.119/emergencies/yellow-fever/maps/arc hive/en/ on 21.10.2020.

2

THE MOSQUITO

An introduction

Frances M. Hawkes and Richard J. Hopkins

Mosquitoes are some of the most intensely studied creatures on the planet and their role in disease transmission and nuisance biting makes them worthy of such attention. There are over 3,500 species of mosquito on earth, being found everywhere except in Antarctica. Yet, from this great diversity, only a small handful can carry the pathogens that cause human disease and it is these species which have been studied most thoroughly. For the purposes of public health, this substantial body of research has helped us to understand mosquito-borne disease transmission and informed the development of mosquito and disease control methods. A fascinating spinoff of that body of research has been to reveal a complex biology, showing the mosquito's incredible and unusual behavioural, anatomical and physiological traits.

Animal behaviours are linked to the intricate displays of brightly coloured tropical birds, the long-range migrations of grazing mammals, the semaphore flashing of fireflies in a darkened landscape, together with an infinite variety of other activities and colourful patterns across the animal kingdom. Mosquitoes, like all animals, are driven by a fundamental set of needs. The behavioural organization of an individual animal species is at the core of understanding the ecology of that species. In Dutch Biologist Nikolaas Tinbergen's classic 1963 paper, "On aims and methods of ethology," he defines four categories of explanations of animal behaviour: causation, evolution, development and function (Tinbergen, 1963). In pragmatic terms, these categories can then be regarded as either "proximate" or "ultimate" causes of a behaviour. The patterns of behaviour exhibited by mosquitoes are complex and driven by sensory systems that are adapted to the environments they inhabit and the ecological niches they exploit. Their life cycle, anatomy, physiology and behaviour make these creatures both an extraordinary object of study and crucial to human culture.

DOI: 10.4324/9781003056034-2

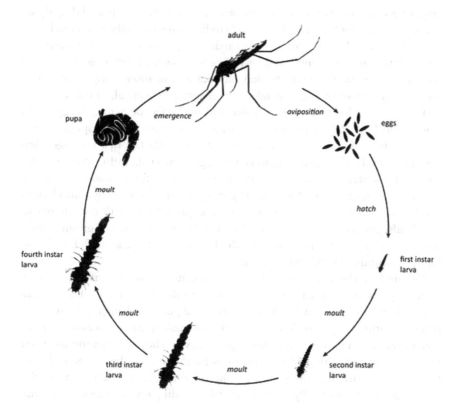

FIGURE 2.1 The mosquito life cycle. Image courtesy of Louise Malmgren/NRI.

Mosquitoes are holometabolous insects. This means that, just as caterpillars develop into butterflies, mosquitoes undergo a complete metamorphosis, hatching from eggs into larvae, then into a pupal phase (where the juvenile form liquifies and reforms into the adult body), finally hatching as fully adult flies (Figure 2.1). All mosquitoes therefore start life as an egg with a gravid female mosquito laying as many as 250 of them in each clutch. Since the mosquito's juvenile stages are aquatic, eggs must be deposited in or near water, or somewhere where water may return after flood or rainfall. The female's choice of location for laying eggs is a critical factor for determining the offspring's survival in the immature stages (eggs, larvae and pupae). Once an egg has been laid then the immature must develop in the site selected by its mother. Broadly speaking, mosquito eggs are of two types: rapid-hatch eggs which are laid directly on or adjacent to the water surface, which hatch within a couple of days; and delayed-hatch eggs typically laid adjacent to water or on moist soil or vegetation some metres distant from water. Delayed-hatch eggs can survive for long periods—months or years—being resistant to desiccation and undergoing extremes of temperature that may include freezing winters. Egg laying varies widely by mosquito species, from single eggs to small rafts of eggs cemented to each other and placed directly on the water or else laid nearby, always ready to hatch as soon as the water level rises.

A gravid female mosquito aims to hatch her eggs in a water resource that is sufficiently rich in nutrients and long-lasting to allow the larvae to grow, develop and produce pupae from which adult mosquitoes can successfully emerge. Her selection of a laying site is dependent upon various chemical, visual, olfactory and tactile cues that influence the behaviour of the female before an egg is laid (Ignell and Hill, 2020). For some *Anopheles* mosquitoes, water vapour itself is attractive to gravid females (Okal et al., 2013), while tall riparian vegetation has been found to be a deterrent to laying eggs (Low et al., 2016). Whatever the egg-laying strategy of the species, the female's search for a location to lay her eggs may last several days. Mosquito flight is generally favoured by warm humid conditions, and if the wind is too strong then mosquitoes will not attempt to fly. Whilst generally associated with flights relatively close to the ground, some gravid females have been captured hundreds of metres in the air with little being known about these long-range movements.

Dictated by the availability of aquatic habitats, mosquitoes are found in a wide range of environments from the tropics to the Arctic circle. Their larvae can be found wriggling in vast marshlands, flood plains and wherever else water collects continuously or periodically, such as in small tree holes or human-made containers, which have become ideal reproductive niches for many species. Even the water-filled leaf axils of such plants as bromeliads can be mosquito larvae habitat. After hatching, the young mosquito larva harvests nutrients from the water. Larvae are essentially detritivores, filter feeding on decomposing organic matter, bacteria and algae for several weeks, spending much of their time at the water's surface to take in air, much like a snorkeler. As they build food reserves necessary to tide them through the intense process of metamorphosis, larvae can be aggressively predated on by fish, amphibians and other aquatic invertebrates. Moreover, once emerged as adults, mosquitoes transfer huge volumes of biomass into the terrestrial food web, in turn contributing to the diets of insectivorous mammals, birds and other invertebrates. So fundamental are mosquitoes in the food chain that when their numbers were controlled in the Camargue region of southern France, breeding success of the house martin, *Delichon urbicum*, was reduced by some 25% compared to untreated areas (Poulin et al., 2010).

After progressing through four larval stages, or instars, the mosquito is ready to pupate. Pupae physically resemble so many commas swimming in the water, and though they do not feed, they are highly mobile and respond to the slightest threat by tumbling down through the water to escape potential predation. When the mosquito pupa is fully developed, it will rise to the surface of the water one last time. Here the adult mosquito is ready to emerge, and so straightens its body, splits open its exoskeleton and emerges upright into the air (Figure 2.2)

After resting briefly on the surface of the water, the adult mosquito must take a short shaky flight to find a refuge, typically in surrounding vegetation, where it rests to allow its newly pumped-up wings to dry and properly harden.

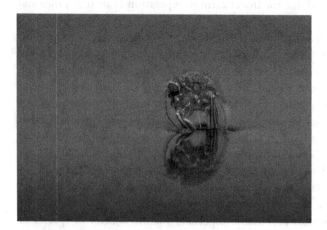

FIGURE 2.2 An emerging male *Culex pipiens.* Photo by Anders Lindstrom/SVA.

As a consequence of the wide range of their larval habitats, there is a correspondingly large variation in emergence patterns of different mosquito species. Whilst the number of mosquitoes that are able to grow in and emerge from the water in a tin can will always be small, the numbers emerging from larger bodies of water can be massive and dramatic. This is most apparent for species such as the inland floodwater mosquito, *Aedes vexans*, a highly cosmopolitan mosquito found in many countries with a range covering every continent except Antarctica and South America. Although capable of transmitting a range of human pathogens, *Aedes vexans* is best known for its role as a nuisance mosquito, hence its binomial name: the Latin *vexāre* means to torment or harass. This mosquito does not lay its eggs directly in the water but in the moist soil above the waterline. After a period of drying, these eggs can survive for years waiting for the water level to rise and be sufficiently warm. If the water is too cold or clear, the eggs will not hatch. When suitable waters do come to inundate meadows or river flood plains, *Aedes vexans* eggs can hatch across vast areas; hundreds of larvae can be found in a litre of floodwater, equating to over 100 million larvae per hectare (Becker et al., 2010), the subsequent emergence of adult mosquitoes reaching biblical proportions. Such population levels of this, and other floodwater species, can become so extreme as to deter all normal human activities. *Vexāre* indeed.

Once emerged as adults, both male and female mosquitoes feed extensively on sources of plant-based sugars, such as those found in nectar and fruit juices. Only the adult female mosquito seeks a blood meal, which has the requisite nutrients to support egg development. When the female does feed on blood it does not necessarily select humans as the source of this blood, and indeed humans are rarely a mosquito's main blood source. Other mammals, birds or reptiles will also satisfy the palate of some mosquito species. It is when the mosquito selects a human for its blood meal that the insect earns its reputation as an annoyance and harbinger of disease.

It might also be noted that while the majority of mosquito species follow this general dietary pattern, there is a notable exception in the genus *Toxorhynchites*. This group includes the world's largest mosquito, *Toxorhynchites speciosus*, whose wingspan may be four times larger than most other species. The idea of a giant mosquito may seem somewhat terrifying; however, the 90 or so species in this genus are particularly noteworthy because the adults do not take any blood meals at all and feed exclusively on plant sugars. This is on account of the predatory nature of the larvae, which kill live prey—including other mosquito larvae—in order to acquire sufficient reserves of protein for egg development when adult. So aggressive are the predatory (and even cannibalistic) appetites of *Toxorhynchites amboinensis* larvae that this species has been cultivated and distributed as an effective form of mosquito biocontrol, especially for the control of species of mosquitoes that typically breed on shipping containers and which are associated with the transmission of dengue and Zika virus (Collins and Blackwell, 2000).

The secret life of a mosquito

Whilst for most people, mosquitoes are defined by an incessant whining that disturbs their sleep at night or by an intense swollen itch on their ankle, there is far more to mosquito biology than their interactions with humans. These are but brief moments in their admittedly rather short lives—in the tropics most individuals will seldom survive longer than a month as adults. Throughout the course of their adult life, mosquitoes must perform a series of complex searches for resources at different times and in different places across the landscape. They interact not only with their blood-meal host, but with plants that are also sources of food, with a mate, and with places and structures for resting and laying their eggs. The resources that each individual insect searches for vary in their spatial and temporal availability and are sometimes to be found in widely differing environments. The behaviour of a searching adult mosquito is driven by external cues in the form of chemical and visual signals that the insect must process to guide its searches.

The organs that the mosquito uses to inform the searches are all remarkable in their own way. Stimuli that are visual, chemical and aural all play important roles at some point in the life of the adult mosquito. The compound eyes of night-active mosquitoes are amongst the most sensitive to low light levels in the animal kingdom and the structure of the nocturnal mosquito eye is uniquely adapted to maximize this sensitivity. Such eye sensitivity enables visually guided flight in light conditions equivalent to moonless, starless nights, although such sensitivity comes at the expense of visual resolution, with the world appearing as a heavily pixelated image of light and dark patches. The mosquito antenna is another remarkable organ. It can detect odours that distinguish potential hosts, sugar meal sources and egg-laying (oviposition) sites. This antenna not only has humidity and thermal receptors, it is also endowed with one of the most sensitive sound detectors in the insect kingdom, the Johnston's organ. Described by and named after Christopher Johnston (1855), these are the most complex mechanosensitive organs yet found in insects. This doughnut-shaped organ at the base of the antenna detects minute vibrations from sound waves. The Johnston's organ's extreme sensitivity to sound allows a flying mosquito to detect the tones produced by the wingbeats of other flying mosquitoes and distinguish these from tones produced by its own wings. Fascinatingly, conspecific male and female mosquitoes not only detect the sound of each other's wingbeats, they also adjust their own wingbeat frequency to match that of their potential partner during flight, producing a harmonious duet in a prelude to mating (Gibson and Russell, 2006).

Often, all the resources that a mosquito needs can be found in a relatively small area, with conventional wisdom being that mosquitoes, on the whole, travel relatively short distances, generally less than a few hundred metres, with exceptions of up to several tens of kilometres being documented. With the high habitat diversity and host availability found in some environments, there may be little need to travel far. However, research carried out in Africa's Sahel has demonstrated that malaria mosquitoes fly hundreds of metres up, where they may be carried on the wind for distances of around 300 kilometres in a single night (Huestis et al., 2019). The majority of these insects were found to be blood-fed females, so that their travel over long distances may have significant repercussions for transmitting such diseases as malaria and for the ecological aspects of their searching for egg-laying sites during prolonged periods of drought.

In any case, flying between resources and in search of shelter requires a great deal of energy and adult mosquitoes need to feed in order to gather the energy that flight requires. Whilst people generally think of mosquitoes as exclusively blood-feeding, sugar feeding is a cornerstone of adult mosquito life. Newly emerged mosquitoes cannot survive for long without taking in a sugar meal and it is the consumption of sugar that facilitates females in their search for blood. Although female adult mosquitoes in all but a few species require a blood meal to produce eggs, both male and females feed on nectar and other sources of plant sugars to provide energy. Given the choice, the majority of female mosquitoes will consume a sugar meal before they take blood, with floral nectar being by far the most important of the sugar sources for mosquitoes. Although the phrase "sugar feeding" is commonly used, it is perhaps a misnomer for the process of mosquitoes feeding on plants, since mosquitoes gain greater value from a plant's other nutrients than simple carbohydrates. "Phytophagy" may therefore be the more appropriate way to describe mosquito feeding (Peach and Gries, 2020). It has even been further demonstrated that compounds present in nectar can differentially affect the development of malaria parasites within the mosquito to such an extent that their feeding on certain plants can suppress the malaria cycle in the insect phase (Hien et al., 2016).

Since floral meals are the most significant contributor to mosquito phytophagy, then how do mosquitoes find this key food source? In general, it is common amongst phytophagous insects that their attraction to the plant is governed by a gestalt of signals available to guide the insect to the correct plant. It is almost certainly the case for mosquitoes seeking nectar to fuel their flights that their search is based on a range of signals coming from flowers. The visual cues associated with flowers and insects have been extensively explored for day-flying pollinators, such as bees, but less is known about floral visitation by nectar-foraging mosquitoes. Broadly speaking, nectar-foraging mosquitoes often visit flowers that are white or pale yellow to the human eye. For nocturnal species of mosquito, this can be linked to the fact that many flowers that make nectar available at night are often pale flowers, which have a strong contrast against the dark landscape, thereby offering stronger visual cues for the pollinators. In addition to visual cues, floral odours, metabolic heat and the nocturnal respiration of carbon dioxide are all associated with floral location by mosquitoes (Peach et al., 2019). Floral feeding by mosquitoes has been relatively understudied compared to other aspects of mosquito biology. It can be concluded that mosquitoes do feed on extrafloral nectaries and on fruit juices, and that mosquitoes will utilize a broader range of plant material than just flowers when flowers are scarce.

Such nectar-feeding habits mean that mosquitoes may have a role in pollination. Mosquitoes appear able to pick up small clusters of pollen during nectar feeding, thereby facilitating plant pollination, even if there are very few documented cases of obligate pollination by mosquitoes. The blunt-leaved orchid, *Platanthera obtusata*, which can be found in the bogs, swamps and wooded fens of northern North America, is one such mosquito-pollinated plant, with *Aedes communis* attracted to the orchid's chemical compounds (Lahondère et al., 2020).

While locating plant-based sugars is one occupation of male mosquitoes, their other chief activity is mate-seeking. The growing importance of research about male mate-seeking stems from an interest in mating disruption or using modified males to spread characteristics which disrupt a mosquito's ability to act as a vector of disease (Takken et al., 2006). Like most insect species, male adult mosquitoes typically emerge slightly ahead of females by a day or so, requiring that extra time to become sexually mature. When females emerge, they are often ready to mate almost immediately. It is common for many mosquito species to have mating "swarms" formed predominantly by the males, usually around dusk. These swarms often form close to visible structures or other conspicuous landmarks, although the exact mechanisms that guide the positioning of these mating swarms are poorly understood. Most female mosquitoes will mate just once during their lifetime, storing the sperm to fertilize all subsequent eggs they produce. Alongside the genetic material that allows sexual reproduction to take place, various proteins are also transferred from the male to the female during mating. This transmitted chemical concoction triggers changes in female behaviour, switching from mate-seeking to searching for blood to nourish her eggs.

Commonplace misconceptions regarding the seemingly indomitable ability of mosquitoes to locate and bite us—and us *specifically*, rather than anybody else—arise from an awareness that our body odour or something of our scent is somehow detectable and traceable by mosquitoes. Olfaction is indeed the critical mechanism that females use to locate a suitable blood meal. The mosquito's primary scent-sensing organs are the antennae. These paired appendages are covered with hundreds of tiny hairs called sensilla, each capable of detecting airborne molecules, including various chemical odours emanating from animal skin (Sutcliffe, 1994). Breath also releases important telltale chemicals and mosquitoes carry a pair of sensory palpi next to the antennae crucial for detecting those, too.

Like other blood-sucking insects, adult female mosquitoes are highly attracted to carbon dioxide. Produced during respiration by every vertebrate animal and exhaled in the breath, carbon dioxide is an extremely reliable indicator of the presence of living animals and, thus, potential blood meals. Of course, carbon dioxide is also a natural component of the atmosphere, but malaria mosquitoes can detect changes in concentration of as little as 0.01%. Such minute changes in concentration are sufficient to trigger flight in mosquitoes at rest (Healy and Copland, 1995). Trails of the molecule can also be identified by mosquitoes from some distance, with *Anopheles melas* able to detect plumes of carbon dioxide at 18 metres (Gillies and Wilkes, 1969). This first detection of carbon dioxide initiates a complex sequence of behaviours that ultimately lead the insect to its prey.

For some species of mosquito, carbon dioxide appears to be all that they require to locate the source of a blood meal; the stronger the signal, the better. In the case of *Culex tarsalis*, the greater the volume of carbon dioxide released, the more mosquitoes are attracted to the source (Reeves, 1953; Allan, Bernier and Kline, 2006). For *Anopheles* species that can carry malaria, their attraction to carbon dioxide can have important implications for the spread of mosquito-borne disease. For example, women in the later stages of pregnancy exhale about 21% more carbon dioxide per breath, meaning that, other factors remaining equal, the number of *Anopheles gambiae* attracted to pregnant women can double (Lindsay et al., 2000). Since such women are at greater risk of complications from malaria, this particular aspect of mosquito behaviour can produce dangerous consequences to those most vulnerable.

While the carbon dioxide in the air is a generic clue that a host may be nearby, it provides no definitive information about which kind of animal is producing the gas. For opportunist species, such as the Caribbean tree hole mosquito, *Aedes mediovittatus*, any blood-carrying animal is targeted, be it sheep, rat, pig, horse, cow, goat, cat, dog, chicken or human (Barrera et al., 2012). Other mosquitoes are even more catholic in their diet, with *Culex erraticus*, for example, also feeding on reptiles, amphibians, as well as birds, large-hooved mammals and humans (Clements, 1999).

But several medically important mosquito species are extremely specific in their preferred host. Indeed, a key factor in making *Anopheles gambiae* a highly efficient malaria vector is its faithful choice of humans for a blood meal, a trait known as anthropophily. Once infected with human malaria parasites after the first feeding, a female mosquito can feed several more times, potentially transmitting parasites to a new human host each time (a cow, to consider a different vertebrate, cannot become infected with human malaria and so suffers no ill-effects if fed upon by mosquitoes carrying human malaria; from the human point of view, every blood meal taken from non-human vertebrates is one less chance to spread infection). *Anopheles gambiae* evolved its extreme specialization to humans through ongoing association with agricultural communities, which provided it with reliable sources of food and niches for resting and oviposition (Besansky et al., 2004). How, then, can this species that is so discerning in its host, distinguish between all animal sources of carbon dioxide and pinpoint a human? And is every person's scent equally appetizing to a hungry mosquito?

An animal's emanations of sweat, breath and bacteria are composed of a complicated array of volatile compounds. Around 350 different chemicals have been identified in human skin odours alone (Bernier et al., 2000). *Anopheles gambiae*'s sensitive antennae detect those chemicals that are tied most closely to humans alone. Chemical analysis and direct recording of electrical signals from live *Anopheles gambiae* antennae revealed the identity of these compounds (Cork and Park, 1996). Yet even if a mosquito can detect an odour compound, it does not always respond to it, making behavioural research into their responses to chemical stimuli a delicate operation, with results that may vary according to an odour's concentration, volume or the presence of other odours at the same time. Key, behaviour-influencing compounds include carboxylic acids, lactic acid and ammonia (related to sweat production and its incubation, respectively), and octenol, which is more abundant in cattle, for example, than humans and may therefore aid *Anopheles gambiae* in discriminating between them. All of these odours stem from communities of bacteria that live harmlessly on our skin but vary from person to person, and it is these individual differences that affect attractiveness to mosquitoes, regardless of the gender or age of the person (Verhulst et al., 2011); thus, certain unfortunate people are genuinely more attractive to malaria mosquitoes than others, simply by virtue of their unique skin microbiota (Qiu et al., 2006). Moreover, recent evidence suggests that an infection of *Plasmodium* parasites enhances one's production of volatile chemicals attractive to malaria mosquitoes (Robinson et al., 2018). In this way, *Plasmodium* seems to be luring mosquitoes in for a blood meal that will serve to propagate the plasmodium.

How valid are claims that consuming garlic or spicy foods, or vitamin B supplements, might disguise a person's odour fingerprint, and make it less appealing to mosquitoes? There is limited evidence that a person's diet can alter his or her attractiveness to a mosquito—although the results of a study about beer consumption offer some intriguing news: controlling for individual variation and baseline attractiveness, researchers found that those drinking a litre of beer caused more malaria mosquitoes to fly towards them than those drinking a litre of water (Lefèvre et al., 2010). Researchers speculate that ingesting alcohol causes changes in breath and volatile odours that are more attractive to *Anopheles gambiae*—with implications for beverage choice when needing to confront this particular mosquito.

Beyond the dangers presented by a handful of disease vectors and nuisance biters, most other mosquito species will rarely, if ever, bite a person. Much less is known of the details of life histories and ecological interactions of these other species, as they have not been deemed so worthy of research. However, some investigations are beginning to reveal the stunning complexity in other mosquito–host interactions.

Cold-blooded hosts, such as toads, frogs, salamanders, lizards and even mudskippers (amphibious fish), are important blood sources for many mosquitoes in the genera *Mimomyia*, *Uranotaenia* and *Deinocerites*. Since body heat has been shown to be an important signal for other mosquitoes locating hosts over short distances, these colder hosts present a challenge. It turns out that several mosquito species, including Japanese *Uranotaenia yeyamana*, American pale-footed *Uranotaenia lowii* and European *Uranotaenia unguiculata*, are apparently sensitive to the sounds of their hosts, since recordings of certain frog calls have been shown to attract these mosquitoes (Borkent and Belton, 2006; Tamashiro et al., 2011; Camp et al., 2018).

While the idea of mosquitoes feeding on frogs and toads may seem peculiar, there are very few groups of animals off the menu to at least one or two species of mosquito. Researchers have recently identified the mystery host animals of *Uranotaenia sapphirina*, a mosquito from eastern North America characterized by attractive stripes of iridescent blue scales, tracing it to various annelid worms and leeches (Reeves et al., 2018). Even fish blood has been extracted and identified from the gut of engorged *Aedes baisasi* mosquitoes (Tamashiro et al., 2011). DNA sequencing of blood meals has been used to verify that these mosquitoes also feed on various species of eel, goby, mudskipper, rockskipper (or blenny) and triggerfish common to mangrove lagoons and rocky reefs (Miyake et al., 2019). Many of these fish are amphibious or air-breathing and some eels will wriggle out of the water and across muddy ground, while others inadvertently expose their upperparts to air when feeding in shallow waters. *Aedes baisasi* is able to exploit these brief moments of vulnerability.

Whatever a mosquito's choice of host animal, the insect must undertake the risky business of landing on and puncturing the host's skin. The mouthparts of all insects are derived from common structures, with adaptations to suit their particular diets, be they nectar, grain or, in the case of mosquitoes, blood. A mosquito's long and slender mouthparts, collectively known as a proboscis, are supremely adapted to the task of blood feeding and give the mosquito a reputation as a flying syringe—yet the underlying anatomy is far more sophisticated than a simple needle. Once the female has landed on a suitable host, she begins to probe, repeatedly driving her mouthparts into the host. Using a pair of blade-like mandibles, which in other insects may grasp or slice food, the mosquito pins the host skin firmly in place. A second pair of serrated maxillae proceed to saw through the surface of the skin. These appendages are so sharp that the host is often quite unaware of their action. Once the skin is pierced, the mosquito inserts two hollow tubular structures through the skin to search for a blood vessel from which to draw the vital fluid. The first tube, called the labrum, moves freely, bending and curving as it probes the tissue until it detects a suitable capillary (Choumet et al., 2012). When a vessel is located, the labrum pierces it and begins drawing up the host's protein-rich blood. Meanwhile, the second tubular structure, called the hypopharynx, injects the mosquito's saliva into the surrounding tissue. This saliva contains over 100 proteins that keep the blood flowing while slowing the immune and defensive responses of the host (Vogt et al., 2018). The proteins include also anesthetics that numb the area surrounding the bite, anti-inflammatories to maintain blood pressure, vasodilators to keep blood vessels wide and anti-clotting agents to keep the blood flowing near the feeding site.

It is the host's inflammatory immune response to mosquito saliva that results in the painful, itchy welts associated with the insect's bite. Yet, the impressive array of chemicals within mosquito saliva may also include compounds of significant value in developing the next generation of pharmaceutical medicines. Researchers have found that anophelin, the salivary protein produced by *Anopheles gambiae* as an anti-coagulant, can be modified for helping to dissolve human blood clots, thereby opening up new possibilities for developing novel drugs that can prevent stroke and deep vein thrombosis (Watson et al., 2018).

A mosquito's reliance on blood feeding is the characteristic that allows mosquitoes to transmit pathogens from infected to healthy hosts. Pathogens are taken up by mosquitoes incidentally when the latter are imbibing a blood meal. These viruses and parasites, which accumulate in the mosquito's salivary glands, are then injected into new hosts along with saliva during the probing phase. However, this is not the full story, since only a small fraction of the 3,500 mosquito species can transmit human pathogens, mostly limited to those of just three genera: *Anopheles*, *Aedes* and *Culex*. Only mosquitoes of the genus *Anopheles* can transmit human malaria parasites, and only three species of over 500 described anophelines are responsible for the majority of malaria transmission. It is worth remembering that most species of mosquitoes rarely, or never, bite humans, having specialized instead to take blood meals from other mammalian, avian, reptilian or amphibian hosts.

Moreover, the simple exchange of blood and saliva is insufficient for making a mosquito into a vector, at least not instantaneously. Most mosquito-borne pathogens must undergo a process of replication or development within the body of the mosquito, which can take up to 23 days for *Plasmodium vivax* (Thomas et al., 2018), but can be as quick as two days in the case of dengue viruses, depending on environmental conditions (Chan and Johansson, 2012). Should the insect feed on another host before this process is complete, she will not yet be able to pass on viable infective agents. Yet proof that the mosquito can successfully imbibe blood from infected hosts, and then inject pathogen-laden saliva into uninfected hosts, is shown by the nearly 700 million cases of mosquito-borne illnesses occurring each year (World Mosquito Program, 2020).

It would be a mistake to assume that the presence of the pathogen is unproblematic to the mosquito, for even the immune system of the vector will attempt to tackle the invading pathogen (Rodrigues et al., 2010). A female mosquito consuming a meal from a malaria-infected human can ingest thousands of gametocytes (the stage of malaria parasites found in infected human blood). By digesting these gametocytes and exposing them to other toxic processes, her immune system can reduce their numbers from thousands to the tens (Smith et al., 2014). Moreover, white blood cells belonging to the host animal and ingested by the mosquito during feeding will also continue to target the malaria parasite for hours after entering the mosquito gut (Lensen et al., 1997). But even this two-pronged attack can fail to halt the malaria parasite's growth. Despite these gametocyte elimination processes, a small number may still survive to form oocysts (the parasite's next developmental stage) on the outside of the mosquito's gut lining. When mature, these burst open, each releasing thousands of sporozoites, which migrate to the mosquito's salivary glands ready to infect the next suitable host. The successful development of just one oocyst is, therefore, all it takes for the mosquito to become infectious.

Vectors, too, can be stricken by the effects of the pathogens which infect them following a blood meal. Dengue virus, for instance, detrimentally affects the fecundity and fitness of its principal vector, *Aedes aegypti*. Dengue-infected mosquitoes lay fewer or no eggs, with adult longevity being halved (Sylvestre et al., 2013). Malaria parasites can also upset the normal reproductive processes in anophelines. By promoting cell death in the lining of the insect midgut, the rodent malaria, *Plasmodium yoelii*, is found to cause *Anopheles stephensi* to reabsorb ovarian follicles, essentially destroying the next clutch of eggs the female would have produced (Hopwood et al., 2001).

In other considerations, certain parasites have been shown to manipulate their hosts for enhancing their own chances of survival. Malaria parasites have highly complex associations with their mosquito and vertebrate hosts, and it has been suggested that these single-celled protozoa may also influence mosquito physiology and behaviour to increase the probability of their survival and transmission. The introduction of a malaria parasite into a mosquito vector undoubtedly changes the mosquito, although whether such changes are truly an adaptive manipulation or simply a side effect of infection can be difficult to determine (Hurd, 2003). Nonetheless, several studies suggest that parasites produce physiological and behavioural changes in mosquitoes that favour their onward transmission.

It has been determined that wild *Anopheles gambiae* mosquitoes infected with the most deadly human malaria parasite, *Plasmodium falciparum*, take blood meals from more than one person in a single night, whereas uninfected mosquitoes are more likely to feed on a single individual. Such multiple feeding behaviour increases the number of contacts between the infected mosquito vector and human hosts, thereby increasing the transmission potential of the parasite (Koella et al., 1998). Laboratory studies also emphasize the complexity of the vector–host relationship. Research has shown that *Anopheles gambiae* mosquitoes infected with *Plasmodium berghei* (a strain of rodent malaria) were willing to probe a mouse's skin more often than uninfected mosquitoes (Choumet et al., 2012). Although the source of this behaviour is unknown, it may nonetheless confer advantage to the parasite by increasing the likelihood that a mosquito successfully feeds on blood and passes the parasites to the next host.

Ultimately, we realize that the unflattering reputation of mosquitoes may be well-earned. Their visceral parasitic strategy for acquiring nutrition can certainly appear more gruesome, and less honourable, than other predators going about their lives in the animal kingdom. That they stalk us and frequently attack in stealth, often under the cover of darkness, and target specific individuals may be perceived at some level as both devious and personal. That their feeding aggravates us, disturbs our rest, creates an itch that can stay for days and may even infect us with debilitating and potentially deadly disease elevates mosquitoes to the level of the positively dastardly. It may therefore seem unsurprising for those of us involved in the study of this insect to be asked, "What is the point of a mosquito?" Although scientists aim to avoid teleological explanations for natural phenomena, some of the less commonly studied aspects of mosquito biology already demonstrate biotic interactions that are much more complicated than those of a simple blood-sucking pest and carrier of disease. Although we are just beginning to uncover some of their more cryptic behaviours, much work remains to be done. Thousands of mosquito species have evolved marvelous and intricate biological adaptations for generating diverse behavioural and ecological traits that are still unknown to science. The activities of mosquitoes in the ecosystem are as sophisticated and specialized as that of any other creature, and indeed more complex than many. The study of mosquito biology may reveal biochemical, anatomical and behavioural secrets that may not only enrich our understanding of nature but also become a source of bioinspiration in future sciences and technologies, from the design of pain-free microneedles (Gurera et al., 2018) to algorithms for flying drones (Nakata et al., 2020). Critically, the overwhelming majority of insects that fall within the Culicidae do not pose a threat to human health or comfort, so caution must be exercised when discussing "mosquitoes", *generically*, as carriers of disease. For the mosquitoes that are vectors of disease, it is the pathogens and parasites they harbour which cause us morbidity and mortality, and in some cases not without cost to the infected mosquito itself. This is key. While malaria cannot persist without mosquitoes, mosquitoes can persist without malaria, or dengue, or Zika. When driven to distraction by the whining of a mosquito or the itch from their bite, many will not realize that "that wretched mosquito" is but one of myriad species each occupying a unique niche in the environment. Appreciating these subtleties in how we frame debates about "mosquito eradication" can inform a more nuanced discussion, where these key differences call for differences in our response.

Bibliography

Allan, S.A., Bernier, U.R. and Kline, D.L. 2006. Laboratory evaluation of avian odors for mosquito (diptera: culicidae) attraction. *Journal of Medical Entomology*, 43(2), pp. 225–231.

Barrera, R. et al. 2012. Vertebrate hosts of aedes aegypti and aedes mediovittatus (diptera: culicidae) in rural Puerto Rico. *Journal of Medical Entomology*, 49(4), pp. 917–921. Available at: http://ovidsp.ovid.com/ovidweb.cgi?T=JS&PAGE=reference&D =emed10&NEWS=N&AN=22897052.

Becker, N. et al. 2010. *Mosquitoes and Their Control, Second Edition*. Heidelberg: Springer. doi:10.1007/978-3-540-92874-4.

Bernier, U.R. et al. 2000. Analysis of human skin emanations by gas chromatography/ mass spectrometry. 2. Identification of volatile compounds that are candidate attractants for the yellow fever mosquito (Aedes aegypti). *Analytical Chemistry*, 72(4), pp. 747–756. doi:10.1021/ac990963k.

Besansky, N.J., Hill, C.A. and Costantini, C. 2004. No accounting for taste: Host preference in malaria vectors. *Trends in Parasitology*, 20(6), pp. 249–251. doi:10.1016/j. pt.2004.03.007.

Borkent, A. and Belton, P. 2006. Attraction of female Uranotaenia lowii (diptera: culicidae) to frog calls in costa attraction of female Uranotaenia lowii (diptera: culicidae) to frog calls in Costa Rica. *Canadian Entomologist*, 138, pp. 91–94. doi:10.4039/N04-113.

Camp, J.V. et al. 2018. Uranotaenia unguiculata Edwards, 1913 are attracted to sound, feed on amphibians, and are infected with multiple viruses. *Parasites and Vectors*, 11(1), pp. 1–10. doi:10.1186/s13071-018-3030-2.

Chan, M. and Johansson, M.A. 2012. The incubation periods of dengue viruses. *PLoS ONE*, 7(11), pp. 1–7. doi:10.1371/journal.pone.0050972.

Choumet, V. et al. 2012. Visualizing non infectious and infectious anopheles gambiae blood feedings in naive and saliva-immunized mice. *PLoS ONE*, 7(12). doi:10.1371/ journal.pone.0050464.

Clements, A.N. 1999. *The Biology of Mosquitoes Volume 2*. Oxfordshire: CABI Publishing.

Collins, L.E. and Blackwell, A. 2000. The biology of toxorhynchites mosquitoes and their potential as biocontrol agents. *Biocontrol News and Information*, 21(4), pp. 105N–116N.

Cork, A. and Park, K.C. 1996. Identification of electrophysiologically-active compounds for the malaria mosquito, anopheles gambiae, in human sweat extracts. *Medical and Veterinary Entomology*, 10(3), pp. 269–276.

Gibson, G. and Russell, I. 2006. Flying in tune: Sexual recognition in mosquitoes. *Current Biology*, 16(13), pp. 1311–1316. doi:10.1016/j.cub.2006.05.053.

Gillies, M.T. and Wilkes, T.J. 1969. A comparison of the range of attraction of animal baits and of carbon dioxide for some West African mosquitoes. *Bulletin of Entomological Research*, 59(3), pp. 441–456. Available at: https://www.cambridge.org/core/jour nals/bulletin-of-entomological-research/article/comparison-of-the-range-of-attra ction-of-animal-baits-and-of-carbon-dioxide-for-some-west-african-mosquitoes/ DF0C87E573834F02844F8C07BFB7DFF5.

Gurera, D., Bhushan, B. and Kumar, N. 2018. Lessons from mosquitoes' painless piercing. *Journal of the Mechanical Behavior of Biomedical Materials*. Elsevier Ltd, 84(November 2017), pp. 178–187. doi:10.1016/j.jmbbm.2018.05.025.

Healy, T. and Copland, M. 1995. Activation of anopheles gambiae mosquitoes by carbon dioxide and human breath. *Medical and Veterinary Entomology*, 9(3), pp. 331–336.

Hien, D.F.d.S. et al. 2016. Plant-mediated effects on mosquito capacity to transmit human Malaria. *PLoS Pathogens*, 12(8), pp. 1–17. doi:10.1371/journal.ppat.1005773.

Hopwood, J.A. et al. 2001. Malaria-induced apoptosis in mosquito ovaries: A mechanism to control vector egg production. *Journal of Experimental Biology*, 204(16), pp. 2773–2780.

Huestis, D.L. et al. 2019. Windborne long-distance migration of malaria mosquitoes in the Sahel. *Nature*. Springer US, 574(7778), pp. 404–408. doi:10.1038/s41586-019-1622-4.

Hurd, H. 2003. Manipulation of medically important insect vectors by their parasites. *Annual Review of Entomology*, 48(1), pp. 141–161. doi:10.1146/annurev. ento.48.091801.112722.

Ignell, Rickard and Sharon Rose Hill. 2020. Malaria mosquito chemical ecology. *Current Opinion in Insect Science*, 40, doi:10.1016/j.cois.2020.03.008

Johnston, C. 1855. Auditory apparatus of the Culex Mosquito. *Journal of Cell Science*, 3, pp. 97–102.

Koella, J.C., Sorensen, F.L. and Anderson, R.A. 1998. The malaria parasite, *Plasmodium falciparum*, increases the frequency of multiple feeding of its mosquito vector, anopheles gambiae. *Proceedings of the Royal Society B: Biological Sciences*, 265(1398), pp. 763–768. doi:10.1098/rspb.1998.0358.

Lahondère, C. et al. 2020. The olfactory basis of orchid pollination by mosquitoes. *Proceedings of the National Academy of Sciences of the United States of America*, 117(1), pp. 708–716. doi:10.1073/pnas.1910589117.

Lefèvre, T. et al. 2010. Beer consumption increases human attractiveness to malaria mosquitoes. *PLoS ONE*, 5(3), pp. 1–8. doi:10.1371/journal.pone.0009546.

Lensen, A.H.W. et al. 1997. Leukocytes in a plasmodium falciparum-infected blood meal reduce transmission of malaria to anopheles mosquitoes. *Infection and Immunity*, 65(9), pp. 3834–3837. doi:10.1128/iai.65.9.3834-3837.1997.

Lindsay, S. et al. 2000. Effect of pregnancy on exposure to malaria mosquitoes for personal use only. Not to be reproduced without permission of. *The Lancet*, 355, p. 2000.

Low, M. et al. 2016. The importance of accounting for larval detectability in mosquito habitat-association studies. *Malaria Journal*. BioMed Central, 15(1), pp. 1–9. doi:10.1186/s12936-016-1308-4.

Miyake, T. et al. 2019. Bloodmeal host identification with inferences to feeding habits of a fish-fed mosquito, *Aedes baisai*. *Scientific Reports*, 9(1), pp. 1–8. doi:10.1038/ s41598-019-40509-6.

Nakata, T. et al. 2020. Aerodynamic imaging by mosquitoes inspires a surface detector for autonomous flying vehicles. *Science*, 368(6491), pp. 634–637. doi:10.1126/science. aaz9634.

Okal, M.N. et al. 2013. Water vapour is a pre-oviposition attractant for the malaria vector anopheles gambiae sensu stricto. *Malaria Journal*, 12(1), pp. 1–8. doi:10.1186/1475-2875-12-365.

Peach, D.A.H. et al. 2019. Multimodal floral cues guide mosquitoes to tansy inflorescences. *Scientific Reports*, 9(1), pp. 1–10. doi:10.1038/s41598-019-39748-4.

Peach, D.A.H. and Gries, G. 2020. Mosquito phytophagy – sources exploited, ecological function, and evolutionary transition to haematophagy. *Entomologia Experimentalis et Applicata*, 168(2), pp. 120–136. doi:10.1111/eea.12852.

Poulin, B., Lefebvre, G. and Paz, L. 2010. Red flag for green spray: Adverse trophic effects of Bti on breeding birds. *Journal of Applied Ecology*, 47(4), pp. 884–889. doi:10.1111/j.1365-2664.2010.01821.x.

Qiu, Y.T. et al. 2006. Interindividual variation in the attractiveness of human odours to the malaria mosquito anopheles gambiae s.s. *Medical and Veterinary Entomology*, 20(3), pp. 280–287. doi:10.1111/j.1365-2915.2006.00627.x.

Reeves, L.E. et al. 2018. Identification of Uranotaenia sapphirina as a specialist of annelids broadens known mosquito host use patterns. *Communications Biology*. Springer US, 1(1), pp. 1–8. doi:10.1038/s42003-018-0096-5.

Reeves, W.C. 1953. Quantitative field studies on a carbon dioxide chemotropism of mosquitoes. *American Journal of Tropical Medicine*, 2(2), pp. 325–331. Available at: http://www.ajtmh.org/content/journals/10.4269/ajtmh.1953.2.325.

Robinson, A. et al. 2018. Plasmodium-associated changes in human odor attract mosquitoes. *Proceedings of the National Academy of Sciences of the United States of America*, 115(18), pp. E4209–E4218. doi:10.1073/pnas.1721610115.

Rodrigues, J. et al. 2010. Hemocyte differentiation mediates innate immune memory in anopheles gambiae mosquitoes. *Science*, 239(5997), pp. 1353–1355. doi:10.1038/jid.2014.371.

Smith, R.C., Vega-Rodríguez, J. and Jacobs-Lorena, M. 2014. The plasmodium bottleneck: Malaria parasite losses in the mosquito vector. *Memorias do Instituto Oswaldo Cruz*, 109(5), pp. 644–661. doi:10.1590/0074-0276130597.

Sutcliffe, J.F. 1994. Sensory bases of attractancy: Morphology of mosquito olfactory sensilla-- a review. *Journal of the American Mosquito Control Association*, 10(2 Pt 2), pp. 309–315.

Sylvestre, G., Gandini, M. and Maciel-de-Freitas, R. 2013. Age-dependent effects of oral infection with dengue virus on aedes aegypti (diptera: culicidae) feeding behavior, survival, oviposition success and fecundity. *PLoS ONE*, 8(3), pp. 1–8. doi:10.1371/journal.pone.0059933.

Takken, W. et al. 2006. Mosquito mating behaviour. In Knols, B. and Louis, C. (eds.) *Bridging Laboratory and Field Research for Genetic Control of Disease Vectors*. Springer Netherlands, pp. 183–188. doi:10.1007/1-4020-3799-6_17.

Tamashiro, M. et al. 2011. Bloodmeal identification and feeding habits of mosquitoes (diptera: culicidae) collected at five islands in the Ryukyu archipelago, Japan. *Medical Entomology and Zoology*, 62(1), pp. 53–70. doi:10.7601/mez.62.53.

Thomas, S. et al. 2018. Microclimate variables of the ambient environment deliver the actual estimates of the extrinsic incubation period of plasmodium vivax and plasmodium falciparum: A study from a malaria-endemic urban setting, Chennai in India. *Malaria Journal*. BioMed Central, 17(1), pp. 1–17. doi:10.1186/s12936-018-2342-1.

Tinbergen, N. 1963. On aims and methods in ethology. *Zeitschrift fur Tierpsychologie*, 20, pp. 410–433.

Verhulst, N.O. et al. 2011. Composition of human skin microbiota affects attractiveness to malaria mosquitoes. *PLoS ONE*, 6(12). doi:10.1371/journal.pone.0028991.

Vogt, M. et al. 2018. Mosquito saliva alone has profound effects on the human immune system. *PLOS Neglected Tropical Diseases*, 12(5), pp. 1–27. doi:10.1371/journal.

Watson, E.E. et al. 2018. Mosquito-derived anophelin sulfoproteins are potent antithrombotics. *ACS Central Science*, 4(4), pp. 468–476. doi:10.1021/acscentsci.7b00612.

World Mosquito Program. 2020. *Mosquito-Borne Diseases*. Available at: https://www.worldmosquitoprogram.org/en/learn/mosquito-borne-diseases.

3

UNDERSTANDING MULTISPECIES MOBILITIES

From mosquito eradication to coexistence

Uli Beisel and Carsten Wergin

Extensive loss in biodiversity and warming climates mean that the world faces an unparalleled historical situation of global multispecies suffering. In light of this, it is crucial we widen our discussions about social-cultural change in the Anthropocene from narrow human-centred considerations towards more speculative fields of more-than-human relations. One of the most persuasive methods to account for such entangled lifeworlds is found in "multispecies storytelling," a method that recognizes the human and the more-than-human in onto-epistemic partnership (Haraway, 2016). Multispecies stories challenge anthropocentric narratives that tend to depict the bodies of other species as rhetorically passive resources for human appropriation, whether as consumptive commodities in global economies, or as metaphors and symbols in aesthetics and media. Along these lines, the method of "multispecies ethnography" is a vital tool to study and account for ecological assemblages in ways that aim to highlight and address epistemic inequalities (Kirksey and Helmreich, 2010). Important, though, is that more-than-human relations are not considered a harmonious or romantic endeavour. Rather, often the pressing question for humans in more-than-human encounters is about "how to survive"—a question that is more often than not answered with calls for eradication of non-human disease carriers.

Here we focus on mosquito-borne diseases where the question of human survival and non-human extinction has been prominent for many decades. Our aim is to weave insights about the history of malaria and human–mosquito relations in West Africa together with those of a multispecies ethnography of invasive mosquitoes in Germany. Following threads of multispecies mobility, we show how particular human mobility has come to render mosquitoes killable in colonial West Africa. At the same time, we can see how through globalization and warming climates, mosquitoes remain highly active and mobile. We focus on what is considered number four of the "100 world's worst invasive alien species,"

DOI: 10.4324/9781003056034-3

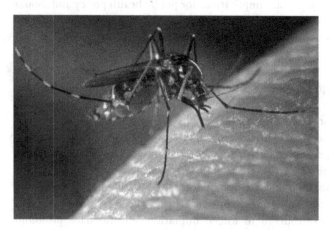

FIGURE 3.1 Asian tiger mosquito (*Aedes albopictus*). Source: Wikicommons.

the *Aedes albopictus* (GISD, 2019, see also Kraemer et al., 2019). *Ae. albopictus*, also known as the "Asian tiger mosquito" due to its striped legs and body, is considered native to the tropical and subtropical areas of Southeast Asia but is today found in many parts of the globe, including Australia, Africa and the Americas (see Figure 3.1). It is an epidemiologically important vector for the transmission of many viral pathogens, including those of yellow fever, dengue and chikungunya. *Ae. albopictus* can also host the zika virus and potentially transmit it between humans.

It is important to note that *Ae. albopictus* are considered by the European Centre for Disease Prevention and Control (ECDC)'s *Ae. albopictus* factsheet as "one of the top 100 invasive species" (ECDC, 2020). It is thus subjected to a rhetoric of "illegality" and "border control" that is enmeshed with global trade, as much as climate change concerns, race and power politics. As Ernwein and Fall show, this border and invasion rhetoric is also utilized in communications about invasive plants (Ernwein & Fall, 2015). In her work, Fall further shows how this rewrites "the nation state as the most pertinent scale for identity politics" (Fall, 2013: 171). For *Ae. albopictus*, this tendency is exemplified by a quote from a recent article about the introduction of mosquitoes from Africa to Europe via the Mediterranean Sea. Finding *Ae. albopictus* caught in traps on Pantelleria, Lampedusa and Linosa, the author presumes links to the arrival of refugees but omits the relevance of global trade for the dispersal of mosquitoes:

> *Aedes albopictus* was found on all three islands under investigation. The consequences on public health with regard to the presence of this mosquito vector *and* the migrant people entering the country from Africa and the Middle East are also discussed (...) The detection of the Asian tiger mosquito on these islands, *which represent the last European strip of land*

facing Africa, has important implications for public health policy and should prompt the national authorities to implement tailored surveillance activities and reinforce plans for preparedness strategies in such contexts.

(Di Luca et al., 2017, emphasis added)

Through this framing, invasive mosquitoes are linked to migrating humans in a problematic way, that is not only dehumanizing and delegitimizing refugees and migrants, but also establishing a wrong, racially charged idea of how invasive mosquitoes travel and extend their habitats. It has been shown in scientific studies that the movement of invasive species is mainly to be linked to trade-related mobility. As the ECDC factsheet also notes, *Ae. albopictus* are known to travel in used car tyres and "lucky bamboo" (ECDC, 2020). Clearly, economic ties and their diverse technologies of transport are the crucial factor. Yet, human mobilities, from leisure tourism to forced migration, all also have profound impacts on public health. In general, with globalization, mobilities have become more dynamic and complex (Sheller & Urry, 2006), but also more controllable due to innovations in transportation, border control, media and communication and surveillance technologies. These technologies are actively used in the control of invasive species, which has in the last decade received more attention under the label of biosecurity (Dobson et al., 2013). However, these measures are usually not successful at keeping mosquitoes out of a territory or country. Biosecurity initiatives are in practice rather aimed to control and contain mosquitoes and minimize the disease risk. So, while mosquito eradication has been attempted several times in history, mosquitoes have proven to be good at utilizing human infrastructures and adaptive to changing ecological conditions.

In order to address the complex socio-ecological dynamics at play, there is certainly a need to consider the Asian tiger mosquito as a learning species—a migratory species that makes use of and stimulates social-cultural change, and in doing so reveals problems typical of those of the Anthropocene, such as the prioritization of the economy over planetary health. The movement of the mosquito further calls into question the quest for local eradication strategies while demanding transdisciplinary research partnerships. Increased sightings of the Asian tiger mosquito in Germany have growing potential to generate anxiety in the wider public, since the animals can theoretically transmit a suite of serious infectious diseases (see also Ernwein & Fall, 2015). At the same time, this mosquito, as a sentinel device older than humans, also offers a form of "radical hope" in our age of global environmental degradation through its capacity to adapt to climate change and counteract violent human efforts to propel it to extinction (Lear, 2006).

In what follows, we draw together historical observations on how anxieties about and reactions to mosquitoes are interlinked, and furthermore, how these have played out in racialized politics of the past. To do so, we initially turn to malaria as a mosquito-borne disease with a well-documented history, recounting certain aspects of the localization of this disease in particular regions of the world and imbued with imperial logics that serve to make mosquitoes objects of eradication. We then consider *Ae. albopictus* and its connection to contemporary questions of mobility, eradication and multispecies coexistence.

Histories of mosquito–human relations

> We believe that when men appeared, mosquitoes were already an ancient
> form of life, with needles sharpened and adapted to the procurement of
> vertebrate blood. Very likely too, the mosquito had already formed its
> close partnership with the protozoan that is the cause of malaria. In what
> vertebrate the plasmodia first existed as parasites we don't know, but it
> seems likely that they were not long, as time is measured, in adapting their
> metabolism to the chemistry of man's cells and fluids. One assumes (...)
> that disease is as old as life.
>
> *(Russell, 1955: 2)*

Malaria is one of the most widely known vector-borne diseases across the globe, and it has been so for millennia. Long before health reports started to compile disease mortalities, Indian Vedic texts called malaria "the King of Diseases." Malaria symptoms were outlined in the writings of Hippocrates in fourth century BC Greece, while genetic tests have linked malaria to the death of King Tutankhamun in Egypt. Centuries before, the Chinese treated malaria fever with the *qīnghāo* plant, whose active ingredient, artemisinin, remains the standard WHO treatment up to present. *Mala aria*, medieval Italian for "bad air," reflects how the fever was believed to emanate from unhealthy air in swamps. The etiological significance of air was overturned in the late nineteenth century when French army physician Charles Laveran, working in Algeria, observed *Plasmodium* parasites in a patient's blood-slides. Ronald Ross, a British Garrison Surgeon working in India, is credited with associating the life cycle of the avian *Plasmodium* parasite with the *Anopheles* mosquito.

Despite the historic evidence for the global distribution of this vector-borne disease, and that of mosquitoes as its main "distributor," malaria remains defined by a particular physical and socio-economic geography. Indeed, conceptions of the Global South by European colonialists were deeply influenced by the experience of mosquito-borne diseases. Many colonial accounts speak of bountiful and, at the same time, barren and nasty lands (Blaut, 1993). Such portrayals are firmly influenced by the experiences of struggling with fever and other illnesses. Both tropes—the bountiful and the nasty—were instrumental for justifying colonialism (cf. Blaut: 77). What became popularly known as "the white man's burden" is thus strongly linked to mosquito-borne diseases, which in turn supported a deterministic view of colonial landscapes and their populations, and helped to establish a contrast between so-called natives and Europeans (cf. Arnold, 2000: 81, see also Carlson, 1984: 15–16; Webb, 2014). In other words, perceived differences in vulnerability to vector-borne diseases opened the door to violence and racial segregation policies, such that African children, for example, were hypothesized to be disease reservoirs for parasites (Ross, 1910).

Segregation measures ramified across the colonies to find white populations fenced off from African housing, a spatial relationship whose legacies one can still trace through housing developments in what has become known as gated communities (Webb, 2014). Such practices of geographical distancing demonstrate a mutual influence between the wish (and ability) to tame the environment and racial discourses, which are rooted in overtones about the "natural" superiority of one population over another. These discourses also locate the mosquito in some areas but not others. Mosquitoes, infectious diseases, as well as native human populations can all be confined to particular environments where the *natural* turns *nasty*, thereby justifying orders to "keep one's distance." The quote from this chapter's introduction demonstrates how racial discourse still impacts our perception of the global spread of mosquitoes. David N. Livingstone adds that in the colonial past, "disease ecology and moral cartography were much closer than distant cousins" (Livingstone, 2002: 173). What is central here is that a rhetoric of invasion and border control attached to the challenges of global containment of *Aedes albopictus* is still manifested in our political and scientific engagements.

Such long-standing socio-political entanglements of race and society provide the background against which mosquito control mechanisms, from containment to extinction, are conceived and exercised. The following paragraphs discuss how this discourse goes hand in hand with rendering mosquitoes killable and extinction-able. As shown, the history of international malaria control interventions was an integral part of colonial practices that were not only informed by a misunderstanding of the transmission of malaria but were also highly racialized. Indeed, as postcolonial scholars such as Chakanetsa Mavhunga have argued, these interventions stand in contrast with African practices of living with mosquitoes, as colonial rule was introducing, "a new dynamic of relations (…) from co-existence to exterminating the insect" (2018: 12).

In the late nineteenth century, the violent politics of extermination and eradication received new technological tools from imperialist science. The scientific documentation of the *Plasmodium* parasite and the malaria transmission mechanism laid the foundations for new technological innovations in malaria control. Based on these discoveries, larviciding, screening and the creation of ditches, for instance, became crucial elements of malaria and yellow fever control as in the building of the Panama Canal (Gorgas, 1915; D'Antonio & Spielman, 2001: 124ff). Further, more elaborate technological innovations were developed during World War II, most notably the malaria drug *chloroquine* and the insecticide DDT, which eventually led the WHO to officially endorse a Global Malaria Eradication Program (GMEP). To appreciate the importance that the GMEP had for the WHO, it is important to remember that the WHO was founded in 1948 and hence was very much a post–World War II institution, with the GMEP being one of its first major projects.

But Africa, the continent with most cases of malaria, was not included in the GMEP, partly because of worries about the holoendemic status of malaria in the vast part of sub-Saharan Africa. Experts feared that an incomplete eradication campaign could diminish the acquired partial-immunity of Africans, and this would have resulted in an even greater malaria mortality than before the campaign. As Dobson et al. (2000) argue, the WHO's decision to exclude Africa was based on racial stereotypes about "African monotony" together with the little-understood relationship between endemicity and immunity. Of course, this decision to exclude Africa from the programme also meant that the eradication campaign was in fact never truly global, as its name claimed.

By many indications, the results of GMEP were generally mixed at best, which can also be seen in the abandonment of the programme after a mere 14 years (Packard, 2007). A crucial obstacle for the eradication campaigns that was not considered at the time was related to the adaptability of both mosquitoes and the disease itself. Before 1945 only a dozen species were known to be resistant to pre-DDT insecticides. However, by 1960 already 139 species were reported to be resistant against DDT (Carson, 1962: 234). Thus, the potency of DDT was compromised by the evolution of mosquitoes (cf. Packard, 2007: 155). Countries that managed to achieve eradication mostly lay in sub-tropical climates with unstable, seasonal disease transmission; the only high-transmission regions that managed to eradicate malaria were island nations. In addition, as shown by historical analyses of malaria elimination in the United States (Humphreys, 2001), in Italy (Snowden, 2006) and in Argentina (Carter, 2007), sustainable reductions in disease incidences came about because of a multifaceted approach, which included not only the killing of the mosquitoes, but comprehensive social, economic and environmental changes. The number of malaria incidences remained low because industrial agriculture brought more distance between humans and mosquitoes, and because there was more investment in healthcare and public welfare. Humphreys quotes a malariaologist of the day, who, judging the effect of the DDT campaign, said that "the best we can claim in this country is that 'we kicked a dying dog'" (2002: 149). Comprehensive social treatment of malaria was a must, if the aim was its disappearance; the GMEP's strong reliance on technical tools spelled failure for its eradication campaign.

Still, many other retrospective analyses continue to regard the WHO's eradication campaign as highly successful. This reading of the GMEP praises chemical tools such as DDT, and marginalizes other more complex evaluations and interventions aimed at human–mosquito coexistence (Kelly & Beisel, 2011). The impact of this other eradication narrative is reflected in contemporary discussions about mosquito control, as well as in the Gates Foundation's push for malaria eradication and as a rationale for the WHO's malaria eradication programme (https://www.who.int/malaria/areas/elimination/en/).

These simplifications of the history of mosquito control in Africa and the first malaria eradication campaign have—by relying on imperial and racial logics—rendered the mosquito killable and eradicable. In addition, while mosquito-borne diseases have been present also on the European continent until the beginning of the twentieth century, disease transmission was successfully interrupted through improved health infrastructures (for the case of Italy, see Snowden, 2006). The modernist success against mosquito-borne diseases in combination with the historical narratives described above, has also established a narrative that locates dangerous, infectious disease-carrying mosquitoes in countries of the Global South, and so enables the narrative of a menacing "invasive species" to be extended to mosquitoes. One also sees that eradicating highly mobile, biologically complex mosquitoes that populated the earth long before humans existed, has not been easy. Indeed, the failures of earlier eradication campaigns would encourage more humble attempts in dealing with these ancient pesky creatures. The next section takes up this issue of identifying more effective contemporary mosquito control measures, especially the control of mobile, so-called invasive mosquito species.

A multispecies mobilities approach to *Aedes albopictus*

What can be learned from the history of mosquito control in Africa when devising mosquito control in Germany? We suggest that this historical framing requires us to attend to situated practices of multispecies mobility in a socio-ecological way. Contemporary interpretations of mosquito–human relations compare these with human encounters with animals, bacteria and other microorganisms within multispecies entanglements (Whatmore, 2002; Hinchliffe, 2007; Kirksey & Helmreich, 2010). Here, analyses focus on the interwovenness, or "material-semiotic knottings" of humans with other forms of life—such as understanding dogs and humans as companion species, and bacteria as constituents of human bodies (Haraway, 2008).

While initial studies centred on the moments "when species meet" (ibid.) or on tracing non-human "presences" in urban centres (Hinchliffe et al., 2005), later studies turned to more troubled forms of multispecies coexistence (Buller, 2008; Collard, 2012; Barua et al., 2013; on insects/mosquitoes: Beisel et al., 2013; Kelly and Lezaun, 2014; Beisel, 2015). As Nading shows for *Aedes aegypti* in Nicaragua, humans, mosquitoes and dengue virus are deeply entangled so that "changes in bodies reverberate through landscapes, and vice versa" (Nading, 2014: 10).

The view of landscapes and infrastructures as shared lifeworlds of mosquitoes and humans provides a way for understanding mosquito–human relationships in a manner wider than the biter–bitten dyad. But how can one track entangled human–non-human mobility in such a way as to limit our impulses stemming from such loaded terms as "invasiveness" and "eradication" and instead search for ways to live together on a mobile and warming planet? Here we sketch a multispecies approach to dealing with what is considered a new arrival in Germany: the *Aedes albopictus* mosquito. Just as humans and goods move, disease vectors and pathogens utilize global connectivities to expand their habitat. As the 2020 SARS-CoV-2 pandemic painfully showed, a better understanding of the mobility patterns of disease agents and their vectors is crucial for the early detection of outbreaks and their successful containment. The geographical distribution of *Aedes* mosquitoes has continuously broadened over the last decades, with the many species in this genus spreading to different countries through human activities and transportation. Alongside these mosquitoes, arboviral diseases also moved to unprecedented places.

The Mediterranean Basin offers a case in point. Since the Late Bronze Age, this region has continued to be a global hotspot for trade, transport and migration. As a result, countries surrounding the Mediterranean Sea share not only goods but also common health threats posed by vector-borne diseases transmitted by mosquitoes (Jourdain et al., 2019). Since at least the 1960s, the Asian tiger mosquito's geographical distribution has continuously expanded, a process which stems from increased global travel and trade, urban development and tourism, and also climate-change phenomena, such as changing land use and management. As a result, diseases like dengue or chikungunya are no longer considered restricted to tropical and subtropical regions, and are developing a strong urban component (Jourdain et al., 2019: 10).[1]

After spreading to the United States via imported second-hand automobile tyres from Asia, *Ae.albopictus* is now found in Mexico's Yucatan Peninsula (Salomón-Grajales, et al. 2012), where dengue is a concern not only for medical entomologists but also for the local tourist industry, which depends on an international draw to its world heritage sites. In 1990–1991, *Ae. albopictus* were again found in used tyres traded from Georgia (USA) to Italy, having previously emerged in Albania in 1979, arriving there in a shipment of goods from China.

Recent surveys showed that these mosquitoes have now spread across the entire peninsula of Italy, parts of Sicily and Sardinia, and into Switzerland. In late 2007, the first *Ae. albopictus* eggs were discovered in southwestern Germany (Pluskota et al., 2008), where they continue to arrive via freight transport from Italy and Switzerland. *Ae. albopictus* migrate along the German A5 motorway and have by now settled in the Rhine-Neckar metropolitan region, which counts approximately 2.4 million inhabitants. In multispecies terms, truck drivers and gardeners have become companion species of mosquitoes. The mosquito's disregard for political and economic borders creates a significant challenge for possible control mechanisms, and places these insects alongside other "hyper-objects" such as CO_2 or micro-plastic, which also demand political decision-making for crossing and transgressing national borders (Morton, 2013).

Meanwhile, dengue and chikungunya remain a health threat in many African countries. Tanzania is a good example: there, *Aedes* mosquitoes are so far mainly associated with major urban centres, but *Ae. aegypti* have recently been shown to have high incidence rates in small towns, too (Kahamba et al., 2020). In early 2005, this species was implicated in a major outbreak of chikungunya in the Indian Ocean, especially in the southern states of India, and in a dengue outbreak in Havelock, a tourist destination in the Andaman and Nicobar archipelago (Sivan et al., 2016).

This entangled globalization of mobile humans and mosquitoes demands a new research focus on transmission that is fostered by transdisciplinary collaboration. In particular, the increased mobility of the *Aedes* mosquitoes highlights crucial linkages between humans and non-humans that remain understudied in the traditional fields of entomology, global medicine and health research. Rather than continuing to focus on imperially minded war on nature, or focusing on false localizations of which mosquitoes are "native" or "invasive," sustainable mosquito control in times of climate change will need to learn to account for the interlinked mobilities of humans, mosquitoes and goods, as well as to be adaptive by developing infrastructures accounting for changing multispecies environments.

Infrastructuring multispecies environments

Societies organize movement through the environment with relatively enduring patterns: namely, infrastructures. However, environments are not passive receivers of infrastructures but actively impact on how the latter come into being. Infrastructuring environments means organizing, knowing and managing a multiplicity of relations (cf. Blok et al., 2016).

As the history of mosquito control aptly shows, the dominance of the eradication approach has not only been more complicated, but also more destabilized through climate change and biodiversity decline. Despite all efforts made in the past, mosquitoes' transgression of political, cultural and economic borders remains a significant challenge with regard to selecting control mechanisms. Most entomologists and disease ecologists prioritize the tracking and monitoring of vector movements. As mentioned earlier, unwittingly aiding vector mobility, travellers, truck drivers and gardeners become *Aedes'* "companion species" (Haraway, 2005). Such entanglements of species are most visible in the diverse ways in which they share infrastructures. This sharing of truck and train routes, planes, or boating facilities challenges conventional assumptions of how human and non-human species live separate lives in a shared environment. Related to this, categorizations into developed regions vs. emerging regions—us vs. them— need to be replaced by mobile documentation and experiences of place-making. One way to confront health threats arising from the spread of *Aedes albopictus* and its adaptations to human environments is therefore to become attuned to how human–mosquito entanglements shift due to new infrastructurations in our shared environments, in order to (re)negotiate the arrival of new vector species by recording how local communities perceive and react to mosquito presence.

An increased emphasis on bottom-up and citizen science research can help deliver new information on these changing human–mosquito relations. Helpful here would be a multi-sited approach of "following the mosquito," for example by travelling with trucks from Italy to Germany (cf. Marcus, 1998). Other fields useful for developing multispecies ethnographic interventions are existing surveillance systems that are drawn upon to confront the global spread of arboviruses. These surveillance technologies are meant to allow for interdisciplinary collaboration and promote cooperation between academic institutions, regional, national and international government agencies. The focus here is on the main routes of introduction, and on infrastructures such as ports, airports or ground crossings like railway nodes and communication and trade routes, as much as on tourist areas. In Germany, such work has already been conducted by the regional health department Rhein-Neckar-Kreis, the Institute of Dipterology and the mosquito control association (KABS), with emerging international partnerships such as TIGER, the Tri-national Initiative Group of Entomology in Upper Rhine Valley (TIGER, 2019).

Due to *Ae. albopictus'* affinity to human environments, further crucial research sites include used tyre storage facilities, greenhouses and green urban spaces such as vacant lots. Studies show that mosquitoes move *between* continents mainly via used tyres and to a lesser extent in lucky bamboo, and that they move *within* continents via the traffic of roadways, as shown by *Ae. albopictus'* proclivity to enter vehicles (Jourdain et al., 2019: 12–13).

Added to these trends of mosquito dispersal are micro-level movements, for example in backyards that share watering cans among neighbours. Collaborative analyses between entomologists, ecologists and anthropologists would shed light on the socio-ecological dynamics that stem from these entangled mobilities of

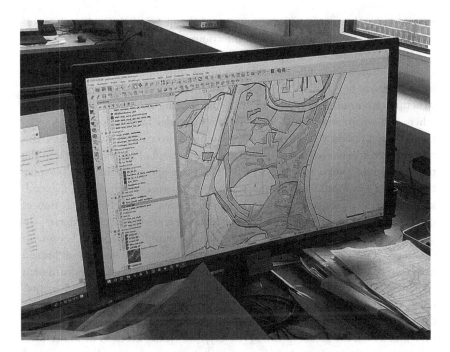

FIGURE 3.2 Computer monitor displaying a section of the Rhine meadows under surveillance. Colour-codes identify the surveillance and control methods used. Source: Carsten Wergin; KABS, https://www.kabsev.de.

SWR > SWR Aktuell > SWR Aktuell Rheinland-Pfalz

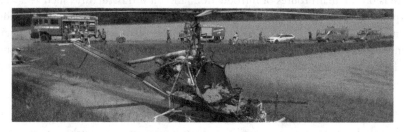

SCHNAKENPLAGE AM RHEIN DROHT

Hubschrauber der Mückenbekämpfer brennt aus

FIGURE 3.3 Burned-out KAPS helicopter. The translated newspaper headline reads: "Danger of mosquito plague along the Rhine: helicopter of mosquito fighters burns out." Copyright: SWR.de, 2019.

mosquitoes and humans, offering answers to the question about the role infrastructures play in the transmission of infectious diseases.

Of final concern are the very infrastructures used to study and control the spread of mosquitoes. The control of moving mosquitoes demands that some infrastructures be similarly mobile, since a focus on infrastructures and infrastructural environments means to trace the shifting mobilities of who moves where and when; and whose (im)mobilities engender fresh movement. A spectacular case in point was when the German mosquito control association KABS encountered trouble in June 2019 when it lost control of their helicopter at the peak of the mosquito season (Figure 3.3). This piece of equipment is used to spray the bacteria-produced toxin *Bacillus thuringiensis israelensis* (*Bti*) that, if digested, kills the larval stages of vulnerable mosquito species. The helicopter is thus of central importance when it comes to impacting potential mosquito habitat.

In sum, a multispecies approach to mosquito control is necessary because of the impossibility of infrastructuring environments based exclusively on human needs, since environments extend across time and space "involving distributed ecologies typically linking thousands of people, computers, sites, and events" (Blok et al., 2016: 13). Embracing the question of how one can (re)present more-than-human agencies, collectives and collaborations in more equitable terms (Wergin, 2018), the global spread of *Ae. albopictus* clearly needs to be understood not as yet another unintended effect of capitalist expansionism, but as part and parcel of the continuous "becoming-with" of human and more-than-human actors. In line with this analysis, one can realize that infrastructuring multispecies environments will bring us into contact with "two essentially contested 'frontiers': those of the global (environment) and the future (of the collective)" (Blok et al., 2016: 14). Rather than trying to eliminate their presence, we suggest that better understanding their entangled mobilities helps us to work towards social-cultural change and planetary health, since the multispecies story of *Aedes albopictus* highlights the close entanglement of health, mobility and migration with the "wicked problems" of climate change, extinction and global environmental degradation.

Conclusion

Many mosquito control interventions have in the past been closely related to the politics of imperial expansion and colonialism. These connections have played heavily on how mosquitoes and human vulnerability to mosquito-borne diseases have been understood. Mosquitoes were not only rendered killable but were also firmly placed in tropical habitats of the Global South, inviting the language of "invasiveness" whenever these creatures moved. Yet one should realize that mosquitoes are older than humans and have always been mobile travellers on this planet. Alongside such facts, one might also remember that most mosquito eradication campaigns have not been very successful. And indeed, where they were successful, careful analysis suggests that changed multispecies infrastructurings were the main factor leading to local demise of the mosquito, and not the techno-fixes of eradication campaigns.

Rather than continuing to set our hopes on a new suite of magic bullets, we suggest that a focus on the entanglements of human and mosquito mobility is urgently needed to detect disease outbreaks early and to develop successful, locally supported control strategies. How are human and mosquito mobilities linked? What methods are most suitable to understand their entanglements and develop more successful control measures? *Ae. albopictus* has shown tremendous resilience in adapting to different geographical and climatic conditions by taking advantage of human-made environments and infrastructures, which has led to its successful global spread. These anthropogenic environments warrant surveillance at points of entry to understand introduction pathways, causes and routes of invasions and connect these to different aspects of its biology and ecology. Yet, a systematic transdisciplinary collaboration that combines research strands on human, vector and viral mobility is still rare.

Such transdisciplinary endeavours point to the fact that humanity is itself an enterprise that needs rethinking. Understanding human–mosquito movements through effective global partnerships among affected communities requires close collaboration between entomologists, social scientists, technologists and the communities themselves for jointly and systematically developing transdisciplinary methodologies based on comparative data analysis of human and mosquito mobilities. Since the fast-paced spread of *Ae. albopictus* is intertwined with international trade and human mobility, we believe that intervention to slow or halt its spread is possible. Its control, however, needs in-depth analyses of multispecies coexistence, rather than a continued focus on eradication of unwanted companion species.

Note

1 For example, an average January temperature of 0°C was usually considered the survival threshold for *Aedes albopictus* diapausing eggs. However, the species was found in Trento (Italy) despite minimum temperatures of −10°C and an average January temperature of −5°C (Jourdain et al., 2019: 14)

Bibliography

Arnold D. 2000. *Science, Technology and Medicine in Colonial India. The New Cambridge History of India.* Cambridge: Cambridge University Press.

Bartumeus F., Costa G.B., Eritja R., Kelly A.H., Finda M., Lezaun J., Okumu F., Quinlan M.M., Thizy D.C., Toé L.P. & M. Vaughan 2019. Sustainable innovation in vector control requires strong partnerships with communities. *PLOS Neglected Tropical Diseases* 13(4): e0007204.

Barua, Maan, Shonil A. Bhagwat, and Sushrut Jadhav. 2013. The Hidden Dimensions of Human–Wildlife Conflict: Health Impacts, Opportunity and Transaction Costs. *Biological Conservation* 157: 309–16.

Becker N., Pluskota B., Kaiser A. & F. Schaffner 2012. Exotic mosquitoes conquer the world. In: H. Mehlhorn (ed.) *Arthropods as Vectors of Emerging Diseases (Parasitology Research Monographs 3).* Berlin: Springer, pp. 31–60.

Beisel, Uli, Ann H. Kelly, and Noémi Tousignant. 2013. Knowing Insects: Hosts, Vectors and Companions of Science. *Science as Culture* 22(1): 1–15.

Beisel U. 2015. Markets and mutations: Mosquito nets and the politics of disentanglement in global health. *Geoforum* 66: 146–155.

Bessaud M., Peyrefitte C.N., Pastorino B.A., Tock F., Merle O., Colpart J.J., et al. 2006. Chikungunya virus strains, reunion Island outbreak. *Emerging Infectious Diseases* 12: 1604–1606.

Blaut J.M. 1993. *The Colonizer's Model of the World. Geographical Diffusionism and Eurocentric History.* New York: Guilford.

Blok A., Nakazora M. & B.R. Winthereik 2016. Infrastructuring environments. *Science as Culture* 25(1): 1–22.

Buller H. 2008. Safe from the Wolf: Biosecurity, Biodiversity, and Competing Philosophies of Nature. *Environment and Planning A* 40(7): 1583–97.

Carlson D. 1984. *Africa Fever: A Study of British Science, Technology and Politics in West Africa, 1784–1864.* Canton: History Publications USA.

Carson R. 1962. *Silent Spring.* Boston, MA: Houghton Mifflin Company.

Carter E. 2007. Development narratives and the uses of ecology: Malaria control in Northwest Argentina, 1890–1940. *Journal of Historical Geography* 33: 619–650.

Cohen S.A., T. Carson & M. Thulemark 2015. Lifestyle mobilities: The crossroads of travel, leisure and migration. *Mobilities* 10(1): 155–172.

Collard, Rosemary-Claire. 2012. Cougar–Human Entanglements and the Biopolitical Un/Making of Safe Space. *Environment and Planning D: Society and Space* 30(1): 23–42. https://doi.org/10.1068/d19110.

D'Antonio M. & A. Spielman 2001. *Mosquito: A Natural History of Our Most Persistent and Deadly Foe.* New York: Hyperion.

Di Luca M., Toma L., F. Severini et al. 2017. First record of the invasive mosquito species Aedes (Stegomyia) albopictus (Diptera: Culicidae) on the southernmost Mediterranean islands of Italy and Europe. *Parasit Vectors* 10(1): 543. Published 2017 Nov 2. doi:10.1186/s13071-017-2488-7

Dobson A., K. Barker & S.L. Taylor. 2013. *Biosecurity: The Socio-Politics of Invasive Species and Infectious Diseases.* Abingdon: Routledge.

Dobson M.J., Malowany M. & R.W. Snow. 2000. Malaria control in East Africa: The Kampala conference and the Pare-Taveta scheme: A meeting of common and high ground. *Parassitologia* 42(1/2): 149–166.

European Centre for Disease Prevention and Control. 2020. *Aedes Albopictus - Factsheet for Experts.* https://www.ecdc.europa.eu/en/disease-vectors/facts/mosquito-factsheets/aedes-albopictus (accessed 31/08/2020).

Ernwein M. & J.J. Fall 2015. Communicating invasion: Understanding social anxieties around mobile species. *Geografiska Annaler: Series B, Human Geography* 97(2): 155–167.

Fall J.J. 2013. Beyond the nativism debate. *Biosecurity: The Socio-Politics of Invasive Species and Infectious Diseases* 167–181.

Faulconbridge J. & A. Hui. 2016. Traces of a mobile field: Ten years of mobilities research. *Mobilities* 11(1): 1–14.

Gorgas W.C. 1915. *Sanitation in Panama.* New York: Appleton.

Haraway, Donna Jeanne. 2005. *The Companion Species Manifesto. Dogs, People, and Significant Otherness.* 3rd printing. Chicago, Ill.: Prickly Paradigm Press, 8.

Haraway D.J. 2008. *When Species Meet.* Minneapolis, MN: University of Minnesota Press.

Haraway D. 2016. *Staying with the Trouble: Making Kin in the Chthulucene.* Durham: Duke University Press.

Hinchliffe Steve. 2007. *Geographies of Nature: Societies, Environments, Ecologies.* London: SAGE.

Hinchliffe F., Kearnes, M.B., Degen, M. and Whatmore, S. 2005. Urban Wild Things: A Cosmopolitical Experiment. *Environment and Planning D: Society and Space* 23(5): 643–658.

Humphreys M. 2001. *Malaria: Poverty, Race and Public Health in the United States.* Baltimore: JHU Press.

Jourdain F., Samy A.M., Hamidi A., Bouattour A., Alten B., Faraj C. et al. 2019. Towards harmonisation of entomological surveillance in the Mediterranean area. *PLoS Neglected Tropical Diseases* 13(6): e0007314. https://doi.org/10.1371/journal.pntd.0007314

Kahamba N.F., Limwagu A.J., Mapua S.A., Msugupakulya B.J., Msaky D.S., Kaindoa E.W., Ngowo H.S. & F.O. Okumu. 2020. Habitat characteristics and insecticide susceptibility of Aedes aegypti in the Ifakara area, south-eastern Tanzania. *Parasites & Vectors* 13(53).

Kelly A.H. & Beisel, U. 2011. Neglected malarias: The frontlines and back alleys of global health. *BioSocieties,* 6: 71–87.

Kelly A.H. & Lezaun, U. 2014. Urban Mosquitoes, Situational Publics, and the Pursuit of Interspecies Separation in Dar Es Salaam. *American Ethnologist,* 41(2): 368–83.

Kirksey, S. and S. Helmreich. 2010. The emergence of multispecies ethnography. *Cultural Anthropology* 25(4): 545–576.

Kraemer M.R., Reiner O., Brady J., Messina M., Gilbert D., Pigott D., Yi K. L. Johnson 2019. Past and future spread of the arbovirus vectors aedes aegypti and aedes albopictus. *Nature Microbiology* 4(5): 854–863.

Lear J. 2006. *Radical Hope: Ethics in the Face of Cultural Devastation.* Cambridge, MA: Harvard University Press.

Livingstone David N. 2002. Race, space and moral climatology: Notes toward a genealogy. *Journal of Historical Geography* 28(2): 159–180.

Marcus George E. 1998. *Ethnography Through Thick and Thin*. Princeton: Princeton University Press.

Mavhunga Clapperton Chakanetsa. 2018. *The Mobile Workshop: The Tsetse Fly and African Knowledge Production*. Cambridge, MA: MIT Press.

Merriman P. & L. Pearce. 2017. Mobility and the humanities. *Mobilities* 12(4): 493–508.

Morton T. 2013. *Hyperobjects: Philosophy and Ecology After the End of the World*. Minneapolis: University of Minnesota Press.

Nading A.M. 2014. *Mosquito Trails: Ecology, Health, and the Politics of Entanglement*. Berkeley: Univesity of California Press.

Packard R.M. 2007. *The Making of a Tropical Disease: A Short History of Malaria*. Baltimore: JHU Press.

Pluskota B., Storch V., Braunbeck T., Beck M. & N. Becker. 2008. First record of stegomyia albopicta (skuse) (diptera: culicidae) in Germany. *European Mosquito Bulletin* 26: 1–5.

Ross P. 1910. *The Prevention of Malaria*. London: J. Murray.

Russell P. 1955. *Man's Mastery of Malaria*. London: Oxford University Press.

Salomón-Grajales J., Lugo-Moguel G.V., Tinal-Gordillo V.R., de La Cruz-Velázquez J., Beaty B.J., Eisen L., Lozano-Fuentes S., Moore C.G. & J.E. García-Rejón. 2012. Aedes albopictus mosquitoes, Yucatan Peninsula, Mexico. *Emerging Infectious Diseases* 18: 525–527.

Sheller M. & J. Urry. 2006. The new mobilities paradigm. *Environment and Planning A* 38: 207–226.

Sivan A., Shriram A.N., Sugunan A.P., Anwesh M., Muruganandam N., Kartik C. et al. 2016. Natural transmission of dengue virus serotype 3 by aedes albopictus (skuse) during an outbreak in Havelock Island: Entomological characteristics. *Acta Tropica* 156: 122–129.

Snowden F. M. 2006. *The Conquest of Malaria: Italy, 1900–1962*. New Haven: Yale University Press.

SWR Aktuell. 2019. *Hubschrauber der Mückenbekämpfer Brennt aus*. https://www.swr.de (Date retrieved: 01 June 2019).

Webb Jr James LA. 2014. *The Long Struggle against Malaria in Tropical Africa*. Cambridge: Cambridge University Press.

Wergin C. 2018. Policy in the Anthropocene. *Glocalism: Journal of Culture, Politics and Innovation* 3: 1–16.

Whatmore S.. 2002. *Hybrid Geographies: Natures Cultures Spaces*. London: Sage.

Web sources

GISD 2019. http://www.iucngisd.org/gisd/100_worst.php
One Health 2019. http://www.onehealthinitiative.com
TIGER 2019. https://tiger-platform.eu/

PART II

Learning from experience

4

THE LONG ARC OF MOSQUITO CONTROL

James L.A. Webb, Jr.

Long before the emergence of *Homo sapiens*, our early hominid ancestors frequently found themselves in close proximity and intimate contact with mosquitoes. Our distant ancestors sojourned nearby bodies of saltwater in order to harvest shellfish and catch marine fish as a source of protein, and by the shores of freshwater rivers, lakes and streams to catch freshwater fish, have ready access to drinking water and hunt animals that came to rehydrate themselves. Mosquitoes likewise were drawn to watery environments. Many species needed salt marshes or the edges of bodies of fresh water in which to lay their eggs, which would develop into larvae, pupae and adult mosquitoes.

In deep time, the biological destinies of human beings and mosquitoes became intertwined. The females of some mosquito species began to take blood meals from humans as well as other animals. Through these blood meals, necessary to nurture their ova, some mosquito species acquired viral and protozoal parasites, eventually evolving the capacity to host these parasites and transmit them. In early tropical Africa, where *Homo sapiens* spent most of its early career, the watery environments were conducive to the spread of mosquito-borne diseases such as malaria, yellow fever and lymphatic filariasis. The disease burden of malaria was so strong that it produced widespread genetic adaptations in human populations (Webb 2009).

In both saltwater and freshwater environments, mosquito populations could be exceedingly dense and constitute a nearly unbearable nuisance as well as a health burden. Our ancestors did what they could: they built smoking fires and in some world regions such as West Africa applied plant repellents to their bodies to try to keep mosquitoes at bay (Iroko 1994). These measures constituted an early chapter in the long struggle of humanity to limit our exposure to mosquitoes. They were only partially effective, however, and had little impact on the transmission of mosquito-borne disease.

DOI: 10.4324/9781003056034-4

Mosquitoes and ecological transformations

During the long transition from gathering and hunting to the cultivation of foodstuffs, human beings transformed local environments to make them suitable for agriculture. In the process, we produced a wide range of unintended consequences, some of which altered our relationships with mosquitoes. In tropical Africa, for example, the clearing of West African rainforest to facilitate the spread of yam vegeculture produced environments that collected rainwater in small puddles that were conducive to mosquito breeding. Some species of *Anopheles* mosquitoes (the genus that can transmit malaria) bred nearby early agricultural villages and evolved to specialize in taking human blood meals, thereby intensifying the transmission of malaria (Webb 2009).

In some world regions, societies undertook large-scale environmental transformations of watery landscapes in order to make them suitable for farming or herding. One prime example is that of the North Atlantic wetlands. Since Roman times, the marshlands of Europe had repeatedly been ditched and/or diked, to drain the wetlands and/or block the inflow of saltwater (Hatvany 2003). These tactics produced varied results. In the notorious marshlands of Kent, England, the diking of the marshlands in the sixteenth century may have inadvertently improved the habitat for *Anopheles atroparvus*, the most important malaria mosquito vector in the British Isles, and consequently increased malaria transmission. But by the second half of the nineteenth century, the incidence of malaria in these wetlands had dropped dramatically. Marsh drainage likely played an important role, although there were other factors involved in the decline, such as improved housing with screened windows and doors and the ready availability of such medicines as quinine and other antimalarial alkaloids isolated from cinchona bark (Dobson 1980). Another contribution to the reduction in malaria transmission was the colonization of the British marshlands, beginning in 1870, by a hybrid species of marsh grass, *Spartina townsendii*. This plant spread throughout the marshlands of the British Isles and along the coasts of Atlantic Europe, stabilizing silt and elevating the wetlands, making them suitable for "reclamation," which generally meant ways to make grasslands available to grazing livestock (Ranwell 1967). Endemic malaria in England was eliminated by the end of the nineteenth century (Dobson 1980).

Vigorous programmes of wetland management and mosquito reduction likewise developed on the other side of the North Atlantic, when European migrants transferred their knowledge of marshland utilization to North America. Some burgeoning seaports saw nearby salt marshes filled in for industrial and urban growth projects. In the area around Boston after the late eighteenth century, for example, some 81% of marshes were converted to other uses (Seasholes 2018). In the agricultural regions of the northeastern seaboard of the United States, farmers drained salt marshes in order to boost yields of coastal marsh grasses for animal bedding, feed, and roof thatching, and in the process significantly reduced mosquito densities which in turn made work on former wetlands more feasible. In the second half of the nineteenth century, some farmers installed tidal gates to drain salt marshes for converting them to freshwater crops (Bourn and Cottam 1950, Crain et al. 2009).

During the economic depression of the 1930s, US governmental programmes such as the Civilian Conservation Corps and the Works Progress Administration offered employment in draining coastal wetlands in the eastern and southern states. Over all, more than 90% of the saltwater marshes between Virginia and Maine had ditches dug into them. The marsh draining work reached all the way down the eastern seaboard to Florida and around the Gulf of Mexico as far as Texas (Patterson 1998, 2009). Such ditch-digging programmes had a dual purpose. Their primary goal, pursued long before the Great Depression, had been to reduce the density of *Aedes sollicitans* and *Aedes taeniorhynchus*, saltwater mosquitoes targeted principally because their aggressive biting habits rendered much of the coastal seaboard uninhabitable; it should be noted that these *Aedes* mosquitoes could also transmit viral pathogens that caused Eastern equine encephalitis and Venezuelan equine encephalitis, even if such infections were generally low, going typically undiagnosed. The secondary goal of drainage programmes was to control malaria (Daiber 1986), although most malaria transmission occurred in ecological zones that were not coastal.

Malaria and yellow fever mosquito control

Since its introduction in the seventeenth century, the principal mosquito-borne disease threat to human beings in the Northwestern Atlantic had been malaria. In this temperate region, transmission of malaria occurred during the summer months. The shores of New England lakes were prime breeding grounds for the *Anopheles quadrimaculatus* mosquito, a competent malaria vector that fanned outbreaks of disease when warm weather brought vacationers and locals to the lakes for recreation (Holmes 1838). Protected riverbanks and eddies also provided good mosquito habitat, and in Canada, particularly in southern Ontario and Toronto, malaria was also a seasonal scourge.

In the late nineteenth and early twentieth centuries, key scientific discoveries revealed the role of mosquitoes in transmitting malaria and yellow fever. In 1880, Alphonse Laveran identified malaria plasmodia in the infected blood of malaria sufferers in Algeria. In 1897, Ronald Ross in British India demonstrated that the anopheline species was the vector for bird malaria, and in 1898, Giovanni Grassi and his Italian colleagues found that other anopheline species were the vectors that transmitted human malaria, and they described the life cycle of the falciparum malaria parasite. In 1900, Walter Reed of the US Army medical corps in Cuba confirmed the hypothesis of Carlos Finlay that mosquitoes transmit the yellow fever virus, and that *Aedes aegypti* mosquito is its regional vector in the Americas (Harrison 1978).

Armed with these new understandings, public health scientists focused their efforts to control malaria and yellow fever on the destruction of mosquito habitat. The fact that malaria was a globally distributed disease meant that there was a large variety of anopheline mosquitoes able to transmit the disease, albeit with a broad range of competency in so doing. Malarial vector species bred in a variety of habitats and relied on various feeding behaviours. The formidable challenges in understanding such vectors helped create the discipline of "tropical medicine." Although malaria existed in wealthier nations of the Global North, including northern regions such as Sweden and Canada, the principal burden of this disease was borne by populations throughout the tropics. In part, this was because the malaria parasites common in the Global North, *Plasmodium vivax* and *Plasmodium malariae*, were less lethal than *Plasmodium falciparum*, common in the Global South, and because the mosquito vectors in the Global North were not as competent in transmitting in the parasites. Similarly, the principal burden of yellow fever was concentrated in tropical regions, although some European and North American cities in the eighteenth to early twentieth centuries also suffered the scourge of yellow plague (Coleman 1987, McNeill 2010). Other widespread mosquito-borne diseases, such as dengue fever and chikungunya fever, were also principally transmitted in the tropics, although they were not scientifically identified until the mid-twentieth century.

The nature of the efforts to control vectors of yellow fever and malaria differed, because their breeding habitats differed. *Aedes aegypti* was a domestic mosquito, which meant that it bred principally in anthropogenically altered environments, often in or near human dwellings. By contrast, the array of malaria mosquito vectors was typically not domestic. They bred in marshes, river eddies, lake and pond edges, tree stumps and even small depressions from footprints which collected rainwater. The struggle against yellow fever involved military or quasi-military programmes, mandating city and town dwellers to destroy mosquito habitat in their immediate surroundings, or else harnessing military forces to carry out these functions within domestic spaces. In early-twentieth-century Havana, for example, the US military carried out a programme of urban "sanitation" that involved fumigating the city centre, together with the oiling or removal of water-collecting vessels with open lids. In Brazil in the 1930s, the public health department, under the leadership of Fred Soper, organized a quasi-military strategy of regularly inspecting domestic spaces to ensure compliance with the orders to eliminate *Aedes aegypti* breeding sites (Stepan 2011).

In the early twentieth century, disease control programmes that targeted malaria-carrying mosquitoes were carried out in many tropical and subtropical regions (Watson 1921, Harrison 1978, Farley 2003). They were most successful when focused on identifying local malarial vectors and on detailed knowledge of their spatial distribution and bionomics, which included their breeding habitats, feeding habits and flight ranges. This focused approach to local epidemiological intervention was known as species sanitation. It was pioneered by Malcolm Watson in the Federated Malay States during the early years of the twentieth century (Watson 1921). During a visit to the Dutch East Indies, Watson taught the basics of the local epidemiological approach using anopheline bionomics to the Dutch scientist Nicolaas H. Swellengrebel, who would use this method to transform anopheline breeding grounds in both the Dutch East Indies and the

Netherlands themselves (Verhave 2011). This method was also taken up with success by the French in Algeria, shortly after the conclusion of the First World War (Sergent and Sergent 1947). Later in his career, Watson brought the techniques of species sanitation to the copper-mining zone in central Africa (Watson 1953). In the southern United States, beginning in the 1930s, the construction of hydro-electric dams had a major impact on local densities of both nuisance and malaria-vector mosquitoes, when authorities carried out control measures such as oiling and brush removal (United States Public Health Service and Tennessee Valley Authority 1947).

Species sanitation was not the only approach to malaria control. Some early malaria specialists took the view that the best approach to controlling malaria was to raise the socio-economic status of the afflicted populations, with the anti-malarial drug quinine being useful in restoring the health and maintaining the economic productivity of those stricken by malaria (Verhave 2011). The Italians,

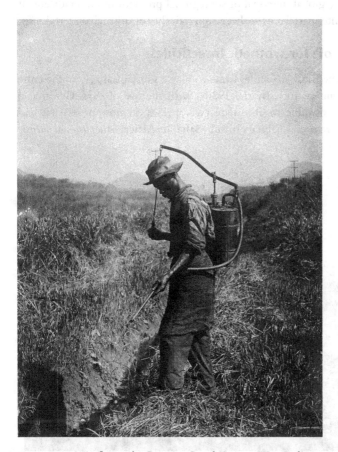

FIGURE 4.1 Miraflores, the Panama Canal Zone: a West Indian man sprays larvicide into a ditch as part of a mosquito control programme implemented during the construction of the Panama Canal. Photograph, 1910.

beginning in 1904, undertook a nationwide campaign to provide quinine to the entire population in order to cure and protect by prophylaxis (Snowden 2006). This was broadly successful in reducing mortality, but was less so in reducing morbidity. Yet even in Italy, by the 1920s, there was a programmatic turn towards mosquito control, with a major focus on the draining of the notoriously unhealthy Pontine marshes near Rome. With assistance from the Rockefeller Foundation, the Italians undertook a marshland drainage programme complemented by the application of Paris Green, an arsenic-based insecticide that killed the anopheline mosquito larvae in the newly dug drainage canals (Russell 1952).

Targeted species sanitation seemed feasible once basic entomological research revealed that the number of truly dangerous mosquito species was very small. Much of the world's heavy burden from mosquito-borne disease was carried by just a few dozen *Anopheles* and even fewer *Aedes* species. These basic facts became well-established early in the era of modern mosquito control, and for this reason there were never any global, regional or subregional programmes to eradicate all mosquito species, quite apart from the sheer impracticality of any such undertakings.

A predominant role for synthetic insecticides

Over the decades, chemical larvicides came to play a substantial role in the control of the anopheline vectors. By the 1930s, with the use of Paris Green as a larvicide, it became possible to eliminate two species of mosquitoes that had spread beyond their regional habitats in sub-Saharan Africa. *Anopheles arabiensis*

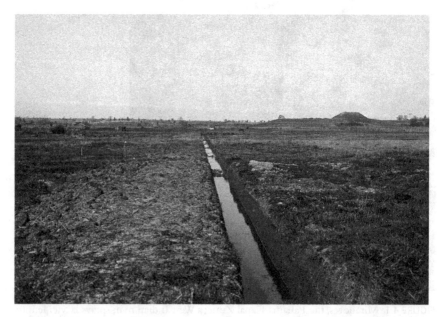

FIGURE 4.2 Nettuno, Italy: a long, narrow drain (to aid mosquito control) in a field. Photograph, ca. 1910–1940.

was eliminated in northeastern Brazil in the 1930s, and following the discovery of DDT during the Second World War, *Anopheles gambiae*, which had infiltrated Egypt from the south, was locally eradicated. Neither of these campaigns used drainage or flooding to accomplish their goals.

These successes in South America and North Africa with Paris Green anticipated the experimentation with DDT during the last phases of the Second World War and in the immediate post-war period. The most significant of the early undertakings was the post-war programme to stop malaria transmission on the island of Sardinia, which then shifted to target the species eradication of the island's malaria vector, *Anopheles labranchiae*. Workers sprayed DDT on breeding sites across the entire island, as well as in the interiors of buildings, as an investigative project to test whether regional eradication of an indigenous mosquito species was possible. The results showed that malaria had largely been eliminated from Sardinia, but not the mosquito. The complete island-wide eradication of *Anopheles labranchiae* proved unattainable. The few remaining covert breeding sites, along with the inadvertent reintroduction of *Anopheles labranchiae* to the island, allowed for the re-establishment of scattered malaria infections, although at dramatically reduced levels (Brown 1991, Hall 2010).

In the United States, malaria had all but disappeared by the end of the 1940s. The construction of dams and the treatment of impounded waters, the draining of wetlands, the relocation of populations from low-lying areas, and the ready availability of prophylactic and curative quinine had achieved most of this success, and in the final years of the decade the application of DDT for mosquito control played a small role (Humphreys 2001). In much of Western Europe, there was a comparable reduction in malaria transmission, owing to the draining of wetlands, increases in agricultural production and standards of living, the screening of houses, and the availability of quinine (Bruce-Chwatt and de Zueleta 1980).

Following a post-war period of experimentation with DDT for malaria control, in 1955 the World Health Organization launched a global campaign based principally on indoor residual spraying with synthetic insecticides—principally DDT—to reduce mosquito densities and to interrupt malaria transmission. The malaria specialists considered it a race against the clock: although it was clear from the start that the wide application of DDT would select for resistance in insects and that it was only a matter of time until mosquito resistance emerged, the logic of the programme balanced upon the notion that rolling out the programme rapidly would be the best hope for interrupting disease transmission globally before resistance emerged (Packard 1998). The Global Malaria Eradication Programme (GMEP) racked up impressive victories, greatly reducing the levels of morbidity and mortality in all world regions outside of sub-Saharan Africa and achieving, on some islands such as Taiwan and most of the Caribbean islands, the complete interruption of malaria transmission. Yet by the time the programme ended in 1969, it was clear that in most other regions, continued spraying with DDT and other residual insecticides would not be able to put an end to malaria transmission. Resistance to insecticides had indeed emerged in some regions; international donors and national governments were unwilling to bear the ongoing costs of the GMEP; malaria specialists deemed the eradication effort in sub-Saharan Africa to be infeasible, owing to an array of insurmountable obstacles (Webb 2011, 2014); and crucially, the GMEP was in political terms judged a failure because it did not achieve its goal of global malaria eradication (Litsios 1996).

A somewhat different scenario played out with regard to yellow fever. Fred Soper, who had directed the regional eradication of *Anopheles arabiensis* in Brazil, the successful yellow fever suppression campaign against *Aedes aegypti* in that country, and the regional eradication of *Anopheles gambiae* in Egypt, was a dedicated advocate of species sanitation who embraced DDT as a crucial larvicide. Soper became director of the Pan American Health Organization in 1947, launching a programme to eradicate *Aedes aegypti* from the Western Hemisphere. It enjoyed large successes, but as political wills and economic resources waned in the early 1960s, *Aedes aegypti* began to fully recolonize and then expand beyond its previous range (Gubler 2004, Stepan 2011, Webb 2016).

DDT, disease control, and environmentalism

DDT, like the earlier lead- and arsenic-based insecticides, worked against a full range of insects, including those which threatened agriculture (Whorton 1974). In the post–Second World War years, farmers began to use the chemical broadly, and during the 1950s and 1960s, the use of DDT in agriculture spread globally. DDT was effective in sharply increasing crop yields and limiting losses owing to insect infestations. This was immensely important in many regions of the world, including those that were struggling to produce enough food for their burgeoning populations as well as those struggling to overcome the devastation of the world war. Yet the apparent "agricultural miracle" of DDT, even early on, had shown intimations of a dark side. There were warning signs that the profligate use of insecticides in agriculture produced broad, untoward ecological consequences. Biologists and wildlife specialists reported that heavy applications of DDT killed fish, birds and rodents in addition to insects. Initially, these reports had limited impact. It was not until the publication of Rachel Carson's 1962 blockbuster *Silent Spring*—a book whose title evoked a future world without birdsong—that a general alarm was rung. The book crystallized the issue of how ecological damage stemmed from the profligate use of pesticides. It played a major role in the birth of environmentalism as a political movement.

The early environmental movement produced tangible results. In 1972, under mounting political pressure, the US government banned DDT for agricultural purposes, reserving it exclusively for use in public health emergencies. This was understandably counted as a major victory by the environmental movement. Yet, ironically, DDT was the least toxic of the chlorinated hydrocarbons used as pesticides, and after its agricultural ban, farmers substituted more dangerous organophosphates (Davis 2014).

The environmental movement also sought more broadly to limit the "destruction" of the environment, and activists advocated for the reversal of earlier land-use transformations, such as the "reclamation" of wetlands through drainage. By the 1980s, the memory of earlier struggles against mosquito-borne diseases had faded. The environmentalists, charged with concerns that human activities were bringing humanity towards a critical tipping point, after which ecological recovery would be increasingly difficult if not impossible, sought to ban synthetic insecticides, including DDT, even for disease control. This put the environmental movement in the Global North on a collision course with public health specialists in the Global South, where malaria was killing one or two million people every year (Murray et al. 2012).

The conflict came to a head in the 1990s, when environmentalists pushing for a universal ban on persistent organic pollutants (POPs) ran up against a consortium of states in the Global South that lobbied for the continued use of DDT and other synthetic insecticides that helped control vector-borne diseases. The result was an accommodation that allowed for ongoing use of DDT and other chemical insecticides in disease control, where needed—in the Global South.

Taking the long view, it is evident that the historical experiences with mosquito-borne disease in the Global North and the Global South underlay the different attitudes towards DDT and other synthetic insecticides. In the Global North, in the last decades of the twentieth century, memories of mosquito-borne disease were distant. In the eighteenth and nineteenth centuries, yellow fever had exacted a significant toll along the Gulf Coast of the United States and had ignited intermittent epidemics along the eastern seaboard. The last outbreak had occurred in 1905 in New Orleans. By the 1940s, malaria in the United States had been defeated. Western Europeans had experienced their last outbreak of yellow fever in the mid-nineteenth century and saw the incidence of malaria drop to near zero in the immediate post–Second World War years. By contrast, mosquito-borne disease in the Global South resurged in the late twentieth century. In the 1980s, malaria deaths increased sharply in tropical Africa, and the annual toll remained high until the second global malaria eradication campaign, launched in the 2000s, cut the number of annual malaria deaths approximately in half through the use of insecticide-treated bed nets, indoor house-spraying with DDT and other residual insecticides, and artemisinin-based medications (Webb 2014). Yellow fever annually took an estimated total of tens of thousands of African lives, until a massive immunization campaign was launched in the 2010s (Garske et al. 2014).

In the twenty-first century, a new mosquito challenge has emerged from the cauldron of climate change. The Asian "tiger mosquito," *Aedes albopictus*, which successfully breeds in small collections of rainwater, has extended its range around the world by virtue of the global trade in used tyres. It exploits both domestic and non-domestic breeding sites, and it is capable of transmitting the same arboviruses (yellow fever, dengue fever, chikungunya and Zika) as *Aedes aegypti*. *Aedes albopictus*, however, has a geographical range far more extensive than that of *Aedes aegypti*. Some specialists fear that the expansion of *Aedes albopictus* may portend the transmission of dengue fever, chikungunya and Zika in eastern North America, Southern Europe, East Asia and Australia.

In recent years, new tools have become available for mosquito control, including the release of "sterile" or otherwise genetically modified mosquitoes, in order to prevent disease transmission. These new approaches to mosquito control have been controversial. Some observers have raised concerns about the potential for deleterious and unintended biological consequences. The ethical and ecological issues are still under discussion. Some limited releases of genetically modified mosquitoes have been carried out, but the practice has not become widely accepted.

The long history of human–mosquito relations will continue to be fraught. In the past, a few targeted efforts to eliminate mosquito vector species have been successful on a regional basis. There has never been, however, any serious proposal for the regional elimination or global eradication of all mosquito species. Because relatively few mosquito species pose threats to human health, any such proposal for regional elimination or global eradication would be misguided as well as ecologically perilous. For the foreseeable future, efforts to suppress mosquito-borne disease transmission will continue to concentrate on the most dangerous species, and in virtually all regions the goal will remain the reduction of these vector populations rather than their local elimination.

Bibliography

Bourn, Warren S., and Clarence Cottam. 1950. *Some Biological Effects of Ditching Tidewater Marshes*. Fish and Wildlife Service, U. S. Department of the Interior, No. 19. Washington, DC: U.S. Government Printing Office.

Bruce-Chwatt, L.J., and J. de Zulueta. 1980. *The Rise and Fall of Malaria in Europe*. Oxford: Oxford University Press.

Carson, Rachel. 1962. *Silent Spring*. New York: Houghton Mifflin Company.

Coleman, William. 1987. *Yellow Fever in the North*. Madison: University of Wisconsin Press.

Crain, Caitlin Mullan, Keryn Bromberg Gedan, and Michele Dionne. 2009. Tidal restrictions and mosquito ditching in New England marshes. In Brian R. Silliman, Edwin D. Grosholz, and Mark D. Bertness (eds.) *Human Impacts on Salt Marshes: A Global Perspective*. Berkeley: University of California Press, 149–169.

Daiber, Franklin. 1986. *Conservation of Tidal Marshes*. New York: Van Nostrand Reinhold.

Davis, Frederick Rowe. 2014. *Banned: A History of Pesticides and the Science of Toxicology*. New Haven: Yale University Press.

Dobson, Mary. 1980. "Marsh Fever"—the geography of Malaria in England. *Journal of Historical Geography* 6, no. 4: 357–389.

Farley, John. 2003. *To Cast Out Disease: A History of the International Health Division of the Rockefeller Foundation (1913–1951)*. Oxford: Oxford University Press.

Garske, Tini, Maria D. Van Kerkhove, Sergio Yactayo, Olivier Ronveaux, Rosamund F. Lewis, J. Erin Staples, William Perea, Neil M. Ferguson, and Yellow Fever Expert Committee. 2014. Yellow fever in Africa: Estimating the burden of disease and impact of mass vaccination from outbreak and serological data. *PLoS Medicine* 11, no. 5: e1001638.

Gubler, Duane J. 2004. The changing epidemiology of yellow fever and Dengue, 1900 to 2003: Full circle? *Comparative Immunology, Microbiology and Infectious Diseases* 27, no. 5: 319–330.

Hall, Marcus. 2010. Environmental imperialism in Sardinia: Pesticides and politics in the struggle against malaria. In Marco Armiero and Marcus Hall (eds.) *Nature and History in Modern Italy*. Athens: Ohio University Press, 70–86.

Harrison, Gordon. 1978. *Mosquitoes, Malaria and Man: A History of the Hostilities Since 1870*. New York: Dutton.

Hatvany, Matthew George. 2003. *Marshlands: Four Centuries of Environmental Change on the Shores of the St. Lawrence*. Quebec: Presses de l'Université Laval.

Holmes, Oliver Wendell. 1838. Dissertation on intermittent fevers in New England. *Boyleston Prize Dissertations for the Years 1836 and 1837*. Boston: C.C. Little and J. Brown.

Humphreys, Margaret. 2001. *Malaria: Poverty, Race, and Public Health in the United States* Baltimore: Johns Hopkins University Press.

Iroko, A. Félix. 1994. *Une histoire des hommes et des moustiques en Afrique*. Paris: Harmattan.

Litsios, Socrates. 1996. *The Tomorrow of Malaria*. Karori, NZ: Pacific Press.

McNeill, John R. 2010. *Mosquito Empires: Ecology and War in the Greater Caribbean, 1620–1914*. New York: Cambridge University Press.

Murray, Christopher JL, Lisa C. Rosenfeld, Stephen S. Lim, Kathryn G. Andrews, Kyle J. Foreman, Diana Haring, Nancy Fullman, Mohsen Naghavi, Rafael Lozano, and Alan D. Lopez. 2012. Global Malaria Mortality between 1980 and 2010: A systematic analysis. *Lancet* 379, no. 9814: 413–431.

Packard, Randall M. 1998. "No Other Logical Choice": Global Malaria eradication and the politics of international health in the post-war era. *Parassitologia* 40: 217–229.

Patterson, Gordon. 1998. *The Mosquito Wars: A History of Mosquito Control in Florida*. Gainesville, FL: University of Florida Press.

Patterson, Gordon. 2009. *The Mosquito Crusades: A History of the American Anti-Mosquito Movement from the Reed Commission to the First Earth Day*. New Brunswick: Rutgers University Press.

Ranwell, D.S. 1967. World resources of *Spartina townsendii* (*sensu lato*) and economic use of *Spartina* Marshland. *Journal of Applied Ecology* 4, no. 1: 239–256.

Russell, Paul F. 1952. The eradication of Malaria. *Scientific American* 186, no. 6: 22–25.

Seasholes, Nancy S. 2018. *Gaining Ground: A History of Landmaking in Boston*. Boston: MIT Press.

Sergent, Edmond, and Etienne Sergent. 1947. *Histoire d'un marais algérien*. Algiers: Institut Pasteur d'Algérie.

Snowden, Frank M. 2006. *The Conquest of Malaria: Italy, 1900–1962*. New Haven: Yale University Press.

Stepan, Nancy Leys. 2011. *Eradication: Ridding the World of Diseases Forever*. Ithaca: Cornell University Press.

United States Public Health Service and Tennessee Valley Authority. 1947. *Malaria Control on Impounded Water*. Washington, DC: U.S. Government Printing Office.

Verhave, Jan Peter. 2011. *The Moses of Malaria: Nicolaas H. Swellengrebel (1885–1970), Abroad and at Home*. Rotterdam: Erasmus Publishing.

Watson, Malcolm. 1921. *The Prevention of Malaria in the Federated Malay States: A Record of Twenty Years' Progress*. London: John Murray.

Watson, Malcolm. 1953. *African Highway: The Battle for Health in Central Africa*. London: John Murray.

Webb, Jr., James L.A. 2009. *Humanity's Burden: A Global History of Malaria*. New York: Cambridge University Press.

Webb, Jr., James L.A. 2011. The first large-scale use of synthetic insecticides for Malaria control in tropical Africa. *Journal of the History of Medicine and Allied Sciences* 66, no. 3: 347–376.

Webb, Jr., James L.A. 2014. *The Long Struggle Against Malaria in Tropical Africa*. New York: Cambridge University Press.

Webb, Jr., James L.A. 2016. *Aedes aegypti* suppression in the Americas: Historical perspectives. *Lancet* 10044, no. 388: 556–557.

Whorton, James. 1974. *Before Silent Spring: Pesticides and Public Health in Pre-DDT America*. Princeton: Princeton University Press.

5

DOMESTICATED MOSQUITOES

Colonization and the growth of mosquito habitats in North America

Urmi Engineer Willoughby

Humans never wanted to cultivate habitats that encouraged mosquito breeding and habitation. However, human settlements and agricultural landscapes often created conditions that attracted mosquitoes, and humans themselves provided a crucial source of blood that enabled the survival and fecundity of several mosquito species. In North America, mosquito populations grew in the context of European colonization and African slavery. Prior to 1500, indigenous mosquitoes lived alongside Native American agricultural communities, as they did in Afro-Eurasia. By the sixteenth century, ecological changes resulting from the Columbian Exchange brought new species of mosquitoes to the Americas. Human migrations and environmental alterations caused by colonization also enabled the expansion of regional, indigenous mosquito populations such as *Anopheles*, which proliferated in the seventeenth through nineteenth centuries. At the same time, ongoing transatlantic commerce, migrations, and urban ports facilitated the growth and dominance of a newly imported species, *Aedes aegypti* (*Ae. aegypti*).

It is possible to discern historical patterns of the emergence and growth of mosquito habitats from accounts of contemporary observers, medical and epidemiological records, and present-day research on mosquito-borne diseases. Historical accounts such as travel journals, diaries and medical literature often include observations of local flora and fauna, including insect life. These provide insights on the presence of mosquitoes, as well as the relative increase or decrease in their abundance. Historical records that indicate the presence of yellow fever and malaria is especially helpful in determining the presence of an established population of a particular species capable of carrying the requisite viruses and parasites: accounts of the earliest recorded epidemics of yellow fever demonstrate the presence of *Ae. aegypti*, while descriptions of intermittent and miasmatic fevers indicate the presence of various *Anopheles* species. Present-day studies of

DOI: 10.4324/9781003056034-5

vector mosquitoes show the global spread of certain *Aedes* species (*Ae. aegypti* and *Ae. albopictus*), and regional dominance of dozens of *Anopheles* species throughout the world. Given the rise of mosquito populations stemming from humanity's propensity to transport these insects and encourage their growth, are humans responsible for the prolific rise of anthropophilic (human–loving) mosquito populations? Since humans accidently enabled the growth of mosquitoes, are they justified in their efforts to control these mosquitoes and even seek to eradicate them? And is it even possible for humans to eradicate a species that has adapted and evolved to live alongside humans?

Settlement

Mosquito populations grew alongside human settlements in native America. Various indigenous species of *Anopheles* mosquitoes lived in the diverse forest, wetland and grassland environments of eastern North America, including *An. quadrimaculatus, An. albimanus, An. pseudopunctipennis* and others (Kiszewksi et al. 2004, 488; Webb 2009, 67). In western North America, native *Anopheles* species included *An. pseudopunctipennis, An. freeborni*, perhaps *An. crucians* (Sinka et al. 2010, 8–9; Mullen et al. 2002, 243). Native North American experiences indicate a familiarity with mosquitoes. It is likely that native agricultural practices, for example, such as the construction of *chinampas* and maize fields, attracted mosquitoes. For centuries, Indigenous farmers in Mexico built *chinampas*, or islands of raised fields within lakes and lowlands. *Anopheles* mosquitoes readily bred in these maize fields, as well as on lake shores, in canals and in swamps surrounding Tenochtitlán and other cities in the Valley of Mexico and the Yucatán. Deforestation and the construction of maize fields throughout the Mississippi Valley likely created mosquito habitats in this lowland valley. It follows that mosquito populations likely decreased with the decline of Mississippian Cahokia and Moundville urban centres in the fourteenth and fifteenth centuries.

The habits of *Anopheles* mosquitoes vary greatly according to species. Some species rarely live near human settlements, while others commonly occupy areas close to human dwellings. Several species' attraction to human settlements appears to arise from their desire to feed on human blood and breed in human-built environments. In the Caribbean and Central America, it is likely that *An. albimanus* populations lived near Indigenous settlements. In mainland North America, several species, including *An. albimanus, An. pseudopunctipennis, An. freeborni, An. quadrimaculatus* and *An. walkeri*, may have adapted to living near Indigenous agricultural settlements in the Valley of Mexico, the Great Lakes region and the Mississippi Valley.

European colonization in the Caribbean and Mexico created additional habitats that attracted *An. albimanus*. Entomological studies demonstrate that this species has developed a strong preference for feeding on human blood and breeding in humanized environments, such as in cleared fields near human settlements, rather than in forested areas away from human communities. It would seem that the construction of roads and use of domesticated animals for transport also contributed to the growth of mosquitoes. Entomologists have shown that *An. albimanus* can breed in very small pools of water, such as in borrow pits, wheel ruts and hoof prints (Sinka et al. 2010, 10).

In mainland North America, European exploration and early contacts with Indigenous peoples and environments also indicate the presence of native mosquitoes. Historical evidence indicates that malaria parasites arrived in North America with the earliest European colonists in the sixteenth and seventeenth centuries. Malaria had been endemic in parts of Europe during this period, especially in coastal regions of Italy, Iberia and England, which emerged as maritime centres. Malaria parasites then found new hosts in native *Anopheles* species in the Americas. Even if there is not much evidence for malaria during the early contact period, it is possible that malaria was at the root of cycles of fever and hunger that caused high mortality and that afflicted newly established colonial settlements and exploratory missions. Moreover, malaria appears to have been part of the cycle of disease and famine that devastated the English settlement at Jamestown in 1607 (Hirsch 1883, 229; Singer 1962, 455–456; Webb 2009, 74). In 1718–1720, the first French expeditions in the Mississippi Delta endured a severe cycle of fever and hunger that are consistent with symptoms of malaria (Usner 1992, 34–36). However, there is not much evidence that malaria was a significant presence or problem in North America until the mid-seventeenth century, when outbreaks appeared more frequently in New England after about 1650. It is possible that malaria played a role in disease epidemics that afflicted Native American populations in the southeast in the sixteenth through eighteenth centuries. However, as Paul Kelton and others have argued, the highest rates of depopulation occurred during the Great Southeastern Smallpox Epidemic that began in 1696, and slave raids exacerbated population loss and disease vulnerability in the region (Kelton 2007, 189–191; Usner 1992, 18–24).

Indeed, *Anopheles* mosquitoes in the Mississippi delta lived alongside a diversity of insects and other species in the wetland environment. French missionary accounts that describe the earliest European experiences in the region demonstrate the presence of large numbers of mosquitoes drawn to the blood of humans who ventured into the swamps. In 1727, the French missionary Father Du Poisson travelled up the Mississippi River from New Orleans to the Arkansas post, and described in great detail his encounters with insects, including mosquitoes— or *maringouins* in vernacular French. Beginning his journey in May, which he described as "the season of the greatest heat, which is increasing every day," he also complained about the lack of food. However,

> the greatest torture—without which everything else would have been only a recreation, but which passes all belief, and could never be imagined in France unless it had been experienced—is the mosquitoes, the cruel persecution of the mosquitoes. … This little creature has caused more

swearing since the French came to Mississippi, than has been done before that time in all the rest of the world.

(Thwaites 1900, 289)

Du Poisson goes on to describe the "millions of mosquitoes" that attacked him and his companions in the morning, afternoon and throughout the night.

As newcomers built new settlements in close proximity to mosquito habitats, settlers provided an abundant food source for mosquito populations. Early colonial settlements may have disrupted some mosquito habitats but they created many new ones. Settlement activities included land clearance, water management, shelter construction and crop cultivation. In many cases, the clearing of land caused deforestation and resulted in the decline of numerous animal species, particularly those that lived in the forest canopy, including rodents, bats and birds that fed on mosquitoes (Moore 2000, 421; McNeill 2010, 48; Watts 1987, 39). At the same time, drainage canals created new freshwater ponds, which provided additional breeding spaces. Accounts of European and Euro-American colonial settlements in North America often described outbreaks of fever, which fit the description of malaria. By the end of the colonial period, malaria was endemic in pockets throughout the eastern Atlantic and Gulf coasts, indicating the presence of *Anopheles*.

Ongoing European and American settlement in the eighteenth and nineteenth centuries helped establish large populations of *An. quadrimaculatus* across eastern North America, which grew in tandem with the establishment of agricultural settlements in the Ohio and Mississippi Valleys. Such presence of *An. quadrimaculatus* became established in rural areas throughout eastern North America, as is indicated by ongoing outbreaks of malaria among early colonists during the territorial expansion of the United States in the early nineteenth century (Nash 2006, 23; Humphreys 2001; Ackerknecht 1945; Chapin 1884). In the 1920s, entomologists found that in the Mississippi Delta region, *An. quadrimaculatus* "greatly predominates over all other species" (Barber et al. 1927, 2494), owing in part to the observation that both *An. quadrimaculatus* and *An. walkeri* populations grew near human dwellings. Both species continue to show a preference for feeding on humans and living in built environments. Entomologists reveal that *An. walkeri* adults "enter dwellings at night to feed on humans and then retire to secretive daytime hiding places" (Carpenter et al. 1955, 55). Similarly, *An. quadrimaculatus* are mainly night-time feeders, and then rest during daylight hours "in dark corners in buildings, underneath houses, in stables, in hollow trees, and other shelters" (Carpenter et al. 1955, 52). *An. Quadrimaculatus* also prefers large natural and artificial bodies of water, including lagoons, lakes, marshes, rice fields and irrigation channels (Sinka et al. 2010, 8–11). It seems that, over the last 500 years in North America, the single most important event to favour multiplication and growth of two key mosquito species was the arrival and expansion of Old World settlers.

Plantation agriculture

The rise of African slavery and plantation agriculture in the Atlantic Americas transformed mosquito–human relationships. The combination of the Atlantic slave trade and plantation agriculture in the Caribbean, Atlantic and Gulf Coast regions led to the growth of North American mosquito populations, including native *Anopheles* species and new *Aedes* species from Afro-Eurasia.

Such human-caused environmental transformations allowed *Ae. aegypti* mosquitoes to become a globally dominant species that lived alongside humans in maritime and urban environments in the seventeenth through nineteenth centuries. Entomologists today consider *Ae. aegypti* to be a "domesticated" species because of its proclivity to inhabit human settlements and thrive in human-built environments. In the wild, *Ae. aegypti* live and breed in forests, laying eggs in tree holes and other cavities. But when exposed to human environments, they typically breed in artificial water containers made of various materials including clay, wood, cement and, more recently, plastic, in close proximity to human residences (Carpenter et al., 1955, 262). *Aedes* originated in sub-Saharan Africa, and spread throughout the globe with European colonial projects in the seventeenth through nineteenth centuries. Although it is unknown exactly when *Ae. aegypti* became an anthropophilic species, it is possible that living alongside early agricultural communities in tropical West Africa, or being transported to the Americas after 1500, accelerated this process. Later, after arriving in the Americas, *Ae. aegypti* travelled across the Pacific on ships and boats to become established in urban environments of coastal Asia and Australia by the close of the nineteenth century (Powell and Tabachnick 2013, 12–13).

The notion of "domesticated" mosquitoes offers an ironic understanding of their evolutionary relationship with humans. Historically, humans have unintentionally supported the growth of numerous animals and plants, usually considered to be pests or weeds, such as lice, rats, cats and jackals, and in some places even bears. The increase of mosquito numbers in humanized environments demonstrates the evolutionary success of mosquitoes, as well as their tenacious ability to resist human efforts to control or eradicate them. Anthropophily benefited mosquitoes that survived by being able to consume human blood meals, even if such mosquitoes did not provide any known benefit to human communities. Due to the role of certain mosquito species as vectors of disease, their attraction to people has caused devastating diseases and mortality to human populations.

Popular sources have depicted mosquitoes as humanity's most dangerous threat, including Bill Gates who has called them "the deadliest animal in the world" (Gates 2016). From the perspective of *Ae. aegypti*, it has increased its temporal and spatial reach by adapting to human environments. One of the key ways in which *Ae. aegypti* modified its behaviour was by developing a preference for blood of humans over non-human primates. Sedentary human communities provided an abundant and stable source of blood—as opposed to feeding on migratory birds or ungulates—so that *Ae. aegypti*'s adaptation to humans allowed it to grow beyond its former geographical reach (Powell and Tabachnick 2013, 11).

Ae. aegypti has been remarkably successful in colonizing the Americas. This mosquito grew on plantations and throughout the infrastructure that supported transatlantic capitalist networks, including densely populated port cities and ships. Because *Ae. aegypti* served as the main vector of the yellow fever virus, it is possible to trace the presence of the species by studying epidemic patterns. Yellow fever incidence in the Atlantic World can therefore reveal links between transatlantic commerce, plantation agriculture, urbanization and the growth of *Ae. aegypti* populations. Such events suggest that *Ae. aegypti* arrived in the Americas in the centuries of accelerated Atlantic trade between 1600 and 1800, with the earliest known outbreak of yellow fever occurring in the 1640s in Barbados, followed by various epidemics in the Caribbean that indicated this mosquito's presence on Atlantic ships and in port cities. By the 1700s, seasonal waves of *Ae. aegypti* were entering South Carolina and the Chesapeake, extending as far north as Quebec (Patterson 1992, 857; Augustin 1909, 652).

That sugar plantations in the Caribbean, Brazil and Louisiana attracted *Ae. aegypti* populations is evidenced by large-scale epidemics during the early phases of establishing plantations and port cities. The earliest known outbreaks of yellow fever were in sugar colonies in Barbados, as well as in Guadeloupe, St. Kitts and Cuba. Descriptions of Caribbean plantations show the ubiquity of mosquitoes and other insects. In Jamaica in 1688, Hans Sloane described how enslaved residents of sugar plantations lit fires to repel "gnats, mosquitoes, and flies." James Goodyear and others explain that sugar cultivation and production served to facilitate the growth of *Ae. aegypti* mosquitoes in several ways. There was clearance of land for sugar fields, which increased deforestation with the demand for wood to fuel sugar mills. To create additional plantations in lowland regions, there was clearance of marshes, swamps and bogs. Drainage canals and ditches also raised susceptibility to flooding, and created new freshwater habitats for mosquitoes. For example, on Louisiana plantations in the nineteenth century, drainage ditches and canals were excavated to keep sugar crops from flooding. French authorities had granted land tracts for plantations that formed 90-degree angles to the river, so that each had river access with a back swamp for drainage, creating additional freshwater ponds and ditches for mosquitoes to lay eggs (Willoughby 2017; Hilliard 1979, 258–263). The plantations also fostered growth of *Ae. aegypti* mosquitoes by creating breeding places in clean water collected in cisterns, water-barrels and clay pots (McNeill 2010, 205; Goodyear 1978, 13).

In addition to fostering *Ae. aegypti* populations, plantation environments likewise enabled the growth of *Anopheles* populations. The drainage ditches, canals and irrigated fields served to create many breeding spaces for this other mosquito species too. In the Caribbean, deforestation and soil erosion in lowland environments created new freshwater swamps, providing ideal breeding places for

An. albimanus due to the species' preference for freshwater habitats with ample sunlight, algae and other organic matter. Other *Anopheles* species fed on a plantation's domesticated animals, providing the mosquito with abundant nutritional resources (McNeill 2010, 55–56).

Rice cultivation was especially important for creating new habitats for *Anopheles* species in the Americas. Rising rates of malaria on rice farms of the Caribbean, Suriname and Brazil implied a rising presence of *Anopheles*. There was a similar pattern in North America, where malaria and mosquitoes followed rice cultivation in South Carolina, Georgia and Louisiana. Before the establishment of large-scale commercial rice production in the 1680s, South Carolina was relatively healthy compared to Caribbean colonies, where there was closer contact between *Anopheles* and people. As J.R. McNeill explains, the wetlands of coastal South Carolina "suited *Anopheles*' habits even before the installation of a rice economy, but the extensive irrigation of fields with shallow and stagnant water, full of organic debris, made good conditions much better." Four floodings each year provided especially favourable breeding grounds for *An. quadrimaculatus*. In South Carolina, plantations required the felling of trees and the construction of ponds and reservoirs, combined with ditches and canals for irrigation and drainage. These new habitats, in close proximity to enslaved African and Afro-American living quarters, provided female mosquitoes with a large supply of human blood and ample space to lay eggs (McNeill 2010, 205; McCandless 2011, 45, 126).

Similarly in Louisiana, subsistence rice production provided an abundance of ideal mosquito habitat. In 1718, the French Western Company ordered the purchase of enslaved Africans who could cultivate rice, along with barrels of rice seed from the African coast (Hall 1992; Dart 1931, 173). Rice farming grew substantially in the 1720s, with the result that by the 1730s, rice was the primary grain of local consumption. Ample evidence shows that it was consumed by European colonists, creoles, enslaved Africans, and African Americans (Hall 1992, 10, 122; Morris 2012, 48). In this period, rice was being cultivated with various methods in the lowlands of South Carolina, Georgia and Louisiana to produce still more *Anopheles* habitat (Gray 1933, 66). These regions became centres of endemic malaria in North America, demonstrating an association between rice cultivation and *Anopheles* growth, mirroring experiences in West Africa and Italy (McNeill 2010, 57; Boccolini et al., 2012). Meanwhile, growing plantation economies in North America also enabled expansion of *Ae. aegypti*, especially in Boston, Philadelphia and New York in summer, and Charleston, Norfolk and New Orleans year around.

Urban environments

Entomologists consider *Ae. aegypti* to be an "urban species" because it prefers feeding on human blood and breeding in artificial containers. The growth of the Atlantic trade system led to the establishment of numerous port cities that connected North America and Europe to ports across the tropical and subtropical Atlantic. Carrying pathogens, *Ae. aegypti* migrated across the Atlantic and around the world, multiplying into large populations wherever people transported it. *Ae. aegypti*, following the path of humans, migrated out of Africa, successfully colonizing most tropical and temperate coasts. By the late eighteenth and early nineteenth centuries, Atlantic ports were developing into large cities with high levels of traffic, dense residential development and diverse human communities with origins in Africa, Europe and the Americas.

Urban growth promoted environments favourable to *Ae. aegypti* through deforestation, urban construction, flooded landscapes and human immigration. Environmental alterations that removed forest cover and created new freshwater habitats provided a base for these mosquitoes. Their populations would then grow in concert with new canals and construction projects.

Outdoor and indoor urban spaces provided still more habitat for *Ae. aegypti*. Preferential breeding spaces of *Ae. aegypti* included any artificial container that could hold clean water, ranging from reservoirs, ponds and cisterns to gutters and drains. In coastal ports that depended on rainwater, cisterns promoted growth of mosquito populations. With the discovery in the early twentieth century of *Ae. Aegypti*'s role in transmitting yellow fever, public health authorities labelled this species the "cistern mosquito" (Boyce 1906, 11). Urban gardens also provided mosquitoes with breeding spaces. Inside homes, adult mosquitoes rested "in closets, cupboards, cabinets, behind doors, and even behind picture frames." Female mosquitoes would then feed at night in lighted rooms (Willoughby 2017, 16; Carpenter et al., 1955, 262).

Newcomers from the Old World (both free and enslaved) provided a large, diverse population of humans for *Ae. aegypti* to feed upon. Although this mosquito species can feed on other mammals, it has shown a preference for human blood over that of domesticated livestock. With *Ae. aegypti* carrying and transmitting yellow fever, the presence of this disease tracks the movement of the mosquito, from Havana to Port-au-Prince, from Charleston to Boston. By the end of the eighteenth century, colonial port cities up and down North America's Atlantic seaboard supported large populations of *Ae. aegypti*, which were becoming naturalized in their new urban habitat. One of the most memorable yellow fever epidemics in US history took place in Philadelphia in 1793, in the aftermath of the Haitian Revolution. The epidemic swept the young United States' first capital city, which became an important national centre of medical institutions.

By the nineteenth century in New Orleans, yellow fever's annual summer visit showed the extent to which *Ae. aegypti* had become established in the city. Here, mosquitoes bred in urban spaces along the waterfront, in residential areas, yards, gardens and cemeteries. Many of the city's unique architectural features, such as the ornamental above-ground cemeteries, proved to be especially attractive to this anthropophilic mosquito. Ongoing immigrant waves of non-immune peoples created ongoing conditions for epidemics: human blood provided mosquitoes with nutrition and city architecture provided them with habitat (Willoughby 2017). The construction of railroads connecting the ports to interior cities further increased the reach of *Ae. aegypti*. The spread of urban *Ae. aegypti* populations after the American Civil War led to the nation's worst yellow fever epidemic, which after breaking out in 1878 radiated up from New Orleans throughout the Mississippi Valley, causing pain and suffering as far north as Chicago and Pittsburgh (Willoughby 2017, 116).

Conclusion

Reviewing the history of how humans domesticated mosquitoes in North America would suggest that it may never be possible for humans to completely eliminate mosquitoes. People did not choose to domesticate these mosquitoes, and efforts to eliminate them over the long term have never been successful. *Homo sapiens* has inadvertently enlarged mosquito habitats, or else created habitats suitable for newly arriving mosquito species. In many cases, efforts to eradicate mosquitoes have revealed the role played by humans in attracting them. For example, in Panama in the early twentieth century, entomologists working to control malaria and yellow fever in the Canal Zone found that some *Anopheles* mosquitoes, including *An. albimanus*, preferred living and breeding in newly constructed landscapes. Human engineering projects attracted mosquitoes that preferred to live near human structures including workers' quarters, construction sites and railroads (Sutter 2007, 743–744). The rapid evolution of mosquitoes to pesticides further emphasizes the role that humans play in cultivating mosquitoes that are more resilient and genetically adapted to man-made chemical poisons.

Although the majority of mosquito species are content to live in the wild, a few species have shown strong preferences for human-modified environments, ranging from small agricultural settlements to large urban metropolises. The attraction of *Anopheles* and *Aedes* to humans and humanized environments would indicate that we may have no choice but to try to learn to live peacefully with mosquitoes. The fact that the settlement of North America involved the domestication of mosquitoes indicates that human societies will probably continue to attract mosquitoes simply by existing. Humans may in the end need to approach mosquito control cautiously and through a more thoughtful approach, while understanding the importance of built environments and wetlands to the life of these disease-carrying insects. As it becomes clear that powerful control measures like pesticides are not sustainable, changes in urban planning and rural land management may be the best way to diminish mosquito populations over time.

Humans and mosquitoes share a long history of coevolution and adaptation, and some mosquito species have learned to depend on *Homo sapiens* for survival. While humans could easily envision a happy future without these irritating and deadly pests, more and more mosquitoes have come to rely on humans for their sustenance and reproduction. As long as humans continue to transform wild and forest lands, it seems likely that humans will continue to be bothered by mosquitoes, with the ecological limits of mosquitoes expanding to merge with human communities. Mosquito numbers grew substantially in the second half of the twentieth century, ushered in by the ecological impacts of globalization, urban development, human population growth and climate change. The effects of climate change have already allowed *Aedes* and *Anopheles* mosquitoes to expand their range in North America, with *Aedes* becoming common in the western United States. If these trends continue, it is probable that humans and mosquitoes will be in even more frequent contact with each other across a widening geographical range.

Bibliography

Ackerknecht, Erwin H. 1945. *Malaria in the Upper Mississippi Valley, 1760–1900. Supplements to the Bulletin of the History of Medicine 4.* Baltimore: Johns Hopkins University Press.

Augustin, George. 1909. *History of Yellow Fever.* New Orleans: Searcy & Pfaff Ltd.

Barber, M.A., W.H.W. Komp, and T.B. Hayne. 1927. The Susceptibility to Malaria Parasites and the Relation to the Transmission of Malaria of the Species of Anopheles Common in Southern United States. *Public Health Reports (1896–1970)* 42, no. 41: 2487–2502.

Boccolini, D. et al. 2012. Impact of Environmental Changes and Human-Related Factors on the Potential Malaria Vector, Anopheles Labranchiae (Diptera: Culicidae), in Maremma, Central Italy. *Population and Community Ecology* 49, no. 4: 833–842.

Boyce, Rubert. 1906. *Yellow Fever Prophylaxis in New Orleans, 1905.* London: Williams & Norgate.

Boyce, Rubert. 1910. *Health Progress and Administration in the West Indies.* New York: E.P. Dutton and Company.

Carpenter, Stanley J., and Walter J. LaCasse. 1955. *Mosquitoes of North America (North of Mexico).* Berkeley: University of California Press.

Chambers, D.M., C.D. Steelman, and P.E. Schilling. 1981. The Effect of Cultural Practices on Mosquito Abundance and Distribution in the Louisiana Riceland Ecosystem. *Mosquito News* 41, no. 2: 233–240.

Chapin, Charles V. 1884. *The Origin and Progress of the Malarial Fever Now Prevalent in New England.* Providence: Kellogg Printing Co.

Christophers, S.R. 1960. *Aedes Aegypti (L.) the Yellow Fever Mosquito: Its Life History, Bionomics and Structure.* Cambridge: Cambridge University Press.

Dart, Henry P. 1931. The First Cargo of African Slaves for Louisiana, 1718. *The Louisiana Historical Quarterly* 14, no. 2: 163–181.

Foster, Woodbridge A. and Edward D. Walker. 2019. Mosquitoes. In Gary Mullen and Lance Durden eds. *Medical and Veterinary Entomology*, 3rd ed. London: Elsevier Academic Press, 261–326. https://doi.org/10.1016/B978-0-12-814043-7.00015-7

Gates, Bill. 2016. Mapping the end of Malaria. In *GatesNotes* on 10 Oct at https://www.gatesnotes.com/Health/Mapping-the-End-of-Malaria on 09.10.2020.

Goodyear, James D. 1978. The Sugar Connection: A New Perspective on the History of Yellow Fever. *Bulletin of the History of Medicine* 52: 5–21.

Gordon, David M., and Shepard Krech III, eds. 2012. *Indigenous Knowledge and the Environment in Africa and North America.* Oxford: Ohio University Press.

Gray, Lewis Cecil. 1933. *History of Agriculture in the Southern United States to 1860*, Vol. I. Washington: The Carnegie institution of Washington.

Hall, Gwendolyn Midlo. 1992. *Africans in Colonial Louisiana: The Development of Afro-Creole Culture in the Eighteenth Century*. Baton Rouge: Louisiana State University Press.

Hilliard, Sam B. 1979. Site Characteristics and Spatial Stability of the Louisiana Sugarcane Industry. *Agricultural History* 53, no. 1: 254–69.

Hirsch, August. 1883. *Handbook of Geographical and Historical Pathology*, Vol. I, translated by Charles Creighton. London: The New Sydenham Society.

Howard, Leland O., Harrison G. Dyar, and Frederick Knab. 1912. *The Mosquitoes of North and Central America and the West Indies*. Washington, DC: Carnegie Institute.

Humphreys, Margaret. 2001. *Malaria: Poverty, Race, and Public Health in the United States*. Baltimore: The Johns Hopkins University Press.

Kelton, Paul. 2007. *Epidemics and Enslavement: Biological Catastrophe in the Native Southeast, 1492–1715*. Lincoln: University of Nebraska Press.

Kiszewski, Anthony et al. 2004. A Global Index Representing the Stability of Malaria Transmission. *American Journal of Tropical Medicine and Hygiene* 70, no. 5: 486–498.

Lee, Chan. 1960. *A Culture History of Rice With Special Reference to Louisiana*. Ph.D. Thesis, Louisiana State University.

Lounibos, L. Philip. 2002. Invasions by Insect Vectors of Human Disease. *Annual Review of Entomology* 47: 233–266.

McCandless, Peter. 2011. *Slavery, Disease, and Suffering in the Southern Lowcountry*. Cambridge: Cambridge University Press.

McCann, James C. 2005. *Maize and Grace: Africa's Encounter with a New World Crop*. Cambrdige: Harvard University Press.

McNeill, J.R. 2007. Yellow Jack and Geopolitics: Environment, Epidemics, and the Struggles for Empire in the American Tropics, 1640–1830. In J.R. McNeill Alf Hornborg, and Joan Martinez-Alier eds. *Rethinking Environmental History: World-System History and Global Environmental Change*. Lanham: AltaMira Press: 199–220.

McNeill, J.R. 2010. *Mosquito Empires: Ecology and War in the Greater Caribbean, 1620–1914*. Cambridge: Cambridge University Press.

Moore, Jason W. 2000. Sugar and the Expansion of the Early Modern World-Economy: Commodity Frontiers, Ecological Transformation, and Industrialization. *Review: A Journal of the Fernand Braudel Center* 23, no. 3: pp. 409–433.

Morris, Christopher. 2012. *The Big Muddy: An Environmental History of the Mississippi and Its Peoples from Hernando de Soto to Hurricane Katrina*. Oxford: Oxford University Press.

Mullen, Gary and Larry Durden eds. 2002. *Medical and Veterinary Entomology*, 1st ed. Elsevier Academic Press.

Nash, Linda. 2006. *Inescapable Ecologies: A History of Environment, Disease, and Knowledge*. Berkeley: University of California Press.

Patterson, K. David. 1992. Yellow Fever Epidemics and Mortality in the United States, 1693–1905. *Social Science and Medicine* 34, no. 8: 855–865.

Powell, Jeffrey R., and Walter J. Tabachnick. 2013. History of Domestication and Spread of *Aedes Aegypti* – A Review. *Memórias do Instituto Oswaldo Cruz* 108, no. Suppl. I: 11–17.

Ries, Maurice. 1962. The Mississippi Fort, Called Fort de la Boulaye. *Louisiana Historical Quarterly* 19, no. 4: 1–73.

Singer, Charles, and E. Ashworth Underwood. 1962. *A Short History of Medicine*, 2nd ed. Oxford: At the Clarendon Press.

Sinka, Marianne E. et al. 2010. The Dominant Anopheles Vectors of Human Malaria in the Americas: Occurrence Data, Distribution Maps, and Bionomic Précis. *Parasites & Vectors* 3, no. 72: 1–26.

Sutter, Paul S. 2007. Nature's Agents or Agents of Empire? Entomological Workers and Environmental Change during the Construction of the Panama Canal. *Isis* 98, no. 4: 724–753.

Thwaites, Reuben Gold ed. 1900. *The Jesuit Relations And Allied Documents: Travels And Explorations of the Jesuit Missionaries In New France, 1610–1791, Vol LXVII, Lower Canada, Abenakis, Louisiana, 1716–1727.* Cleveland: Burrows.

Usner, Daniel H. 1992. *Indians, Settlers, & Slaves in a Frontier Exchange Economy.* Chapel Hill: University of North Carolina Press.

Valenčius, Conevery Bolton. 2002. *The Health of the Country: How Americans Understood Themselves and Their Land.* New York: Basic Books.

Watts, David. 1987. *The West Indies: Patterns of Development, Culture, and Environmental Change Since 1492.* Cambridge: Cambridge University Press.

Webb, James L.A. 2009. *Humanity's Burden: A Global History of Malaria.* Cambridge: Cambridge University Press.

Webb, James L.A. 2014. *The Long Struggle against Malaria in Tropical Africa.* Cambridge: Cambridge University Press.

Willoughby, Urmi Engineer. 2017. *Yellow Fever, Race, and Ecology in Nineteenth-Century New Orleans.* Baton Rouge: Louisiana State University Press.

6

COULD WE/SHOULD WE ERADICATE MOSQUITOES?

The case of the yellow fever vector[1]

Nancy Leys Stepan

It is impossible to write about controlling infectious diseases without having the pandemic of coronavirus in the forefront of our minds. COVID-19 has brought home to all of us very forcefully indeed the incompleteness of our scientific knowledge in the face of novel pathogens, the lack of government preparedness despite repeated forewarnings, and the often fumbling and inconsistent nature of public policies when we are faced with mass public health threats.

Zika provides another example of an uncertain response to an epidemic less universal in scope than coronavirus, but deeply worrying. In 2015 world health experts began to hear about an eruption of an apparently novel viral infection in northeastern Brazil. Zika was not in fact unknown to scientists; but its association in the Brazilian outbreak with microcephaly in newborn infants was unexpected and shocking, and led the World Health Organization (WHO) in early 2016 to declare a Public Health Emergency of International Concern (PHEIC) (Lowe et al., 2018). Zika eventually spread to over 80 countries (Chippaux and Chippaux, 2018). Almost overlooked at the time, but also very troubling, was an outbreak of yellow fever in the states of Rio de Janeiro and São Paulo later that same year—one of the largest such outbreaks in Latin America in decades. And let's not forget the epidemics of chikungunya and especially dengue fever that have plagued the country in recent years (Gubler, 2004).

What distinguishes these viral diseases from COVID-19 is that they involve, either directly or potentially, an insect vector or transmitter, the *Aedes aegypti* mosquito, an age-old "enemy" of public health. In response to Zika, the President of Brazil, Dilma Rouseff, hastily targeted the mosquito, sending in 220,000 soldiers to help with insecticiding, while acknowledging that Brazil was already losing the battle against the insect. This was the country that had once *almost* eradicated this mosquito. So what had happened? Why had vector eradication been given up? Could we do it again? Should we?

DOI: 10.4324/9781003056034-6

After all, most of the more than 3,500 species of mosquito recognized by scientists so far do not transmit diseases to humans. Some species do not bite humans at all, and others are merely a nuisance, with many of them remaining very useful to local ecologies, as pollinators or as food for other animals. So we should learn to live with them.

It's the exceptions that we worry about. Ever since Ross and Grassi proved in 1897–1898 that anopheline mosquitoes transmit malaria, and the Reed Commission established in 1900 that the *Aedes aegypti* mosquito transmits yellow fever, getting rid of these mosquito vectors has been taken to be a legitimate, even necessary, method of disease control. All thought of ecological balance or cooperative living with insects seems to fly out the window once we are in the midst of a mosquito-transmitted epidemic.

It is these dangerous mosquitoes that form the crux of the question asked in this book: "If we *could* rid ourselves of mosquitoes, would we still want to?" This question does an excellent job of focusing attention on critical matters of ecology and ethics in relation to mosquitoes. But as a medical historian who has engaged with the messy details of past efforts to control mosquitoes, I find it difficult to abstract the "could we?" part of the story from the "should we?". Difficult, that is, to disentangle or bracket off eradication or the "getting rid of" process, because embedded in the "could we?" are already many issues of "should we?". How is extermination (or severe reduction) of a mosquito species to be carried out, and at what cost? What eradication methods do we propose? Are there ecological and/or ethical issues associated with these methods? What does "eradication" of a mosquito species imply: local elimination, or worldwide reduction to zero? Is it possible to eradicate an entire mosquito species?

For answers to such questions I turn to what is possibly the best piece of historical evidence available, the extensive pre– and post–World War II campaign to definitively eradicate the *Aedes aegypti* mosquito from the entire continental Americas. I evaluate why, given the existence of an excellent vaccine against yellow fever, the eradication of a mosquito species was chosen as the main method of urban yellow fever control in the Americas, and why the French colonial authorities in West Africa focused largely on mass vaccination instead.

I end the chapter by bringing the issue of mosquito eradication/control back to our ongoing worries about the return and spread of the *Aedes aegypti* mosquito in the Americas, Africa and Asia, keeping in mind the epidemiologically difficult conditions of contemporary urban life. As noted already, *Aedes aegypti* is implicated in the transmission of dengue and chikungunya, as well as yellow fever and Zika. Other *Aedes* species, such as *A. albopictus*, are also capable of acting as vectors for these diseases. Is mass vaccination the path to follow, assuming a vaccine is even available? Or is vector control still a necessary part of disease control? What about social investments and infrastructural improvements?

I use the *Aedes aegypti* eradication campaign here as paradigmatic of a certain style or model of mosquito eradication and/or control. In concluding my chapter, I contrast that style with a potential alternative model, though in the end, I am only able to sketch the outlines of that model.

The background: eradicating malaria mosquitoes

The campaign to eradicate the *Aedes aegypti* mosquito was led by Dr. Fred L. Soper, first in his position as a Rockefeller Foundation (RF) officer in Brazil, where from 1930 until 1942 he directed the RF-Brazilian National Cooperative Yellow Fever Service, and second, in his capacity as Director from 1947 to 1959 of the Pan American Health Organization (PAHO), the American regional office of WHO.

As the arch-eradicationist of his day, Soper was associated with most of the eradication campaigns of the twentieth century, against yaws, smallpox, malaria and yellow fever. In the case of malaria and yellow fever, mosquito reduction was a well-established method of halting disease transmission. Soper's contribution was to try to shift the focus of eradication from the disease, to the vector mosquitoes themselves. Instead of mosquito reduction, Soper aimed for vector extirpation. A larger-than-life character, admirable in his tenacity, Soper was also dogmatic and often wrongheaded. A gift, in short, to medical historians.

A brief look at three experiments with mosquito eradication focused on malaria vectors provide context to Soper's much longer effort to extirpate the urban yellow fever mosquito, *Aedes aegypti*. Malaria at the time was understood to have a very complex etiology, involving multiple factors—ecological, environmental and social, as well as vectorial. In the face of causal complexity, Soper offered instead blunt simplicity, with equivocal results.

First Soper tried to wipe out the highly "efficient" and anthropophilic malaria vector, *Anopheles gambiae*, from an area in the northeast of Brazil (1938–1941), and then again in Upper Egypt (1944–1945), both times in response to severe malaria epidemics. Concentrating his anti-malaria efforts exclusively on eliminating the *gambiae*, using the pre-DDT insecticide house spraying and anti-larval methods perfected for yellow fever, and ignoring all other causes of the epidemics (e.g. troop mobilization, population displacements or other malaria vectors), Soper attributed the end of these malaria epidemics entirely to the disappearance of the *gambiae* species in the two regions (Packard and Gadelha, 1997; Stepan, 2011).

At the time, a malaria expert hailed the vanquishing of the *gambiae* as "one of the greatest accomplishments in all malariology" (Stepan, 2011). Yet in truth, the results were ambiguous. The *gambiae* mosquito was a recent arrival in both Brazil and Egypt, and so not fully integrated into the local ecology. Soper's extermination efforts were noteworthy examples of stopping invasions of a dangerous species—and of potential relevance today, as mosquito species expand into new places as a result of climate change, human mobility and other factors—but not a true test of the possibility of eradicating an indigenous or well-established mosquito species over a large area, let alone the world.

A third species eradication campaign (1946–1950), this time against *Anopheles labranchiae* on the very malarial island of Sardinia, was such a test, indeed a genuine experiment, organized by Soper, with the backing of the Rockefeller Foundation and the post-war Italian government, in a deliberate attempt to rid the island completely of an indigenous malaria-transmitting mosquito species. The campaign was based on the spraying of thousands of tons of the new wartime discovery, DDT, from the air and in homes. At the end of five years, malaria had disappeared, and did not reappear when spraying stopped—seemingly a very satisfactory public health result. But the mosquito itself survived, if only in severely reduced numbers. Considered a test of mosquito eradication, the Sardinian Project proved that completely eradicating a well-established mosquito was very difficult, even impossible, at least by spraying DDT over the kind of terrain where this mosquito was found. Turning this around, the best that could be said was that species eradication was apparently not essential to malaria eradication (Hall, 2010; Stepan, 2011).

From Soper's viewpoint, this was a hard lesson to learn, one reason no doubt why he barely acknowledged it as such. In fact, he continued to refer to the eradication of the main malaria vector in Sardinia as though it were a *fait accompli*, a rare lapse in a person given to accuracy. He chose to ignore the ambiguities of the results and continued to endorse the concept of species eradication, even though the concept was dropped from the most important post-war eradication effort, the WHO's Malaria Eradication Programme (MEP), where the aim was eradication of the disease, not its vectors. As happens so often in public health, Soper had devised his strategy while operating with incomplete knowledge—in these cases, incomplete knowledge of insect ecology.

Eradicating *Aedes aegypti*: the rationale

Soper's anti–*Aedes aegypti* campaign is the least remarked on of his four-vector extermination efforts, but perhaps the most interesting because it was by far the most sustained of its kind, and because it captures so well the ambition as well as the ambiguities of what was aimed for.

Paradoxically, Soper advocated *Aedes aegypti* eradication just when it was being realized that yellow fever is not the kind of disease that could, on biological grounds, be eradicated, the long-standing goal of the RF. Unexpected outbreaks of yellow fever in rural areas of Brazil had led to the belated realization by the mid-1930s that an animal reservoir of the virus existed, the virus being transmitted in rural areas from forest animals, mainly monkeys, to humans by the bite of mosquitoes other than the urban *Aedes aegypti*, such as species of *Haemogogus*. Searching for yellow fever in the main cities and for a single vector, the RF had for years overlooked, or rejected the diagnosis of, yellow fever outbreaks in rural areas. The jungle (or sylvatic) cycle of yellow fever showed that it was wrong to rely on the exclusively urban identity of yellow fever, on which the RF had based its yellow fever eradication strategy.

In rethinking yellow fever epidemiology, it was evident that yellow fever could not be eradicated short of killing off all forest animals harbouring the virus. The RF accordingly abandoned its goal of yellow fever eradication in the late 1930s, leaving as its legacy of decades of anti–yellow fever work, its new 17D yellow fever vaccine.

Soper saw the matter differently. As director of Brazil's national anti–yellow fever service, he had begun in the early 1930s to extend mosquito control to include small rural towns where yellow fever also circulated. Without aiming for it as such, he found that the methods he was using were resulting in the complete disappearance of *Aedes aegypti*. Inspections in town after town showed that the mosquito was gone. From the late 1930s on, as the RF abandoned eradicating the disease, Soper began to promote the idea that public health efforts should shift to complete mosquito eradication (Soper and Wilson, 1942; Soper, 1963) (See Figure. 6.1).

True, jungle yellow fever would remain a constant potential source of the virus, but this yellow fever cycle was sporadic and involved only populations working on the rural borderlands with forests where the animals lived. In the 1930s, Brazil was already an increasingly urbanized country, and it was in the cities that the greatest number of deaths from yellow fever occurred. Soper's public health contribution was to replace mosquito reduction with a new absolute: the complete elimination of a vector that was highly adapted to urban and human life. In this way, urban yellow fever itself would be eliminated.

The trouble, as Soper saw it, with aiming for mere *Aedes aegypti* control (that is, simply reduction of mosquitoes and their larvae to low numbers), as previous yellow fever campaigns had done, was that the authorities invariably relaxed

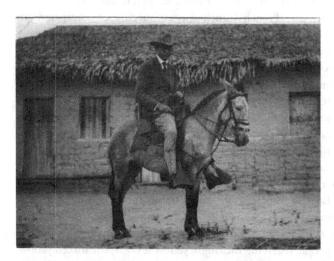

FIGURE 6.1 Fred Soper preparing for an inspection tour of Maranhao, Brazil; 1920s. Image courtesy of the National Library of Medicine.

controls as the urban cases of the disease diminished. The outcome was the eventual return of yellow fever from its rural home to cities, often in explosive epidemics. Why, then, not eradicate the urban mosquito once and for all and stop these cycles?

Soper acknowledged that such an absolutist goal was hard to achieve; it required more money and effort upfront, and more determination. But once achieved, there were huge savings to be had in terms of safety and costs; all controls in urban areas could be given up; with the urban vector wiped off the face of the earth, it could never return to act as a vector again. Making urban areas safe in this way, control and surveillance would be focused eventually on rural areas where yellow fever was only sporadic. The majority of the population, located in cities and towns, would be free of yellow fever forever. To work, however, this new concept of eradication had to be absolute. Any chance that *Aedes aeygpti* mosquitoes might be reintroduced from the outside, into an urban area made free of them for years, would be potentially disastrous, as by this time the city would be filled with highly susceptible people who had never had yellow fever and so never acquired the immunity conferred by a mild childhood infection.

Yellow fever and vaccination

And what about vaccination, usually considered the magic tool of preventive medicine? The isolation of the yellow fever virus in 1927 had provided scientists with an animal model and had led to an intense search for a vaccine. In 1932 French researchers at the Pasteur Institute in Dakar, Senegal, produced a yellow fever vaccine based on one strain of the virus, and in 1937 the Americans, working at the RF laboratory in New York, and relying on the different "Asibi" strain of the virus, produced their own 17D vaccine, used to this day.

Almost immediately, the French launched mass vaccination campaigns in their West African colonies, despite their vaccine's comparatively high numbers of negative neurotropic side effects, notably encephalitis. The scratch method of application in smallpox was well established in Africa, and smallpox vaccination had been made compulsory in the French colonies early, so the yellow fever vaccine was administered by the scratch method, by itself or more often together with smallpox vaccine. The epidemiology of yellow fever was complex in Africa, involving different transmission cycles and several *Aedes* species in addition to *A. aegypti*, factors making mosquito control difficult to carry out beyond selected places like airports. Immunity surveys were still mapping the geography of yellow fever distribution; the population in Africa was still largely rural, and accustomed to mandatory vaccination for smallpox. In the circumstances, mass vaccination was a rational approach to yellow fever control.

Fear of yellow fever outbreaks among the troops mobilized for World War II led to some 14,300,000 people receiving the single yellow fever or the mixed yellow fever–smallpox vaccine, out of a total population of some 16 million in French West Africa (Peltier, 1947). Altogether 53 million people were vaccinated by the

French colonial authorities between 1939 and 1953. In fact, the use of yellow fever vaccination led to the virtual disappearance of yellow fever in francophone West Africa for decades. Nothing like the French colonial vaccination effort was undertaken in British colonial West Africa, where numerous outbreaks of yellow fever occurred (Monath, 1991).

The RF vaccine differed from that of the French in requiring an injection rather than a scratch. The 17D vaccine was tested in Brazil, and by the end of 1938 over a million people in the country had been vaccinated. Initially, this vaccine also produced negative side effects, notably hepatitis, which was only eliminated when human serum, the source of contamination, was removed from the vaccine. Once this problem was solved, vaccination of people exposed to the rural cycle of yellow fever was resumed. Over time, the 17D vaccine would be considered safer than the French vaccine (the latter ceasing production in 1982), but the RF conceded at the time that the low-cost scratch immunization made better sense in large rural populations of French colonial West Africa (Durieux, 1956; Frierson, 2010; Strode, 1951).

As head of the RF-Brazilian yellow fever service, Soper was responsible for supervising the production, testing and distribution of the 17D vaccine in Brazil (Benchimol, 2001). But he had reservations about relying exclusively on the new vaccine; it was expensive to produce and required a cold chain for its distribution. He also worried that demand would outrun supplies. More than this, because yellow fever is often a silent, under-reported disease, Soper was alert to the fact that, unless rural vaccination rates were kept up, the virus could pass unnoticed via its initial rural path into urban areas which, if still infested with *Aedes aegypti* mosquitoes, could have outbreaks of yellow fever before vaccination could be hurriedly introduced to halt its spread. Once administered, a further interval of time (roughly ten days) had to pass before individuals acquired adequate immunity. For these reasons, Soper was always sceptical of controlling yellow fever solely by vaccination. In this respect, Soper may have been right—an issue taken up at the end of this chapter.

Eradicating *Aedes aegypti* in practice

So much for the rationale for *Aedes aegypti* eradication. Crucial to its execution—the "could we?" question—was the confidence Soper had in his methods. As originally established by William Gorgas in Havana in 1901, these involved a mix of the social, biological and chemical, packaged into a top-down, single-disease, military-style campaign: the isolation of those infected, removal of water receptacles near human habitations, and destruction of mosquitoes by chemicals such as crude oil mixed with paraffin and floated on water as a larvicide. Gutters were cleared. Gambusia fish were sometimes introduced to water tanks to eat larvae. Beginning in the 1920s, the arsenic-based chemical, Paris Green, was used in place of oil, in a process called "Greening" by RF personnel. Pyrethrum insecticides were sprayed inside houses

These chemicals had nothing like the potency of DDT, so success with mosquito reduction or actual elimination depended on systematic attention to public health administration: to the routinization of house visits, meticulous larviciding, tight supervision of the "mosquito brigades" of inspectors looking for mosquito infestations, and rigid controls of householders, making sure they kept water receptacles empty or covered to prevent *Aedes aegypti* breeding in them.

This is where Soper excelled, his methods being described as "perfectionism at the end of the line." To the established anti-mosquito techniques, Soper added new ones to make otherwise invisible mosquitoes visible, such as the use of "mother squads" of mosquito inspectors to hunt down hidden breeding female mosquitoes in houses, the carrying out of immunity surveys to identify otherwise unsuspected locations of yellow fever, and the creation of a "viscerotomy" service to conduct post-mortem analyses to detect overlooked yellow fever deaths (Löwy, 1997; Stepan, 2011). Backed by Brazil's authoritarian president, Soper had the tools and resources to pursue *Aedes aegypti* eradication across the country.

The fundamental shift towards the "chemicalization" of anti-mosquito work came with the World War II discovery of the insecticidal properties of DDT. Released for civilian use at the end of the war, DDT was cheap, available, apparently safe, and much more powerful in its residual effects as a larvicide and adulticide than anything before it. It proved irresistible. Having participated in the first uses of DDT against typhus and malaria in Italy during his wartime service, Soper was quick to realize how its superior, long-lasting insecticidal properties would be crucial in his mosquito-killing projects.

Eradicating *Aedes aegypti*: the impossible task

When Soper had begun in the late 1930s to talk about exterminating the *Aedes aegypti* from all of Brazil, "yellow fever experts from Rio to New York laughed at him. They declined to be Soperized" (Stepan, 2011). But to Soper, getting rid of the mosquito was everything. Being elected Director of the Pan American Health Organization (PAHO) in 1947 gave him a wider stage for his eradicationist philosophy, Soper managing to persuade *all* the member countries of PAHO to embrace the eradication programme against *A. aegypti* throughout the continental Americas—even though there had been just one outbreak of urban yellow fever in the Americas in the preceding 15 years, and even if it meant ignoring the negative outcome of the Sardinia experiment.

And at first all went well. In 1958, Brazil became the first country in the Americas to be declared *Aedes aegypti*–free. Soon, country after country was being certified as *Aedes aegypti*–free too. By 1964, the vector had been successfully eradicated in most of South and Central America. Yellow fever disappeared. Thought of as a control effort, this was an impressive result. But thought of as a mosquito eradication campaign, not so.

It turned out that only "most" countries were *Aedes aegypti*–free—there was the rub. Absolute success proved elusive, as continent-wide elimination of the mosquito was not maintained for very long, with constant reinvasion of mosquitoes into areas previously certified as clear. In 1976, the PAHO countries were still at their eradication project, but by this point with only ten countries certified as entirely free of the *Aedes* mosquito. Brazil, the largest endemic center of yellow fever in the Americas, had lost its *Aedes aegypti*–free status.

In regard to these failures, Soper blamed the USA for not doing its part and allowing its *Aedes aegypti* mosquitoes to invade Mexico. The USA had in fact always been reluctant participants in the project. The USA refused to take much action throughout the 1950s, despite having signed on to do so in 1947. The country had not suffered an indigenous case of yellow fever for 40 years, had no jungle reservoirs of the virus, and preferred to rely on the excellent yellow fever vaccine. Only in 1963 did the USA agree to get involved, less because of conviction about feasibility than as a political "goodwill" gesture. Terminating the project in 1968, the USA thought *Aedes aegypti* eradication was unnecessary and anyway unachievable (Sencer, 1969).

The USA's half-hearted participation and then withdrawal from the mosquito eradication project came just as public attitudes towards synthetic organic insecticides were changing. Rachel Carson's target in *Silent Spring* (1962) was DDT's overuse in agriculture; only one chapter in her trenchant book addressed synthetic insecticides in public health. Her main point there was to warn that excessive use of pesticides was creating insect resistance, leading public health officials to seek out new and yet more powerful insecticides, which resulted in yet more insect species acquiring resistance … in a never-ending escalation.

Those involved in anti-malaria and yellow fever campaigns knew this to be true. Yet DDT continued to be used in public health (the USA banned it for agricultural use in 1972). After all, in the many WHO-connected expert reports on insecticides and safety, the conclusion was almost invariably drawn that the benefits of using DDT for public health purposes far outweighed its risks, despite mosquito resistance. Public health use of the new insecticides was, as it were, bracketed or protected as a special case.

But slowly, support for the *Aedes* eradication project was disappearing. One factor was simply programme fatigue, with countries tiring of directing so much effort against *A. aegypti* when mosquito and yellow fever indices were already so low as to be virtually non-existent—yet absolute eradication proved so elusive. The strategy of species eradication was not based on a medical emergency or an overwhelming medical problem but was, as Soper said, a deliberate effort to consolidate the gains of previous decades, and guarantee future freedom from yellow fever to the cities and towns of the Americas. It was a difficult case to make: if control methods had done such a good job, why aim for something so difficult as exterminating every last mosquito? "When could eradication be said to be complete and final," asked a French delegate at a PAHO meeting in 1970, "considering that a few mosquitoes were enough to cause re-infestation?"

(Stepan, 2011). It was proving hard, if not impossible, to prevent constant rein-
festation of already certified countries from across their borders. Simultaneous
extermination of *Aedes aegypti* across the Americas seemed a Sisyphean task.

And yet, old dreams die hard. Soper retired from PAHO in 1959, but the
organization carried on its species eradication mission well into the 1970s. But by
1985 it was time to give up, with PAHO finally admitting that the goal of *Aedes
aegypti* eradication was unrealistic, and shifting its aims to keeping mosquito
indices low. By the late 1990s, even routine control measures were being cut
back in Brazil and elsewhere in the name of cost-saving, with the unsurprising
outcome that *A. aegypti* returned everywhere, to then unleash epidemics of
dengue, and now Zika. Soper's *A. aegypti* campaign had shown that mosquitoes
are among the most resilient of animals; they resist their extermination (see
Figure. 6.2).

Could we/should we, ecologically/ethically?

Turning now to some of the ecological and ethical issues tied up in the "could
we/should we" nexus, Soper's eradication efforts were decidedly "pre-" and
even "anti-" ecological. He famously declared that he regretted the term "ecology" had ever been invented. He knew very little about *Anopheles gambiae* or *A.
labranchiae* when he set out to eradicate them in northeastern Brazil, Upper Egypt
and Sardinia, treating them as though they were the same, in relation to eradication methods, as the very different *Aedes aegypti* mosquito.

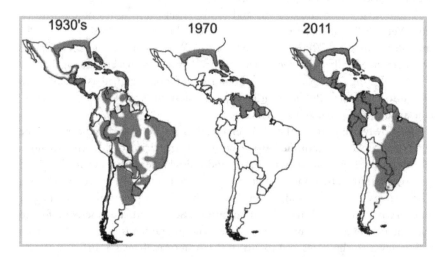

FIGURE 6.2 Map of *Aedes aegypti* distribution in South and Central America in the 1930s,
1970 and 2011. Creative Commons [from Gubler, D.J. 2011. "Dengue,
Urbanization and Globalization: The Unholy Trinity of the 21st Century."
Tropical Medicine and Health, 39(4) Suppl: 3-11. doi: 10.2149/tmh.2011-S05].

Soper knew much more about the behaviour of *Aedes aegypti*, but as was so often the case in eradication campaigns, assumptions about universal ecology meant setbacks when confronting ecological complexity. A case in point was the discovery that in the Caribbean, *Aedes aegypti* could breed high up in tree holes, rendering ineffective spraying regimes that assumed this mosquito only bred near human habitations. The question about the possible ill effects of complete removal of a species from its habitat does not seem to have even been raised.

Nor were ethical questions raised in Soper's eradication projects about the risks of Paris Green and then DDT to humans, animals and the environment more generally. There was no mention about seeking consent to inspect people's homes or spray them with powerful chemicals; instead, mandatory inspections were often imposed on households, with fines for non-compliance. Soper maintained that eradication worked best under authoritarian governments: "if you have democracy, you cannot have eradication," was his view. It was a "command from the top" model that reflected his experience in Brazil under the authoritarian President of the 1930s, Getúlio Vargas. It was not a model that translated well into more democratic settings, where consultation, community participation and citizens' consent are necessary for success. Furthermore, a single disease focus, with its separate and unique organizational structure, also had limits, since integrating the needs of other public health activities was difficult.

Finally, the over-reliance on a biomedical model of public health meant that there was a strong bias against or neglect of social methods of controlling disease, such as installing piped water, screened windows and ensuring regular rubbish collection as ways to ward off mosquito-borne diseases. It is well known that improved housing and socio-economic conditions were and are factors in the secular declines of diseases, but investments to overcome social and economic inequality were by and large absent from post-war campaigns to control and eradicate mosquitoes.

Control versus eradication

So we end with the same question we started with: Could we/should we eradicate mosquitoes?

It seems to me that something has to be done to keep in check the mosquitoes that transmit dangerous human diseases. But what and how? Sending 220,000 soldiers to Brazilian neighbourhoods to deal with Zika was more an exercise in public relations than a thought-out project of public health. Community vector control is judged to be generally unsuccessful as well, so how can our strategies be reconfigured? Why has anti-mosquito work been neglected in Brazil, even though dengue epidemics were, even before Zika, a recurring problem? Why has it been so hard to remodel public health around vector control using appropriate ecological, biological and social methods?

New tools, such as releasing Wolbachia-infected mosquitoes to control dengue, are being tried out as demonstration experiments (Dorigatti et al.,

2018). I doubt that they will escape the "could we/should we" entanglements. What are the effects of releasing bio-engineered mosquitoes on the ecological balance? Are their risks understood? How will members of the public be put in a position to evaluate them? Would some "old tech" methods be better?

I ask these questions in light of the fact that arboviruses represent some of today's most important global health threats, products of intensive human migration, urbanization, globalization, climate change, inadequate vaccination, and failures of former vector control efforts. *Aedes aegypti* is now found worldwide (Gubler, 2011; Ferguson, 2018). Annually, there are 200,000 detected cases of yellow fever and 30,000 deaths, figures WHO regards as underestimates by a factor of 10 to 250 (Tomori, 2004). Africa is the chief worry; after independence, vaccination rates in countries at risk fell off sharply. In 1986–1992, despite the importation of 20 million doses of yellow fever vaccine, Nigeria was unable to control an epidemic. In 2017, WHO announced a new yellow fever initiative, "Eliminate Yellow Fever Epidemics" (EYE) in response to further urban outbreaks in Africa, with the goal of restoring depleted stockpiles of the vaccine over a ten-year period (Brès, 1971; Garske et al., 2014). We must ask, therefore, was Soper right? Is vaccination going to be available and enough, absent other methods of disease mitigation, including improvements in sanitation and urban infrastructure? And what about Zika, and dengue—one with no vaccine, the other with a vaccine of very partial efficacy, and neither with treatment other than palliative care?

Soper always considered "species eradication" his most original contribution to public health. Later, all four of his efforts were judged to be failures, or at best limited in relevance to health policies, in methods and outcomes. As a result, Soper's reputation suffered a dramatic decline after his death. But before we write off Soper as a discredited figure in public health, might we look again, to reassess his work in the light of present-day post-Zika concerns? There is, of course, no going back to the Soper era: new ways to control mosquitoes must be found to suit our own day's political, ecological and scientific circumstances. But could certain "Soperian moments" suggest ways for reimagining some methods of dealing with mosquitoes, short of the utopian dream of complete eradication?

The downsides of Soper's approach are obvious: a chemical and polluting model; a reliance on a universal one-size-fits-all ecology; disregard for social needs such as housing and sanitation; the lack of community participation; little ongoing research; use of military rather than cooperative metaphors; and so on. And meanwhile, post Soper (he died more than 40 years ago), cities like Recife in Brazil, where Zika first erupted, are far larger, more chaotic, more unequal and more trash-filled than ever before. Controlling *Aedes aegypti* is much more difficult than before.

But we must also acknowledge Soper's positive contributions. These would include efficiency in surveillance and tenacity in anti-mosquito efforts; enormous attention to detail; inspections of the inspectors; adequate funding and political commitment (Downs, 1968). Above all, Soper continued his work even in the absence of mosquitoes and/or cases of yellow fever. Such ongoing methods and preventive attitude are rare and are very different from an epidemic-generated, reactive and generally ineffective resort to mosquito reduction (Ooi et al., 2006).

The lesson of history is that revised methods of mosquito control are needed in the short-to-intermediate term (Ferguson et al., 2016, Ferguson 2018). We also need to keep in mind that, originally, the anti-mosquito yellow fever vector programmes aimed not at complete eradication, but at reducing the targeted mosquito indices to a low level, below which the transmission of the pathogen was found not to be sustainable. In the case of yellow fever, reducing the incidence of *Aedes aegypti* mosquito larvae to a presence in 5% or less of houses in a targeted population stopped yellow fever transmission for decades throughout the Americas.

The goal of mosquito reduction, tailored to epidemiological circumstances, along with much more participatory models of public health than in the past, seems to me to combine the positive aspects of Soper's determination to deal with the mosquito as a major factor in disease transmission, with René Dubos's ecological view that takes into account the dynamic and continuous processes by which insects, pathogens and humans interact, adapt and co-evolve (Litsios, 1997). This view achieves a better balance between human health and environmental health as we adjust our policies to confront climate change, which may well spread mosquito-borne infections and accelerate the loss of species.

Controlling mosquitoes raises difficult ethical and ecological questions; but aiming for the reduction of specific mosquito populations, by new means, including social ones, is possible, and less distorting of public health than aiming for vector eradication.

Note

1 Sections of this chapter are drawn from my book on eradication (Stepan, 2011).

Bibliography

Benchimol, J. 2001. *Febre Amarela: A Doença e a Vacina: Uma História Inacaba*. Rio de Janeiro: Editora Fiocruz.

Brès, P. 1971. *Recent Epidemics of Yellow Fever in Africa*. Symposium on Vector Control and the Recrudescence of Vector-Borne Disease. Washington: PAHO and WHO.

Chippaux, Jean-Philippe, and Alain Chippaux. 2018. Yellow Fever in Africa and the Americas: A Historical and Epidemiological Perspective. *Journal of Venomous Animals and Toxins Including Tropical Diseases*, 24(1): 1–14. doi:10.4269/ajtmh.1969.18.341

Dorigatti, Ilaria et al. 2018. Using *Wolbachia* for Dengue Control: Insights from Modelling. *Trends in Parasitology*, 34(2): 102–113. doi:10.1016/j.pt.2017.11.002

Downs, Wilbur G. 1968. The Story of Yellow Fever Since Walter Reed. *Bulletin of the New York Academy of Medicine*, 44(6): 721–727.

Durieux, C. 1956. *Mass Yellow Fever Vaccination in French Africa South of the Sahara. WHO Monograph Series No. 30, Yellow Fever Vaccination*. Geneva: WHO, 115–122.

Ferguson, Neil M. 2018. Challenges and Opportunities in Controlling Mosquito-Borne Infections. *Nature*, 559: 490–497. https://doi.org/10.1038/s41586-018-0318-5

Ferguson, Neil M. et al. 2016. Countering the Zika Epidemic in Latin America. *Science*, 353(6297): 353–354. doi:10.1126/science.aag0219

Frierson, Gordon. 2010. The Yellow Fever Vaccine: A History. *Yale Journal of Biology and Medicine*, 83: 77–85.

Garske, T. et al. 2014. Yellow Fever in Africa: Estimating the Burden of Disease and Impact of Mass Vaccination from Outbreak and Serological Data. *PLOS Medicine*, 11(5): e1001638. doi:10.1371/journal.pmed.1001638

Gubler, D.J. 2004. The Changing Epidemiology of Yellow Fever and Dengue, 1900–2003: Full Circle. *Comparative Immunology, Microbiology & Infectious Diseases*, 27: 319–330.

Gubler, D.J. 2011. Dengue, Urbanization and Globalization: The Unholy Trinity of the 21st Century. *Tropical Medicine and Health*, 39(4): 3–11. doi:10.2149/tmh.2011-S05

Hall, Marcus. 2010. Environmental Imperialism in Sardinia: Pesticides and Politics in the Struggle against Malaria. In Marco Armiero and Marcus Hall, eds. *Nature and History in Modern Italy*. Athens: Ohio University Press, 70–86.

Litsios, Socrates. 1997. René J. Dubos and Fred L. Soper: Their Contrasting Views of Vector and Disease Eradication. *Perspectives in Biology and Medicine*, 41(1): 138–149.

Lowe, Rachel et al. 2018. The Zika Virus Epidemic in Brazil: From Discovery to Future Implications. *International Journal of Environmental Research and Public Health*, 15(1). doi:10.3390/ijerph15010096

Löwy, Ilana. 1997. Epidemiology, Immunology, and Yellow Fever: The Rockefeller Foundation in Brazil, 1923-1939. *Journal of the History of Biology*, 30: 397–417.

Monath, Thomas P. 1991. Yellow Fever: Victor, Victoria? Conqueror, Conquest? Epidemics and Research in the Last 40 Years & Prospects for the Future. *American Journal of Tropical Medicine*, 45(1): 1–43.

Ooi, E.E., Kee-Tai Goh, and Duane J. Gubler. 2006. Dengue Prevention and 35 Years of Dengue Control in Singapore. *Emerging Infectious Diseases*, 12(6): 887–893.

Packard, R.M., and P. Gadelha. 1997. A Land Filled with Mosquitoes: Fred L. Soper, the Rockefeller Foundation, and the *Anopheles Gambiae* Invasion of Brazil. *Medical Anthropology*, 17(3): 215–238.

Peltier, Maurice. 1947. Yellow Fever Vaccination Simple or Associated with Vaccination against Smallpox of the Population of French West Africa by the Method of the Pasteur Institute of Dakar. *American Journal of Public Health*, 37(8): 1026–1032.

Sencer, David J. 1969. Health Protection in a Shrinking World. *American Journal of Tropical Medicine & Hygiene*, 18(3): 341–345. doi:10.4269/ajtmh.1969.18.341

Soper, F.L. 1963. The Elimination of Urban Yellow Fever in the Americas through the Eradication of *Aedes Aegypti*. *American Journal of Public Health* 53(1): 7–16.

Soper, F. L., and D.B. Wilson. 1942. Species Eradication: A Practical Goal of Species Reduction in the Control of Mosquito-Borne Disease. *Journal of the National Malaria Society*, 1: 5–24.

Stepan, Nancy Leys. 2011. *Eradication: Ridding the World of Diseases for Ever?* London: Reaktion Books.

Strode, G.K. 1951. *Yellow Fever*. New York: McGraw-Hill.

Tomori, Oyewale. 2004. Yellow Fever: The Returning Plague. *Critical Reviews in Clinical Laboratory Sciences*, 41(4): 391–427.

7

FIGHTING NUISANCE ON THE NORTHERN FRINGE

Controlling mosquitoes in Britain between the World Wars

Peter Coates

"Mosquito pest conference—in England!" This incredulous headline appeared in a London-based magazine, *West Africa*, which covered news items about Britain's West African colonies.[1] Whether in the 1920s or at other times in the twentieth century, the British tendency has been to think that mosquito problems were "far away." The 34 species of mosquitoes native to Britain, admittedly, is a modest, even trifling number compared to the global total of circa 3,500 species. And most of Britain's mosquitoes do not even belong to the disease-transmitting family. Britain's mosquitoes are categorized as nuisance mosquitoes—after all, *West Africa* referred to the mosquito as (mere) pest. Just five British mosquitoes are Anopheline and only one, *Anopheles atroparvus*, Europe's major malaria carrier, breeds in big enough numbers and sufficiently close to humans to serve as an efficient vector of one of malaria's main parasites, *Plasmodium vivax* (West Africa 1927, BMCI, AMWL; Manchester Guardian 1929: 8; Snow 1998: 9; Marshall 1938: 2).[2]

But a comparatively small number of lethal varieties does not mean that the mosquito chapter of British domestic history is unimportant. A century and a half ago, the connection between Britain and mosquitoes was stronger. *Anopheles atroparvus* was apparently the species that transmitted a native strain of malaria known as ague. Endemic for centuries to the coastal marshlands of Essex and Kent, and watery lowlands including the fenlands of East Anglia and the Somerset Levels in southwest England, ague—aka marsh fever—killed or debilitated thousands of young, old, undernourished, sick and poorer residents of wetland regions (Dobson 1998: 312, 321). By 1900, ague had pretty much died out, not because the parasite's mosquito vector had been eliminated, but thanks to extensive drainage, advances in public health care and improved sanitation. Increased separation of human dwellings from livestock and a growing cattle population also transformed mosquito biting habits by providing alternative sources of blood meals (Peacock

DOI: 10.4324/9781003056034-7

1859: 453, 478; James 1929: 71–87; MacArthur 1951: 76–79).[3] Combined with decreasing virulence of the malaria parasite, growing resistance in the human patient and greater availability of quinine, lowland England saw this scourge disappear.[4] Once ague was gone, the mosquito, itself, effectively disappeared from domestic British history—although British imperial history is another matter.

This chapter explores questions of control, and the desirability and feasibility of elimination from the unlikely perspective of Britain's interwar mosquito experience.[5] The case study considered here is the British Mosquito Control Institute, or BMCI, established in 1925. This non-medical enterprise started out five years earlier as the Hayling Mosquito Control in the English Channel's resort of Hayling Island near Portsmouth, to combat a particular nuisance mosquito that was making local residents' and vacationers' lives miserable. The Institute's locally successful "anti-mosquito crusade" from 1921 to 1924 (*Daily Mail* 1925: 15), subsequently expanded under a new name in purpose-built premises (1925–1939), is examined within a wider geographical framework that includes campaigns to eliminate deadly varieties of mosquito, from Italy's Pontine Marshes to the Panama Canal and various parts of Britain's empire (Birmingham Post 1927; Morning Post 1925a). "From Nairobi to Hayling Island is a far cry," ruminated a local journalist, "but it sounds in our ears" (Portsmouth Gazette 1930).

The deadly-disease–carrying mosquitoes of Nairobi can be regarded, from a strictly biological standpoint, as a human population reduction agent; or, as entomologist Daniel Strickman of the US Department of Agriculture observed bluntly a decade ago, "The ecological effect of eliminating harmful mosquitoes is that you have more people" (Fang, 2010: 432). But even if there were no human lives to be saved in combatting non-lethal mosquitoes in Hayling Island, one should not underestimate the efforts expended against what Sir Ronald Ross referred to as, at first sight, a "wholly insignificant creature" (Ross 1926: 481). Ross, who began his malaria research in India 30 years earlier, and was now director-in-chief of London's Ross Institute and Hospital for Tropical Diseases, made this remark at BMCI's opening day on 31 August 1925. To gain a deeper understanding of the non-lethal mosquitoes that inflicted such "injuries" as depressed real estate value and lost tourist revenue, I situate the BMCI's exploits within parallel efforts across the North Atlantic to control nuisance mosquitoes in coastal New Jersey. I then compare control strategies adopted at Hayling Island with larger-scale, more heavily chemicalized interventions beyond Britain after the first deployment of DDT in 1942 and the subsequent worldwide war against malaria. Such comparisons allow us to engage with themes of imperialism, macro- and micro-strategies of control as well as species sanitation. We will find a consensus among applied entomologists in Britain regarding the desirability of controlling nuisance mosquitoes, but a recognition that doing so was not always feasible.

It should also be pointed out that mosquitoes need not carry deadly diseases to be lethal to humans or non-humans. Technically non-lethal varieties claim the occasional human death from, say, septicaemia when a bite becomes inflamed and infected, resulting in blood poisoning. A. Moore Hogarth, the founder and chairman of the London College of Pestology, recorded 21 deaths over a seven-year period in Britain (1921–1928) that were "definitely traced or at least reasonably attributed to mosquito bites" (Hogarth 1928: 40–42). The focus here, though, is on the "discomfort" and "general annoyance" mosquitoes of the inter-war period inflicted (Marshall [undated A], MP, LSHTM[6]; Simpson[7] in Hogarth 1928: 15).

In search of comfort

The British press reported with gusto the declaration of war on the pesky mosquito on Hayling Island in 1920 and did not flag in its coverage of the subsequent waging of warfare against the insect "enemy" (Daily Express 1920; Turnbull 1925: 228; Morning Post 1925b; Evening Standard 1925). This coverage cannot be fully appreciated without reference to malaria contracted in Britain during the latter stages of World War One by soldiers and civilians who had never set foot abroad. The sites and distribution of locally contracted cases from August 1917 onward closely matched the incidence of indigenous malaria in 1860, with the highest numbers along the south and southeast coasts (Ministry of Health (MoH) 1949, Appendix IV, 33).[8] In north Kent, for example, at the military camps and hospital near Sheerness, Isle of Sheppey, and at Grain Fort, Isle of Grain, Anopheles mosquitoes were "generally abundant" in the "marshland and stagnant pools, intersected with dykes [that] surround the station" as well as indoors (Parsons 1919: 95–112; Newman 1919: 11). Ministry of Health officials reckoned demobilized troops brought in the parasite from the Salonika campaign, as well as from Mesopotamia, Egypt and German East Africa (Macdonald 1919: 179–180, 184, 193; Ross 1919: 324; James 1920: 83–93).

Medical authorities worried that infected soldiers or "carriers" bitten by local Anopheline mosquitoes would spread malaria across Britain during demobilization, at a time when *A. maculipennis* was "ubiquitous and extraordinarily numerous" (James 1920: 81–83, 85) (Figure 7.1). An official source logged 178 documented cases of malaria of "indigenous" origin in southeast England in 1917 with none classified as severe, being all "Benign tertian" and with no deaths (Grove 1919: 44–50). This hardly constituted a major public health problem. Yet the report's author was troubled by Anopheles' presence "sometimes in notable abundance, practically in any part of England where the conditions are favourable to their breeding" (Newsholme 1918: A2).

Inspired by successful control of yellow fever and malaria in the Canal Zone of Panama with drainage and larvicide—and similar initiatives in Egypt and Sudan—the Royal Army Medical Corps' First London Sanitary Company was assigned to control "dangerous areas" such as north Kent. The detachment not only applied chemical larvicides to self-contained pools and sheep-dipping wells, it also fumigated farm steadings and cleaned cobwebby attics and lime-washed stables where *A. maculipennis* hibernated. Mainly, though, its job consisted of routine maintenance work neglected by civil authorities during wartime such as clearing the "quagmire of vegetation" from ditches, dykes and ponds,

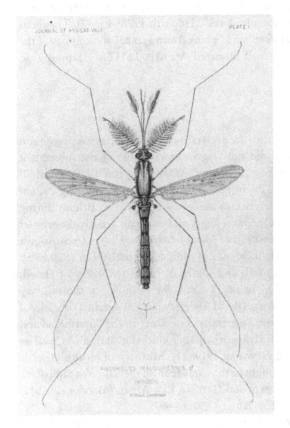

FIGURE 7.1 Male mosquito, *Anopheles maculipennis* (*atroparvus*), 1901. Credit: Wellcome Collection. Attribution 4.0 International (CC BY 4.0).

"brushing the shores" and filling in derelict canals that multiplied mosquito habitat. Collectively, these tasks were described as anti-*malaria* measures, not anti-*mosquito* measures (Macdonald 1919: 175, 249, 245–246, 248, 251, 255; Buchanan and Newsholme 1919: iv; Macfarlane 2012). The objective was "limitation" and "reduction," not eradication, a modesty of ambition that characterized anti-malaria measures as "petty." The informing "principles" were to limit the extent of "open water" and otherwise diminish water bodies' suitability as breeding grounds (Macdonald 1919: 248–249, 254).

The gravity of the menace[9]

With locally contracted cases of nonindigenous malaria drying up once all troops were back, and the First London Sanitary Company clipping the wings of Anopheles in north Kent, a new war on a different kind of mosquito began along the marshy coast of Hampshire. This 1920 campaign is rumoured to have started when the BMCI's founder, John F. Marshall, a trained mechanical engineer, barrister and, later, self-taught entomologist, found that guests at his Hayling Island villa were complaining of being bitten by mosquitoes while playing tennis and afterward "eating their cucumber sandwiches on the lawn" (Service 2003, BMCI, AMWL).[10] Hogarth recalled that Hayling Island had become "almost uninhabitable" and was "rapidly ceasing to exist as a pleasure-resort" (Hogarth 1928: 48). Marshall reported that residents usually "vacate their homes in July and August, and leave the island as far as possible to the mosquitoes" (Marshall 1930, MP, LSHTM).[11] He related how "a visitor arriving at a house adjoining the Salterns [on the edge of the saltmarshes] for a projected stay of some weeks [September 1922] was compelled to depart on the next day" (Marshall 1924, Marshall, LSHTM). When Sir Ronald Ross first visited the island in August 1922, he underestimated the gravity of the problem. Until, that is, Marshall

> took me to a sheltered spot in his garden where there were innumerable mosquitoes. It was then that I suddenly found two or three of them engaging in extracting blood from the back of my neck. I have seldom had such an experience, even in the West Indies.
>
> *(Daily News 1925)*

Garden parties were not the only outdoor activities mosquitoes ruined. And Hayling Island was not the only place afflicted. Various sources testify to the severity of the mosquito "scare" along England's south coast during the 1920s, and how, to quote *Country Life* magazine, a bite could destroy the "whole idyll of a summer evening" (Manchester Guardian 1925; Times [London] 1926; Country Life 1926: 4). According to the Ministry of Health's advisor on tropical diseases, Colonel S.P. James, who was also a member of BMCI's governing council, "the abundance of these insects in nearly every rural district … is greater than in many exceedingly malarious places in the tropics" (James 1929: 75).[12]

High society's mosquito "problem" stemmed from greater numbers combined with closer human–insect contact. Expansion of breeding grounds also encouraged larger populations. "The Salterns" area of southeastern Hayling Island had been reclaimed from the nearby estuary by building earthen sea walls, but such coastal defences had slid into disrepair over the decades. This neglect restored stagnant, brackish waters that made excellent breeding grounds for *Aedes (Ochlerotatus) detritus*, one of two British saltwater varieties, which, of the 17 local mosquito species, was soon identified as the main culprit (Marshall 1924, MP, LSHTM; MoH 1949: 18–19; Nature 1949: 16). Breeding sites for nuisance varieties such as *A. detritus* were not only restored; they also resulted from unintended environmental transformations. Humans had enlarged mosquito empires across the tropical world through jungle clearance and various landscape disrupting "earth-works" (James 1920: 16–17; Sutter 2007: 743–745).

And wartime and post-war Britain was no exception to the human enlargement of mosquito breeding sites, as Willoughby's chapter attests. Water accumulated in pockets left by wartime bombings and latrines dug at military camps. Newly fashioned recreational landscapes were also mosquito-friendly, with golf's rising popularity leading to a multiplication of courses that incorporated water features, or outdoor camping spreading empty sardine tins and jam jars (Hogarth 1928: 5758; MoH 1949: 18: MoH 1962: 5, 21). Greater numbers of people travelling and spending time out of doors exposed more human flesh, and so promoted more human–mosquito encounters (Hogarth 1928: 48).

Marshall's Institute was not only the first attempt in the United Kingdom to combat nuisance mosquitoes. It also furnished the UK's only opportunity "for studying the various details of a mosquito control organization in actual and continuous operation," not least by showcasing the particular challenges of undertaking these studies in a residential area (Marshall 1924: 10). Existing publications (in English) about mosquitoes and their control were focused largely on disease-carrying mosquitoes in "foreign parts," and so practically irrelevant to controlling Britain's non-lethal varieties (Marshall 1928: 4). (Figure 7.2) Those

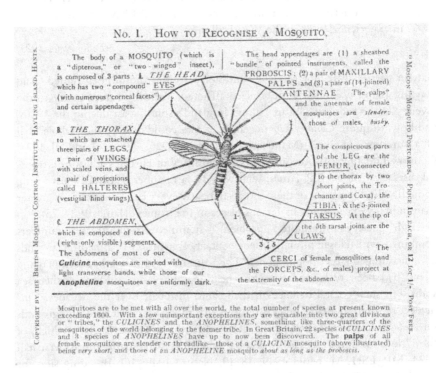

FIGURE 7.2 "How to recognise a mosquito" in John F. Marshall, *A Mosquito Summary* (Hayling Island: British Mosquito Control Institute) [undated], p. 1. Credit: In the possession of Jolyon Medlock, Public Health England. Reproduced courtesy of Jolyon Medlock.

who oversaw the Institute's activities were nonetheless steeped in the context of the tropics: "men learned in the ways of mosquitoes in India, the Gold Coast, or at Khartoum, where it is not merely a nuisance" (The Children's Newspaper 1928, Marshall, LSHTM). When the BMCI began to identify and study the habits of Britain's non-Anopheline mosquitoes, it would borrow heavily from the methods of the tropics.

One example of the transfer of knowledge from tropical to temperate was the formation of a small local workforce known as a Mosquito Brigade, a practice Ross pioneered in the Indian Medical Service. The task of these brigades was to wipe out or treat with petroleum all sources of standing water, not only all marshes, ponds and ditches, but also puddles and water accumulated in tree boles, sites that would not have been considered as breeding environments when the miasma theory held sway (Ross 1902; Christophers and Bentley 1908: 21–22). Ross-style brigades came to play a particularly vital role on Hayling Island because local public authorities felt non-lethal mosquito control was not their responsibility. In many countries, as Marshall pointed out, the owner of the land on which mosquitoes breed is required by law to bear part of the costs of control, besides providing controllers access to the land. Hogarth pointed out that in New South Wales, Australia, powers to enforce mosquito destruction had been vested in local governments since 1906 (Hogarth 1928: 111–113; O'Gorman 2017: 496). However, in Britain, despite the Public Health Act of 1876, which included "any pool, ditch, gutter, watercourse, sink, cistern, cesspool or drain so foul or in such as state or so situated as to be nuisance or injurious or dangerous to health," local municipalities had been reluctant to act on mosquito control (Westminster Gazette 1927; Yorkshire Post 1927). The official line the town council adopted in a south-coast resort in nearby Dorset was that "there are no mosquitoes in Weymouth." Disputing this, one of Hogarth's correspondents insisted that the council was actually "afraid of the existence of mosquitoes getting known" for fear of putting off visitors, and so, "takes no steps to destroy them" (Hogarth 1928: 50). Marshall also suspected that many seaside resorts adhered to a do-nothing policy because they figured that "first-time" blissfully mosquito-unaware visitors would come in sufficient quantities to compensate for those who did not return because of the nasty mosquito surprises awaiting them (Marshall 1928: 37).

Another obstacle faced proponents of control. Not only was permission required to "drain away [a private landowner's] mosquito-infested waters" but funding for control work needed to be secured (Marshall 1928: 37). BMCI (an incorporated organization) and its predecessor, the Hayling Mosquito Control, were unofficial initiatives, funded entirely from private sources (largely Marshall's personal wealth), since the Ministry of Health had no mandate to spend public funds on non-lethal mosquitoes (Marshall 1928: 10). Given the government's lack of support, "education of local public opinion in support of the work" was particularly essential (Marshall 1927: 9). One local headmaster, for example, organized an annual "Mosquito Control Class" where he enlisted schoolchildren to collect samples (Marshall 1928: 10; Lancet 1925).

A pleasure-killing pest across the Atlantic

The existence of a type of juvenile Mosquito Brigade at Hayling Island demonstrates how a local temperate-zone mosquito campaign was shaped by more lethal threats faced by its distant tropical counterparts. Beyond Britain's tropical colonies, the Institute's awareness and frame of reference also extended to American efforts to combat disease-bearing mosquitoes, especially in Cuba, Panama and the Philippines where yellow fever and malaria had raged (*Daily Mirror* 1925; Observer 1925: 5). Yet mosquito control within US borders provides a closer parallel with BMCI's efforts. Only rarely did Marshall, or the press and medical journals, acknowledge that the main precedent for controlling "general annoyance" mosquitoes was from the United States' northeast coast (Marshall, undated A: 3, Marshall, LSHTM; Marshall 1925b: 6, 17; British Medical Journal [BMJ] 1930: 328).

Organized efforts to deal with comparable saltwater mosquitoes, such as *Aedes sollicitans*, the white-banded salt marsh mosquito, began in coastal marshlands of states such as New Jersey in the early 1900s. "Magnificent dwellings," lamented a realtor in the 1890s,

> find no purchasers because ... as soon as dark sets in, piazzas must be abandoned to escape the annoyance of these little nuisances. In almost any car in any morning train to the city during the summer, somebody may be heard talking of mosquitoes.
>
> *(Smith 1904: 462, in Patterson 2009: 12)*

Fifteen years later, Hayling Island residents and visitors expressed identical sentiments regarding what Americans dubbed the "pleasure killing pest" (Chicago Daily Tribune 1914). Indeed, Marshall's organization was a British equivalent of the village improvement societies and town protective associations that emerged in New Jersey from 1901, eventually broadening into state-level organizations such as the New Jersey Mosquito Control Association.

Like their British counterparts, Americans who fought *Aedes sollicitans* thought that eliminating this nuisance would deliver economic benefits, including more tourists and higher property values. Tensions within US mosquito-control circles were often framed as comfort versus disease: those concerned with public health wanting to curb lethal mosquitoes complained that politicians were more responsive to businesspeople moaning about lost profits (Patterson 2009: 88–89). As in England, awareness of a mosquito problem did not guarantee action. Weymouth town council's disinclination to acknowledge a local mosquito problem is a pattern of denial and inaction also observable in areas of the USA where mosquitoes were malarial. In northern California, irrigation infrastructure boosted land values but created excellent breeding conditions for anophelines, particularly where rice was cultivated and there were concomitant water seepages and leaks. Until 1915, many American realtors opposed public funding of mosquito control for fear that such efforts would only draw attention to the problem and deter prospective buyers (Patterson 2009: 83, 107, 122).

A "practically intolerable"[13] nuisance

In 1924, prompted by the growing number of mosquito-bite–related illnesses, and even deaths, together with accumulating complaints about interference with outdoor pursuits, the council of Hogarth's College of Pestology offered a prize for the best essay on Britain's "Mosquito Menace." The competition attracted almost 500 entrants from across the world. The winner, P.G. Shute, an assistant to Colonel James and a veteran of anti-mosquito campaigns in the tropical British Empire, received his gold medal from Ross in the presence of various luminaries at a luncheon in London. Shute's central recommendation for combating *Aedes detritus* was to shrink its breeding grounds through drainage and infilling.[14] Two other points emerged at the lunch that day. Firstly, the need to instil in public authorities, and a rather ignorant and apathetic public, an awareness of "the real urgency of the mosquito evil in this country" (Hogarth 1928: 18). The second imperative was to equip those whose enlistment would be crucial to the success of a coordinated campaign—Boy Scouts, Girl Guides and "village naturalist circles"—with the means "readily to distinguish and identify at least the more common and mischievous species of British mosquitoes" (Hogarth 1928: 18; Liverpool Evening Express 1928).

Despite this sense of urgency and their liberally employed rhetoric of warfare (Marshall 1925a: 475), Marshall and his associates did not exaggerate the threat that British mosquitoes posed. They scrupulously distinguished between species such as *A. detritus* and the Anopheline "tribe." They were also clear that nothing less than the disintegration of Britain's modern sanitary system would be required to re-establish malaria as a "native disease" (Hogarth 1928: 37). Nonetheless, for the likes of Hogarth, Marshall and Ross, "seaside" mosquitoes' non-lethality was no reason to accept they were an unavoidable part of life—as was the weather or taxes, about which you could complain ad nauseam, but just had to live with.

Marshall saw no possibility of coexistence at Hayling Island. Either he and his fellow residents had to go, or their little tormentors had to go (Olver 2014). It was a stand-off. Sir Richard Gregory, editor of *Nature*, who presided over the Institute's opening ceremony in 1925, also took the crusading "us or them" position:

> Man to-day is "up against" the mosquito, and has to fight in order to live at all. In many places, it is a question of mosquito or man, and if the insect is permitted to breed without any control ... man must finally leave the place.
>
> *(Daily Telegraph 1925: 12)*

One reporter offered the following headline of Gregory's talk: "Man against the insect: scientist says we must conquer or die" (Daily Express 1920; Western Mail 1925). Ross's opening address adopted a similar tone. Emphasizing the direct value to the world's tropical regions of the research conducted at this unlikely place, he cast mosquitoes of all kinds (indeed all pestiferous insects that preyed on us, our crops or livestock) as an insufferable affront to human authority:

> Nothing in human history is more remarkable than the contrast between the comparatively rapid and easy victory of man over the great beasts and reptiles and his total helplessness throughout the ages in the face of attack by the tiniest of living things. The empire of the disease-bearing insects has, indeed, been very widely extended in many regions at the same time that ancient and modern weapons were swiftly exterminating the dangerous brutes.
>
> *("Mosquito control," Daily Telegraph, 2 September 1925: 8)*

Ross gave his speech al fresco, before an audience of some 350, in the very garden where he was famously tormented in 1922 (and where Marshall's guests were unable to enjoy their refreshments). His former molesters' absence testified to the Hayling campaign's unambiguous success (*Times* 1925). By the summer of 1923, unsolicited testimonies from locals had already pointed to the remarkable elimination of mosquitoes. A happy repeat visitor reported to Marshall in August 1926 that during her current two-month stay, "I have not seen a mosquito with the exception of those in your [Institute's] cages" (Marshall 1924: 12; BMCI, 8th report 1930). The BMCI had apparently worked out not only which kind of mosquito was biting townsfolk and vacationers, but it had unleashed a multi-pronged assault on the larvae and breeding grounds of *Aedes detritus*.

"No stagnating sea water, no mosquito nuisance"[15]

The work at Hayling Island (covering under seven square miles) was targeted rather than indiscriminate, based on the conviction that control strategies should be micro-strategies, carefully tailored to the habits and micro-habitats of individual mosquito species rather than blanket spraying, as would occur in Sardinia after 1945 (Hall 2010). A researcher summed up the nuanced approach adopted on Hayling Island: "it is idle to blame the domestic water butt if the insects are coming from a pond in a neighbouring wood" (BMJ 1930 : 328). Marshall's team quickly learnt they were dealing with enormous diversity in species, hatching habits and breeding places (BMCI 17 May 1928, MP, LSHTM). Initial collecting activities in the autumn of 1920 disclosed that the "local nuisance" was almost exclusively caused by *Aedes (Ochlerotatus) detritus*, a species particularly active in daytime that was also exceptional among British mosquitoes for other reasons. It was not until the following summer, after experiments in a makeshift laboratory revealed that *A. detritus* would breed in stagnant water comparable in salinity to seawater, that Marshall and his staff figured it out. *A. detritus* was a "long-distance" species with an unusual flight range of up to five kilometres whose breeding grounds were situated two kilometres westward and eastward of its biting grounds in the central residential district (Marshall 1928: 9).

They also discovered that, exceptionally among British mosquitoes, *A. detritus* eggs and larvae can survive the winter. Eggs laid in dry marshland vegetation remained in suspended animation until submerged by tidal action or otherwise wetted. If the weather was mild, the production of adults could continue from April to November—a remarkably long hatching-out period for British mosquitoes (BMJ 1930: 328-329). The campaign's key finding? Successful control at the local level depends on establishing the precise identity of the problem-causing mosquito and thorough study of its attributes (Marshall 1927, BMCI, AMWL; Marshall, Nature 1942: 2). As Marshall explained:

> Each species displays great discrimination as regards the special situations which it selects for its breeding, and its choice depends upon a number of factors which it no doubt understands better than we do. Certain species appear to possess a sufficient knowledge of engineering to enable them to lay their eggs in depressions ... which, although dried up at the time when eggs are deposited, are destined to collect water in the wetter months.
>
> *(Marshall, undated B: 3, Marshall, AMWL)*

This approach belongs, of course, to an era before DDT was available as a super-weapon in the mosquito controller's arsenal. Marshall's views on DDT are not recorded and we can only speculate over whether he would have embraced it wholeheartedly should it have been available in the 1920s. Gordon Patterson divides mosquito control in the USA into two eras before general uses of DDT were banned in 1972: the pre-DDT period of mechanical control (c. 1900 to 1942) and the period of chemical control (1942–1972) (Patterson 2016: 2). Adapting this periodization to the UK, the mechanical era is the same (c. 1900–1942) but the chemical era lasts longer, until 1986. Nuisance mosquito control before DDT was pursued in Britain through a blend of short- and long-term measures. The former consisted of larvae suffocation by spreading paraffin and crude oil or other chemicals on the water surface[16] as well as biocontrol (in other words, leaving larvae-gobbling fish to do the job in certain water bodies). Long-term measures comprised "abolition" of existing and potential macro- and micro-level breeding grounds whether "natural" or "man-made" (MoH 1949: 20-26). The main methods adopted at Hayling Island, after *A. detritus* breeding grounds were pinpointed, were through drainage and infilling of marshlands ("a permanent cure" (Turnbull 1925: 228)).

Targeting of breeding grounds rather than mosquitoes themselves—a method also adopted, among others, on the Pontine marshes after 1922 but mainly during the 1930s—was in stark contrast to the favoured strategy of some local authorities in England at the time: spraying stagnant waters within or close to residential areas. This was not just a waste of money, said the critics. Spraying's ineffectuality undermined public confidence in anti-mosquito activities more generally (Manchester Guardian 1929: 8; Country Life 1925: 430; Caprotti 2006: 145–155; The Field 1924: 502–503).

If a heavy-handed, heavily chemical, top–down approach that ignores species' particularities and specificities on the ground can be characterized as hard, and its more measured opposite as soft, then the Hayling Island approach was "an intimate strategy of detection and destruction of breeding sites" (to borrow a phrase from a study of divergent control strategies in two cities in Arizona, Tucson and Phoenix (Shaw et al. 2010: 375)). Biocontrol methods are not necessarily "soft" if they involve the introduction of a non-native species such as the mosquitofish, *Gambusia*. However, just as Hogarth had noted that industrial pollutants were killing off larvae-gobbling fish, helping explain nuisance mosquitoes' proliferation in southern England in the early 1920s, Marshall warned, in proto-ecological reasoning, against indiscriminate application of chemical larvicides and paraffin that might inflict collateral damage, wiping out the mosquito's "benevolent" "natural enemies" such as fish. Marshall and colleagues instructed their "mosquito brigades" that established water bodies such as cattle ponds and ornamental lakes contained natural allies in the form of fish and other amphibians that feast on eggs and larvae (Hogarth 1928: 57).[17]

In his writings, Marshall never referred to Surgeon Major William C. Gorgas, who led US sanitation campaigns in Cuba and Panama in the early 1900s. But Gorgas's appreciation of the heterogeneity of a potential breeding site, characterized as "on-the-ground, labor-intensive, and environmentally complex" (Shaw et al. 2010: 376), was something that also informed Marshall's every move. Gorgas famously remarked (allegedly, c. 1900) that to combat mosquitoes, one needed to think like a mosquito (Soper 1965: 860; Macdonald 1965: 871; Stepan 2011: 92). Marshall would have echoed these sentiments.

If only we could, should we?

Despite mission accomplished on Hayling Island—subject to regular inspection, maintenance of drainage works and treatment of stagnant water—Marshall accepted that "permanent eradication of mosquitoes from even a limited area is … a matter of impossibility" (Marshall 1928: 27). This reflected respect for the indomitability of an opponent that has been around in the same form and life cycle for at least 80–105 million years and an appreciation of the limits of the science and technology, at least in the pre-DDT era. In today's discourse of ecosystem services and benefits, the presence of nuisance and disease-carrying, if sublethal, mosquito varieties within a wetland represent a potential disservice (Dwyer et al. 2016: 555, 557, 559–560; Knight et al. 2017: 431–440).

Marshall's views on whether the mosquito—*A. detritus* specifically, or more generally—possessed any positive merit are hard to discern from the written record. There is one solitary glimpse but its value as a gauge of what Marshall actually thought may be compromised by its whimsical tone and context. As he told a local Rotary Club in 1923:

> I have noticed that scarcely a week passes without my being asked to give a reply to the query: "what good, if any, do mosquitoes do in the world?" I must confess that, up to the present, I have been unable to give any satisfactory answer to this conundrum: but the next time I am asked this question I am going to say: "The mosquito is a two-winged insect to which I am indebted, up to now, for two highly enjoyable visits to Gosport."
>
> *(Marshall 1923, BMCI, AMWL)*

That does not mean that Marshall adhered to the view, as articulated recently by Janet McAllister of the Centers for Disease Control and Prevention in Fort Collins, Colorado, that "we haven't wanted anything from mosquitoes except for them to go away" (Fang 2010: 433). Nor can we extrapolate that he would be willing to contemplate any available means to rid the world of mosquitoes. And there is no suggestion that he ever wrestled with the profound moral implications of whether it was right to commit specicide, by deliberately wiping out a species. His organization, after all, was not called the British Mosquito Elimination Institute. Despite what he told members of Gosport's Rotary Club, I doubt he would have been happy with total elimination: that would have left nothing for him to study. Journalists wrote of "extermination" as the goal or ideal (Liverpool Courier 1925). But Marshall knew this was unattainable, since unending warfare was required to avoid a return to "the bad old days of 1920" (J.H.P., undated).[18]

In his speech opening the BMCI—in which he name-checked various "white man's graves" (London Evening News 1931) that mosquito control had made safe and habitable, Panama, Havana, Hong Kong, the Malay states and Ismailia—Ross looked ahead to what sounded like a mosquito-tamed utopia: "And the day may come – indeed, I am sure it will come – when all those fertile tracts of the world which are now dominated and ravaged by King Malaria and King Mosquito will be laid open to civilisation" (Marshall 1928: 16; Ross 1926: 486; Times 1925). In fact, his was not an unambiguous call to rid the entire earth. Ross's vision was confined to areas desirable for agricultural development and settlement by white Europeans where malaria was prevalent. Regardless of feasibility, it was simply unnecessary to eradicate mosquitoes wherever they were found. As Ross explained with reference to the control of *A. aegypti*, and "How Panama was made healthy,"

> Our work for the general extermination of insect pests is designed chiefly for the protection of cities and towns. We cannot expect—indeed, there is no need—to drive mosquitoes and the like out of jungles and marshy tracts away from civilisation.
>
> *(Observer 1925)*

This viewpoint, with its implicit distinction between "country" or "wild" anophelines and peri-domestic varieties such as *A. aegypti*, should not be confused, though, with an enlightened ethos of coexistence through live-and-let-live: whereas native peoples could coexist with mosquitoes in the tropics, the same could not be expected of Europeans. As long as there were uninhabited tracts, or places thinly and sporadically populated by non-Europeans, then there would always be places where the mosquito's empire would remain uncontested.

Restoring agency to a creaturely nuisance

The "social evil"—to borrow a term popular in 1920s Britain (Country Life 1927: 108)—caused by non-lethal varieties inhabiting the northern frontiers of the mosquito's global imperium has now been effortlessly eclipsed by the far graver evil of its deadly compatriots. And yet the merely annoying mosquito that ruins a camping trip (rather than an English picnic with cucumber sandwiches) provides the springboard for the most recent book on "our deadliest predator." Timothy Winegard's opening gambit is the scenario of an unwitting American vacationer slumping into a lawn chair to relax with a chilled beer after an exerting hike: "Before you can enjoy your first satisfying swig, however, you hear that all-too-familiar sound" (Winegard 2019: 7). Here is Winegard's hook: who would have thought that an insect most of us know as a pesky intrusion on a summer's evening has played such a profound role throughout human history? Reviewers of Winegard's book have highlighted the "tiny" mosquito's "outsize role" and "outsized effects" in our history (Mirsky 2019; Hemingway 2019). The challenge that the irritating, party-pooping mosquito posed to what Hogarth referred to as "the pleasures of outdoor life" in southern England in the early 1920s (Hogarth 1928: 17) is patently trivial compared to the worldwide, centuries-long, life-and-death struggle against its distant deadly relatives. The predicament *A. detritus* created was especially paltry within the wider context of the post-1919 outbreak of malaria epidemics across southern and eastern Europe. In 1923, in the Soviet Union alone, an estimated 18 million people out of 110 million were afflicted by malaria, resulting in over 60,000 deaths (Gachelin and Opinel 2011: 432). Still, the case of one obscure mosquito species along the southern coast of England provides an intriguing example of an insect pest whose role was far from undersized.

Acknowledgements

The research for this chapter was pursued as a co-investigator on "Taking the bite out of wetlands: Managing mosquitoes and the socio-ecological value of wetlands for wellbeing" ("Wetland Life") (2016–2020), funded by the Valuing Nature Programme (UK) https://valuing-nature.net/about (NERC [Natural Environment Research Council] grant reference number NE/NO13379/1).

Notes

1 The headline was prompted by a gathering of medical officers and sanitary inspectors in Surrey (Britain's first) to plan mosquito control in that county for the coming summer. BMCI, AMWL refers to the papers of the British Mosquito Control Institute (BMCI), Hayling Island, Hampshire, in the Sir Ronald Ross Collection, Archives and Manuscripts, Wellcome Library for the History and Understanding of Medicine, London (BMCI, AMWL).

2 *Anopheles atroparvus* was originally identified as *A. maculipennis* (Marshall 1938: 2).

3 *A. maculipennis/Anopheles atroparvus* is zoophilic and lives and hibernates in pigsties, stables and cowsheds.

4 At the time, improved drainage that eliminated bad air and bad waters was offered as the main explanation for ague's demise, but drainage inadvertently created new breeding places in the shape of ditches and canals (Malaria Commission 1927: 28–29).

5 Britain is not mentioned in Evans (1989).

6 MP, LSHTM refers to: John Frederick Marshall Papers, Library and Archives, London School of Hygiene and Tropical Medicine, London (LSHTM).

7 William John Ritchie Simpson was author of studies such as *Maintenance of Health in the Tropics* (1916) and a founder of the London School of Hygiene and Tropical Medicine.

8 Only in summer are England's temperatures warm enough for an infected mosquito to complete its parasitic cycle (15–20 days). Temperatures and humidity levels are highest along the southern and southeast coasts.

9 This subheading is taken from the title of Chapters 3 and 4 in Hogarth, *British Mosquitoes and How to Eliminate Them* (1928).

10 For details of Marshall's life and career (he was heir to a family business fortune), see Snow and Snow (2004: 23–28).

11 The Institute, housed in new premises adjacent to Marshall's residence ("Seacourt"), consisted, on the ground floor, of a demonstration museum, laboratory, a drawing and record office, a photographic room, dark room and mechanical workshop, and, on the first floor, a library, projection room, secretarial offices and research areas. After 1925, Hayling Mosquito Control continued to exist as the Hayling Island Branch of BMCI, which remained responsible for local control measures, whereas BMCI concentrated on research (pure and applied), advisory and educational work (BMCI 1928: 3, MP, LSHTM; Marshall 1925a). After 1939, BMCI's work shrank to local mosquito control.

12 James was a retired lieutenant colonel in the Indian Expeditionary Force (IEF) "D," and former IEF assistant director of Medical Services (Sanitary). BMCI's governing council's membership list reads like a roll-call of the great and the good of British imperial and tropical science.

13 Marshall 1925b.

14 Shute's essay ("Mosquito eradication") was reproduced as Appendix A in Hogarth 1928: 125–127.

15 Hayling Mosquito Control, undated, MP, LSHTM.

16 Chemical larvicides, such as disinfectant (cresol) and copper sulphate, were deployed where windy conditions tore apart the surface film of oil or vegetation broke it up, allowing air to reach larvae (Marshall 1921: 1).

17 1920s British mosquito researchers were curious about biocontrol practised elsewhere, such as transplantation of top-water minnow from North Carolina to waters in the northern USA and Central America, and French proposals for stocking young eels (Observer 1922; London Evening News 1926). Recognition of certain aquatic species' larvae consumption did not extend to a larger awareness of the place of mosquito larvae and adults at the bottom of a food pyramid. Researchers have recently revisited the mosquitofish's reputation as a "reliable ally" in mosquito control (Fang 2010: 433).

18 On the pursuit of control and elimination as different goals, see Cockburn 1961.

Bibliography

Birmingham Post, 1927. *New Force against Mosquitoes*. 31 March.

BMCI (British Mosquito Control Institute), 1928. Mosquitoes and Their Control. Exhibit 12, Conversazione, The Royal Society, Burlington House, 17 May. John Frederick Marshall Papers, Library and Archives, London School of Hygiene and Tropical Medicine, London. MP, LSHTM.

BMCI, 1928. Reports presented by the Council and the Director at the Second Annual General Meeting, London, 18 June. BMCI: Hayling Island. MP, LSHTM.

BMCI, 1929–1930. Eighth Report of the Proceedings of the Hayling Island Branch of the British Mosquito Control Institute. 1 January 1929 to 1 January 1930. MP, LSHTM.

BMCI, 1930. Report of the Director, 4th Annual General Meeting. London, 9 December 1930. BCMI: Hayling Island. MP, LSHTM.

British Medical Journal, 1930. *Mosquitoes in Britain*. *2/3634*. 30 August, 328–329.

Buchanan, G.S. and Newsholme, Arthur. 1919. Reports and Papers on Malaria Contracted in England in 1917. In *Reports to the Local Government Board on Public Health and Medical Subjects*. London: HMSO.

Caprotti, Federico, 2006. Malaria and Technological Networks: Medical Geography in the Pontine Marshes, Italy, in the 1930s. *The Geographical Journal* 171/2, 145–155.

Chicago Daily Tribune 1914. *Mosquito fight begun in Chicago spreading afar. Other states take up campaign against pleasure-killing pest*. 16 July, 13.

Christophers, S.R. and Bentley, C.A. 1908. *Black-water Fever: Scientific Memoirs by Officers of the Medical and Sanitary Departments of the Government in India, New Series, No. 35*. Simla: Government of India.

Cockburn, T. Aidan. 1961. Eradication of Infectious Diseases: "control" is an Unending Operation. After "eradication," No Further Effort Is Required. *Science*, 133/3458, 1050–1058.

Country Life, 1925. *Notes*. *57/1472*. 21 March, 430.

Country Life, 1926. *Country Notes. 60/1537*. 3 July, 4.

Country Life, 1927. *Pardonable Irritation. 66/1592*. 23 July, 108.

Daily Express, 1920. *New war against Mosquitoes*. 28 August.

Daily Mail, 1925. *Control of Mosquitoes: Plans to Exterminate Them*. 10 August, 15.

Daily Mirror, 1925. *Perilous Parasites*. 31 August.

Daily News, 1925. *Snack from Neck of Scientist: Hayling Island Warfare*. 1 September.

Daily Telegraph, 1925. *Man Versus Mosquito: Controlling a Pest*. 1 September, 12.

Dobson, Mary, 1998. *Contours of Death and Disease in Early Modern England*. Cambridge: Cambridge University Press.

Dwyer, P.G. Knight, J.M. and Dale, P.E.R., 2016. Planning Development to Reduce Mosquito Hazard in Coastal Peri-Urban Areas: Case Studies in NSW, Australia. In *Balanced Urban Development: Options and Strategies for Liveable Cities*, eds. B. Maheshwari et al. Basel: Springer International, 555–574.

Evans, Hugh, 1989. European Malaria Policy in the 1920s and 1930s. *Isis* 80/1, 40–59.

Fang, Janet, 2010. A World Without Mosquitoes. *Nature* 466, 432–434.

Gachelin, Gabriel and Opinel, Annick. 2011. Malaria Epidemics in Europe after the First World War: The Early Stages of an International Approach to the Control of the Disease. *História, Ciências, Saúde–Manguinhos* 18/2, 431–469.

Grove, A.J. 1919. Anopheline Mosquitoes in England. V. English Mosquitoes. In *Reports to the Local Government Board on Public Health and Medical Subjects*, 44–50.

Hall, Marcus. 2010. Environmental imperialism in Sardinia: Pesticides and Politics in the Struggle Against Malaria. In *Nature and History in Modern Italy*, eds. Marco Armiero and Marcus Hall. Athens: Ohio University Press, 70–86.

Hayling Mosquito Control. Undated. The Facts about the Salt-Water Mosquito Ochlerotatus Detritus (The Nuisance). Circular No. 7, MP, LSHTM.

Hemingway, Janet. 2019. A New Tome Traces the Outsized Effects the Mosquito Has Had on Human History. *Science*, 30 July, https://blogs.sciencemag.org/books/2019/07/30/the-mosquito/

Hogarth, A. Moore. 1928. *British Mosquitoes and How to Eliminate Them*. London: Hutchinson.

J.H.P., undated. Where the Mosquito Meets His Fate: Avengers at Hayling Island; a War That Never Ends. MP, LSHTM.

James, S.P. 1920. *Malaria at Home and Abroad*. London: John Bale.

James, S.P. 1929. The Disappearance of Malaria from England. *Proceedings of the Royal Society of Medicine* 23, 71–87.

Knight, J., Dale, P. Dwyer, P. and Marx, S. 2017. A Conceptual Approach to Integrate Management of Ecosystem Service and Disservice in Coastal Wetlands. *AIMS Environmental Science* 4/3, 431–440.

Liverpool Courier, 1925. *Mosquito Peril to Man. Institute to Wage War of Extermination*. 1 September.

Liverpool Evening Express, 1928. *The Mosquito*. 17 January.

London Evening News, 1926. *Sticklebacks to Rescue*. 9 August.

London Evening News, 1931. *Those Mosquitoes*. 13 August.

London Evening Standard, 1925. *War on England's Mosquitoes: How Hayling's Summer Swarms Were Removed*. 31 August.

MacArthur, W.P. 1951. A Brief History of English Malaria. *British Medical Bulletin* 8, 76–79.

Macdonald, Angus. 1919. Report on Indigenous Malaria and on Malaria Work Performed in Connection with the Troops in England during the Year 1918. In *Observations on Malaria by Medical Officers of the Army and Others*, ed. Ronald Ross. London: War Office/HMSO, 178–258.

Macdonald, George. 1965. Eradication of Malaria. *Public Health Reports* 80/10, 870–879.

Macfarlane, R. 2012. Item of the Month, April 2012: On Indigenous Malaria. 25 April, http://blog.wellcomelibrary.org/2012/04/item-of-the-month-april-2012-on-indigenous-malaria/

Malaria Commission. 1927. Principles and Methods of Antimalarial Measures in Europe. In *Second General Report of the Malaria Commission*, doc. C.H./Malaria/73. Geneva: League of Nations Health Organisation.

Manchester Guardian, 1925. *English Mosquito Scare*. 11 June, 18.

Manchester Guardian, 1929. *The Mosquito in our Midst*. 29 August, 8.

Marshall, J.F. 1921. The Destruction of Mosquito Larvae in Salt or Brackish Water. Hayling Mosquito Control, Circular No. 6, Marshall, LSHTM.

Marshall, J.F. 1923. Lecture to Gosport Rotary Club, 19 July, British Mosquito Control Institute [Unit] (BMCI), Hayling Island, Hampshire, Sir Ronald Ross Collection, Archives and Manuscripts, Wellcome Library for the History and Understanding of Medicine. BMCI, AMWL.

Marshall, J.F. 1924. A Report on the Anti-Mosquito Operations Carried out by the Hayling Mosquito Control during the Period October,1922 to February,1924 Inclusive (15 March). Marshall, LSHTM.

Marshall, J.F. 1925a. Fighting the English Mosquito: The Hayling Island Institute. *Illustrated London News*, 12 September, 475.

Marshall, J.F. 1925b. Coastal Mosquitoes and Their Control. A Paper Read before the Zoology Section of the British Association for the Advancement of Science [Southampton Meeting], 27 August, Marshall, LSHTM.

Marshall, J.F. 1927. Account of the Origin of the British Mosquito Control Institute (presented to the Council of the Institute. 30 March 1927, BMCI, AMWL.

Marshall, J.F. 1928. *Principles and Practice of Mosquito Control: Being a Handbook to the British Mosquito Control Institute*. Hampshire: Hayling Island.

Marshall, J.F. 1930. The Organization of Mosquito Control Work. Presidential Address, Zoology Section, South Eastern Union of Scientific Societies, Portsmouth Congress, May. Marshall, LSHTM.

Marshall, J.F. 1933. Mosquito Control in Dorset (letter to the editor). Portsmouth Evening News, 11 September 1933. Marshall, LSHTM.

Marshall, J.F. 1938. A Revised List of the British Mosquitoes, with Some Notes Regarding Those Discovered in England since the Year 1918 (No. 30), 2.

Marshall, J.F. 1942. Mosquito-Breeding in Static Water Supplies. *Nature* 149, 2.

Marshall, J.F. Undated a. *The Organization and Operation of a Mosquito Control*. Marshall, LSHTM.

Marshall, J.F. Undated b. *A Mosquito Summary*. BMCI: Hayling Island, AMWL.

Ministry of Health, 1949. *Memorandum on Measures for the Control of Mosquito Nuisances in Great Britain*. London: HMSO.

Ministry of Health, 1962. *Memorandum on Measures for the Control of Mosquito Nuisances in Great Britain*. London: HMSO.

Mirsky, Steve. 2019. The Outsize Role of Tiny Mosquitoes in Human History. *Scientific American*, October, https://www.scientificamerican.com/article/the-outsize-role-of -tiny-mosquitoes-in-human-history/

Morning Post, 1925a. *Hayling Island Mosquito Control: New Stage in the Work*. 16 March.

Morning Post, 1925b. *Routing the Mosquito: The Hayling Island war; World's Interest in British Methods*. 31 August.

Nature, 1949. *Mr. J.F. Marshall, C.B.E. (obituary), 165*. 7 January, 16.

Newman, George. 1919. Reports and Papers on Malaria Contracted in England in 1918 (June 1919). In *Reports to the Local Government Board on Public Health and Medical Subjects*. London: HMSO, New Series, No. 123, 1–42.

Newsholme, Arthur. 1918. Reports and Papers on Malaria Contracted in England in 1917 (June 1918. In *Reports to the Local Government Board on Public Health and Medical Subjects*. London: HMSO, New Series, No. 119, Appendix 2.

Observer, 1922. *The Fish Cure for Mosquitoes: Successful Experiments in America*. 12 November, 9.

Observer, 1925. *The Campaign against Insect Pests: Interview with Sir Ronald Ross*. 30 August, 5.

O'Gorman, Emily. 2017. Imagined Ecologies: A More-Than-Human History of Malaria in the Murrumbidgee Irrigation Area, New South Wales, Australia, 1919–1945. *Environmental History* 22, 486–514.

Olver, Chris. 2014. Malaria in the UK (25 April). Library and Archives Service Blog, LSHTM, https://blogs.lshtm.ac.uk/library/2014/04/25/malaria-in-the-uk/

Parsons, A.C. 1919. Practical Notes on Mosquito Surveys of Camps and Barracks during 1917 and 1918. In *Observations on Malaria by Medical Officers of the Army and Others*, 95–112.

Patterson, Gordon. 2009. *The Mosquito Crusades: A History of the American Anti-Mosquito Movement from the Reed Commission to the First Earth Day*. New Brunswick, NJ: Rutgers University Press.

Patterson, Gordon. 2016. Looking Backward, Looking Forward: The Long, Torturous Struggle with Mosquitoes. *Insects* 7, 1–14, https://doi.org/10.3390/insects7040056

Peacock, T.B. 1859. On Recently Prevalent Malarious Affections. *Medical Times and Gazette* 19, 399–400, 453–455, 478–479.

Portsmouth Gazette, 1930. *Today.* 5 March.

Ross, Ronald. 1902. *Mosquito Brigades and How to Organize Them.* London: George Philip.

Ross, Ronald. 1919, An Interim Report on the Treatment of Malaria – Abstract of 2,460 Cases. In *Observations on Malaria by Medical Officers of the Army and Others,* 323–327.

Ross, Ronald. 1926. The Importance of Mosquito Control. *Science Progress in the Twentieth Century (1919–1933)* 20/79, 481–486.

Service, Mike W. 2003. Ross Letters, Press Cuttings, Hayling Island Institute. 22 October, BMCI, AMWL.

Shaw, Ian Graham Ronald, Robbins, Paul F. and Jones, John Paul III. 2010. A bug's Life and the Spatial Ontologies of Mosquito Management. *Annals of the Association of American Geographers* 100/02, 375.

Smith, John. 1904. *Report of the New Jersey Agricultural Experiment Station upon Mosquitoes Occurring within the State, Their Habits, Life History, Etc.* Trenton: New Jersey Agricultural Experiment Station.

Snow, Keith R. 1998. Distribution of Anopheles Mosquitoes in the British Isles. *European Mosquito Bulletin* 1, 9–13.

Snow, Keith R. and Snow, Susan E. 2004. John Frederick Marshall and "The British Mosquitoes." *European Mosquito Bulletin: Journal of the European Mosquito Control Association* 17, 23–28.

Soper, Fred L. 1965. Rehabilitation of the Eradication Concept in the Prevention of Communicable Diseases. *Public Health Reports* 80/10, 855–869.

Stepan, Nancy Leys. 2011. *Eradication: Riding the World of Diseases Forever?* London: Reaktion.

Sutter, Paul S. 2007. Nature's Agents or agents of Empire?: Entomological Workers and Environmental Change during the Construction of the Panama Canal. *Isis* 98/4, 724–754.

The Children's Newspaper, 1928. *Hayling Island's War: Conquering the Mosquito.* 29 September, Marshall, LSHTM.

The Field, 1924. *Hayling Island Mosquitoes.* 25 September, 502–503.

The Lancet, 1925. *British Mosquito Control Institute.* 5 September.

The Times, 1925. *British Mosquito Conquered: Work at Hayling Island; new Institute Opened.* 1 September, 14.

The Times, 1926. *Mosquitoes in Epping Forest: A Summer Nuisance.* 13 August.

Turnbull, R.E. 1925. Controlling the Mosquito in Britain: Campaign Methods. *Illustrated London News,* 4 August, 228.

West Africa, 1927. *Mosquito Pest Conference – in England!* 12 March.

Western Mail, 1925. *Mosquito or man? Case of Survival of the Fittest.* 1 September.

Westminster Gazette, 1927. *New War on the Mosquito: Legislation Need Emphasised.* 31 March.

Winegard, Timothy. 2019. *The Mosquito: A Human History of our Deadliest Predator.* New York: Penguin.

Yorkshire Post, 1927. *British Mosquito Pest: Health Ministry official Suggests Legislation.* 31 March.

PART III
Know thy enemy

8

THE MOSQUITO AND MALARIA

Would mosquito control alone eliminate the disease?

Willem Takken

In the third decade of the twenty-first century, malaria continues to be one of the world's most devastating infectious diseases, mostly in low-income countries. The disease is caused by *Plasmodium* parasites, which are transmitted between humans by mosquitoes of the genus *Anopheles*. The World Health Organization reported 228 million cases in 2018, with around 405,000 deaths. The majority of these cases occurred in tropical Africa, and most deaths were children below age five (WHO 2019). With so many new annual infections and deaths, the disease levies enormous burdens, particularly in malaria-endemic countries. It is estimated that an African household spends on average 10% of its annual income on malaria prevention and control, and that the combined economies of Africa lose US$4 billion per year due to the disease (Sachs and Malaney 2002, Shretta et al. 2016, Sarma et al. 2019). For example, the average annual cost of malaria to society was recently estimated at US$7.80 per uncomplicated case and US$107.64 per severe case in an endemic area of Mozambique (Alonso et al. 2019). Using these figures and considering all cases to be uncomplicated, malaria prevention and treatment currently cost the world some US$1.7 billion per year.

Human malaria is caused by five species of the genus *Plasmodium*, of which *Plasmodium falciparum* and *Plasmodium vivax* are most prevalent, and most responsible for the disease. *P. falciparum* is the main malaria killer, being especially virulent in non-immune people, particularly young children (White et al. 2014). The parasite has a complex life cycle, starting when infectious sporozoites are injected into the human bloodstream by the bite of an anopheline mosquito. The parasite then undergoes a series of developments in the human host to eventually develop male and female gametes, which can be found in the peripheral blood (Figure 8.1). This development process can vary from 10 to 20 days, depending on the *Plasmodium* species and condition of the human host. After male and female gametes are ingested by an anopheline mosquito, the gametes fuse into a

DOI: 10.4324/9781003056034-8

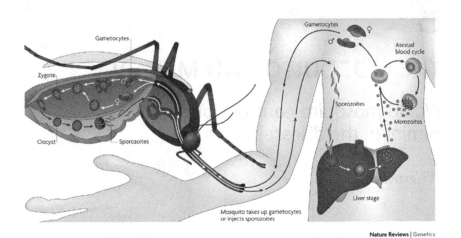

FIGURE 8.1 *Plasmodium* life cycle (Source: Su et al., *Nature Reviews Genetics* 8: 497-506, 2007).

zygote, which subsequently develops into an oocyte. Next, oocytes migrate to the interior wall of the mosquito's midgut where they grow out into oocysts in which the sporozoites develop. After 7 to 10 days, mature oocytes burst, with the sporozoites migrating to the salivary gland, from where another mosquito bite can start the transmission cycle again (Warrell and Gilles 2002).

It was the discovery of Sir Ronald Ross in 1897 that malaria parasites developed in the mosquito which led to the realization of the importance of this creature to malaria transmission: without anopheline mosquitoes, human malaria could not exist (Ross 1900). Before Ross's discovery, malaria was generally treated by administering quinine and prevented, if possible, by temporarily vacating residences during the "fever season" for healthier areas or else draining nearby pestilential swamps thought to carry the "bad air" of malaria (Webb 2009).

Malaria epidemiology and R0

Following his discovery of the life cycle of *Plasmodium*, and the role of mosquitoes in this process, Ross developed one of the earliest epidemiological models for the prediction of a vector-borne disease (Ross 1910). The model was based on the basic reproductive number, R0, and gave a central role to the mosquito vector. The model was further developed by McDonald (MacDonald 1957), and rapidly became a standard for the design of malaria control and prevention programmes (Figure 8.2).

The basic reproductive number, R0, represents the rate with which malaria spreads through a human community and is defined as the expected number of cases directly generated by one case in a population where all individuals

$$R = \frac{ma^2 bp^n}{- r(\ln p)}$$

Legend:
- ma = human biting rate
- b = proportion of mosquitoes developing parasites following infective blood meal
- n = extrinsic incubation rate
- p = daily survival rate of mosquito
- 1/r = days of infectivity per case

FIGURE 8.2 Basic reproductive number of malaria (adapted from Smith et al., *PLOS Biology* 5: 531–542, 2007).

are susceptible to infection (Anderson and May 1992, Wilson et al. 2020). It is assumed in this equation that no other individuals are infected by the pathogen or immunized to the disease. When R0 is greater than 1, the number of infected individuals will increase, whereas when R0 is less than 1, the disease will die out. The mosquito is represented in the model by its human biting rate *ma* and its daily survival rate *p*. Indirectly, the *Plasmodium* infections in the mosquito, represented by factor *b* (viz. the proportion of mosquitoes developing parasites), also relate to the role of the mosquitoes in the model.[1] Given the central role of mosquitoes in the basic reproductive number, it follows that effective vector control can lead to a rapid decline of new infections, meaning that vector control is one of the pillars of combatting malaria. In the history of malaria control, many efforts have been directed at eliminating the mosquito vectors to halt the spread of the disease.

Short history of malaria control

Until the development of affordable (synthetic) malaria drugs, the disease was treated primarily with quinine, a drug originating from the Peruvian cinchona tree that acted on the parasite itself (Rocco 2003). Following the discovery of the role of the mosquito in malaria's transmission cycle, control strategies were reoriented towards reducing human–mosquito contact. At first this was done with environmental management through the removal or modification of breeding sites. Famous examples of these were the anti-malaria works at the Panama Canal (Dehne 1955) and the environmental management methods in Malaysia and Indonesia (Watson 1921, Takken et al. 1990) where the breeding sites of malaria mosquitoes (swamps) were drained and predatory mosquito-eating fish were released in rice fields. These methods were quite effective and led to strong reductions or even local elimination of malaria.

In the 1920s, Paris Green, an inorganic insecticide containing copper acetoarsenite, was developed for mosquito control. The compound was successfully used to eradicate the invasive African malaria mosquito *Anopheles arabiensis* (*Anopheles gambiae sensu lato*) from Brazil (Killeen et al. 2002) and in 1944 it was used on a widescale for malaria control in Italy (de Zulueta 1998).

During the Second World War, the synthetic insecticide dichlorodiphenyl-trichloroethane (DDT) was introduced as a novel, effective, mosquito control tool as it could be used to kill adult mosquitoes by treating the resting sites of the mosquitoes, especially walls and ceilings in houses and stables. At the same time, the synthetic malaria drug chloroquine was developed, and both tools were used in tandem for the dramatic control of malaria in many parts of the world. Initial results were so successful that the World Health Assembly launched a global malaria eradication campaign in 1955. The campaign was highly successful in eradicating malaria from temperate climate zones, but its application in tropical climate zones proved more complicated: the enormous scale of the malaria endemic combined with a rapid development of insecticide resistance and a growing scarcity of financial resources drew the global campaign to a halt. In 1969 the campaign was officially ended, with malaria persisting in large parts of the world, many considered as low-income countries, where malaria continued to cause heavy burdens. In many countries, malaria mosquitoes had become resistant to DDT, rendering this compound and its derivatives obsolete.

The discovery in the 1970s of a new class of insecticides, the synthetic pyrethroids, led to a renewed interest in malaria vector control. It was found that bed nets treated with these new synthetics, or Insecticide-Treated Nets (ITNs), gave far better protection against malaria than untreated nets. The insecticide on the nets killed mosquitoes landing on the net, as well as deterring them (Alonso et al. 1991, Lindsay et al. 1993). Large-scale trials with ITNs in several African countries proved so successful that the World Health Organization included them in its Roll Back Malaria programme (WHO 2005).

The new global malaria eradication campaign launched in 2007 appeared hopeful, and led to a 50% reduction of global malaria, of which at least 78% was due to vector control with ITNs and indoor residual spraying (IRS) (Bhatt et al. 2015). This rapid decline of malaria since the launch of the Roll Back Malaria programme in 2000 was, however, put to a halt after 2015, with little further progress reported since then (WHO 2019). One of the reasons for this halt in progress is the rapid and widespread development of insecticide resistance, a repeat of what happened in the DDT era (Hemingway et al. 2016, Ranson and Lissenden 2016). Should the high degree of insecticide resistance in many anopheline populations be a reason to abandon vector control, even with methods that go beyond insecticides? After all, it was through vector control that the earliest successes of malaria control were achieved, with only limited successes derived from anti-malarial drugs (Bhatt et al. 2015).

The Global Vector Control Response

Despite significant reductions in malaria achieved under the Roll Back Malaria programme, an increase in programme costs and the rapid rise in insecticide resistance, a new approach to disease vector control was required. The WHO's Global Vector Control Response (GVCR) was launched in 2017 aiming for Integrated Vector Management (IVM), which is a toolbox of mosquito control methods designed to suppress or eliminate malaria vectors (WHO 2017). The toolbox includes environmental management, house improvement, biological and rationale methods as well as insecticides. With this greater emphasis on non-chemical methods, while strategically employing novel insecticides, it is expected that resistance can be delayed and insecticides can be utilized over a longer period. The GVCR encourages intersectoral collaboration and social aspects of vector control through community engagement.

The World Health Assembly adopted the GVCR unanimously in May 2017, with member states subsequently playing an active role in adapting this latest push for improving health through their national malaria control programmes.

Current tools for malaria vector control

- Environmental management: mosquitoes depend on aquatic sites for egg-laying and larval development. Drainage of such sites can be highly effective, but often requires engineering works which can be costly. Irrigated rice fields offer special potential as breeding sites for anopheline mosquitoes. Intermittent irrigation is another effective method for periodic killing of immature mosquitoes (Liu et al. 2004) and can be conducted at small and large scales. At the community level, removal of small puddles and water bodies in the peridomestic area has been practised as a method for malaria vector control (van den Berg et al. 2018).
- Housing improvements: many *Anopheles* species, in particular those that feed readily on humans, have developed the habit of using houses as feeding and resting sites. The most important African malaria vectors, *Anopheles gambiae sensu stricto, An. coluzzii* and *An. funestus,* are highly anthropophilic and take nearly all blood meals indoors during nocturnal hours. This is the reason why bed nets are such effective tools for malaria prevention (see below). Screening of doors and windows, and screening or closure of eaves, has been shown to prevent mosquito entry, and even to reduce malaria risk (Kirby et al. 2009). Housing improvement is considered an important component of malaria control and currently several studies are under way to develop this into a practical tool (Lindsay et al. 2002, Tusting et al. 2017, Mburu et al. 2018).

- Biological control: natural products or organisms that kill mosquitoes are used for biological control. These include predatory fish, pathogenic fungi and bacteria. Of the last organisms, *Bacillus thuringiensis israelensis* (*Bti*) and *Bacillus sphaericus* have been particularly popular for malaria vector control (Fillinger et al. 2009, Tusting et al. 2013, Afrane et al. 2016, Dambach et al. 2019). Such bacteria can be described as biological insecticides.
- Bio-rationale methods: these approaches for control are based on disrupting the growth and development of mosquitoes as well as their communication systems. The most widely used bio-rationale (or "biorational") tools are insect growth regulators (IGRs). These are products that mimic juvenile hormones and interfere with the growth and development of an insect. In mosquito control, common products are methoprene (Altosid®), pyriproxyfen and diflubenzuron (Dimilin®), and they are mostly used as larvicides. IGRs have been widely used for the control of nuisance mosquitoes as well as for the control of mosquitoes transmitting viruses like dengue, chikungunya and Zika. By contrast, insect growth regulators are rarely used for malaria control.
- Chemical control: despite the widespread presence of insecticide resistance in many species of malaria mosquitoes, insecticide-impregnated bed nets continue to provide good protection, albeit to a lesser degree than in the period before insecticide resistance (Yang et al. 2018). It is less clear if there will still be a role for indoor residual spraying (IRS) in future malaria programmes, as this method does not provide protection against mosquito bites, unlike bed nets, once the mosquitoes have become resistant. The Innovative Vector Control Consortium (IVCC), which consists of a network of private and public organizations, is working on the development of novel classes of insecticides and novel strategies for application of insecticides, as by combining several different classes of insecticides or combining an insecticide with a synergist (Hemingway 2017, Gleave et al. 2018). It is expected that within a few years, new chemical products will be available to replace current insecticides (Knapp et al. 2015, Killeen 2020).
- Behavioural control: mosquitoes respond to visual, acoustic and chemical cues for intra- and interspecific interactions. Knowledge of these cues can be used to manipulate the behaviour of the mosquitoes, leading to reduced vector densities and possibly vector eradication. Some behavioural control depends on mosquito gender, as outlined below.

Male mosquitoes: males form swarms when searching for a mate using aggregation cues. These swarms can be manipulated by acoustic and chemical cues aimed at mating disruption (Cator et al. 2011, Wooding et al. 2020). Male mosquitoes feed on nectar, and toxic sugar baits have been developed to alter the mosquitoes' nectar-feeding behaviour, leading to significant reductions in mosquito populations (Traore et al. 2020).

Female mosquitoes: female anophelines feed primarily on vertebrate blood. Vertebrate hosts are located with odorous cues emitted by the host

(Takken and Knols 1999), and synthetic odour cues that mimic a human have been employed to mass trap host-seeking mosquitoes with the aim for reducing their biting intensity and, subsequently, *Plasmodium* transmission rate. In a recent study in Kenya it was shown that mass trapping with odour-baited traps led to a 30% reduction in malaria prevalence (Homan et al. 2016). Female mosquitoes can also be manipulated to lay their eggs in selected sites, using odorant cues that attract gravid females (Lindh et al. 2015, Eneh et al. 2016, Schoelitsz et al. 2020). Such sites can be laced with a biological larvicide (*Bti*), as an alternative and efficient way of larval control.

Push-pull: repellents are compounds that deter mosquitoes so that they move away from feeding and resting zones. Currently, there is much interest in the pyrethroid compound transfluthrin, as this acts not only as an insecticide, but also as a strong repellent, disrupting the mosquito's ability to land and/or bite. Transfluthrin can be impregnated into fabrics and nettings, producing mosquito-free zones (Syafruddin et al. 2020). When repellents are combined with an attractant, a push–pull system can be created that is under investigation as a novel tool for malaria control (Menger et al. 2015, Hiscox et al. 2019, Mmbando et al. 2019).

- Genetic control: advanced technologies in molecular and cellular biology have made it possible to identify and manipulate mosquito genes that regulate specific traits of their biology (Adolfi and Lycett 2018). For example, genes that regulate reproduction can be knocked out leading to sterilization of mosquito populations. It is also possible to modify genes that increase susceptibility of *Plasmodium* infections, thus rendering mosquito populations vulnerable and unable to transmit the malaria parasite. A third genetic method relies on introducing a gene that regulates host-seeking behaviour, so that mosquitoes no longer recognize their preferred blood host. Some of these technologies are in advanced stages of development, but some are also under strong ethical scrutiny, meaning that these technologies should not be applied in the field until proven safe and acceptable to society (James et al. 2018).
- Community engagement: for decades, malaria control was undertaken as a vertically led programme, often run by national or regional public health offices. Communities were generally ill-informed as it was thought that any form of effective malaria control, conducted by the health office, was acceptable because it would lead to less morbidity and fewer deaths, and therefore was of unquestionable benefit to those communities. Public health officials were often poorly trained in public information technologies, and the community typically learned very little through their health centres about how they could obtain malaria treatment and which vector control tools would be applied. Communities were often not consulted beforehand about their own wishes or needs.

Much has changed since insecticide-treated bed nets were introduced globally (Nabarro 1999). Bed-net users needed to be instructed how to use the nets, and also how to care for their nets, with nets being especially needed for children under five years old. Public information campaigns were organized, which led to the awareness that involving the community in malaria control could be hugely beneficial. Also, the advent of the internet, mobile phones and other tools of communication have led to radical changes in the exchange of public health information. Indeed, community engagement has become one of the four pillars of the GVCR and no malaria intervention programme today can do without it (Mutero et al. 2015, Oria et al. 2015, Gowelo et al. 2020).

Future trends and prospects

Malaria is a pernicious disease that can only be managed by integrating several tools designed to kill the parasite in malaria patients, and by preventing new infections by interrupting the transmission of *Plasmodium* parasites. As the mosquito is responsible for malaria transmission (by biting twice!), mosquito control or elimination remains central to any programme of malaria prevention until a vaccine becomes available. As discussed, insecticide-impregnated bed nets and indoor residual spraying combined with good disease diagnostics and treatment are currently the best options for malaria control (WHO 2019). Great efforts are being made to develop malaria vaccines (Wilson et al. 2019), but until effective vaccines are widely available, our best options are to continue with efforts of mosquito control combined with proper disease management (Ashley et al. 2018). Rapidly advancing resistance against common malaria drugs is a serious cause for concern (Menard and Dondorp 2017, Uwimana et al. 2020), and illustrates the urgency of developing an effective vaccine.

The control of mosquito vectors remains a solid strategy for preventing malaria. The insecticide-based methods are considered a temporary solution, as the selective pressures caused by these insecticides on the target mosquito population will inevitably result in new forms of genetic or behavioural resistance (Hemingway 2018). It is now well accepted that Integrated Vector Management should be the leading strategy for controlling malaria vectors, and this strategy is emphasized in the Global Vector Control Response (WHO 2017). New in this programme is the emphasis on, firstly, community engagement, to obtain better support from the target communities and, secondly, monitoring and surveillance, to better understand the dynamics and extent of malaria disease and its mosquito vectors.

This chapter focuses on the mosquito vector, because of its central role in the transmission of malaria parasites. In the opinion of the author, it is unlikely that malaria vectors can be eliminated completely from a region or continent because of their high resilience against interventions. It should be realized that in all places where malaria has been successfully eliminated (Europe, North America), the mosquito vectors are still around. Malaria vectors were combatted to reach temporary low levels of population density so that the parasite reservoir could be more easily cleared with case management. Similarly, in many cases today, it is feasible to reduce mosquito populations to such low densities that the *Plasmodium* reservoir drops below a threshold and can be cleared from the human population. In such areas, "anophelism without malaria" (Aitken et al. 1954), can be the mainstay for many years, with active surveillance detecting the occasional and accidental malaria reintroduction. In most malaria-endemic areas, however, this total clearance of disease appears difficult, and the malaria control strategy should be aiming for low levels of transmission, possibly with known hotspots for targeted clearance, and adequate and effective public health teams for case management and health information.

By selecting the correct tools from the available toolbox, malaria can be controlled effectively. It is expected that further development of new tools may lead to more effective management and control of malaria, possibly leading to local elimination of the disease.

As this volume goes to press, the world has been deeply affected by the emergence and impact of COVID-19. The resources for dealing with this pandemic have had serious consequences for the control programmes of other infectious diseases, in particular the neglected tropical diseases such as malaria. Indeed, it was recently predicted that if malaria activities such as case management and distribution of Long-Lasting Insecticide Nets (LLINs) is halted, the malaria burden could more than double within one year (Sherrard-Smith et al. 2020). As these malaria prevention activities are highly dependent on the availability of scarce resources, this is one more reason to switch to a control programme that is based on the IVM principle, which is more sustainable and makes malaria-endemic countries less dependent on external resources.

Acknowledgements

I thank the stimulating discussions with Steve Lindsay and Ann Wilson, which have greatly contributed to the thoughts and opinions expressed in this chapter.

Note

1 Many readers will recognize the R0 from news about the COVID-19 pandemic; however, it is important to realize that in many malaria endemic areas, R0 is frequently greater than 5, which allows for a very rapid spread of the disease, and is proof of the difficulty faced by malaria control programmes, where R0 must be reduced to less than 1.

Bibliography

Adolfi, A., and G.J. Lycett. 2018. Opening the toolkit for genetic analysis and control of *Anopheles* mosquito vectors. *Current Opinion in Insect Science* 30: 8–18.

Afrane, Y.A., N.G. Mweresa, C.L. Wanjala, T.M. Gilbreath, G.F. Zhou, M.C. Lee, A.K. Githeko, and G.Y. Yan. 2016. Evaluation of long-lasting microbial larvicide for malaria vector control in Kenya. *Malaria Journal* 15: 577–577.

Aitken, T.H.G., J. Maier, and H. Trapido. 1954. The status of anophelism and Malaria in Sardinia during 1951 and 1952. *American Journal of Epidemiology* 60: 37–51.

Alonso, P.L., S.W. Lindsay, J.R. Armstrong, M. Conteh, A.G. Hill, P.H. David, G. Fegan, A. de Francisco, A.J. Hall, F.C. Shenton, et al. 1991. The effect of insecticide-treated bed nets on mortality of Gambian children. *Lancet* 337: 1499–1502.

Alonso, S., C.J. Chaccour, E. Elobolobo, A. Nacima, B. Candrinho, A. Saifodine, F. Saute, M. Robertson, and R. Zulliger. 2019. The economic burden of malaria on households and the health system in a high transmission district of Mozambique. *Malaria Journal* 18: 360. https://doi.org/10.1186/s12936-019-2995-4

Anderson, R.M., and R.M. May. 1992. *Infectious Diseases of Humans: Dynamics and Control*. Oxford: Oxford University Press.

Ashley, E.A., A. Pyae Phyo, and C.J. Woodrow. 2018. Malaria. *The Lancet* 391: 1608–1621.

Bhatt, S., D.J. Weiss, E. Cameron, D. Bisanzio, B. Mappin, U. Dalrymple, K.E. Battle, C.L. Moyes, A. Henry, P.A. Eckhoff, E.A. Wenger, O. Briet, M.A. Penny, T.A. Smith, A. Bennett, J. Yukich, T.P. Eisele, J.T. Griffin, C.A. Fergus, M. Lynch, F. Lindgren, J.M. Cohen, C.L.J. Murray, D.L. Smith, S.I. Hay, R.E. Cibulskis, and P.W. Gething. 2015. The effect of malaria control on *Plasmodium falciparum* in Africa between 2000 and 2015. *Nature* 526: 207–211.

Cator, L.J., B.J. Arthur, A. Ponlawat, and L.C. Harrington. 2011. Behavioral observations and sound recordings of free-flight mating swarms of *Ae. aegypti* (Diptera: Culicidae) in Thailand. *Journal of Medical Entomology* 48: 941–946.

Dambach, P., T. Baernighausen, I. Traore, S. Ouedraogo, A. Sie, R. Sauerborn, N. Becker, and V.R. Louis. 2019. Reduction of malaria vector mosquitoes in a large-scale intervention trial in rural Burkina Faso using *Bti* based larval source management. *Malaria Journal* 18: 311.

de Zulueta, J. 1998. The end of malaria in Europe: An eradication of the disease by control measures. *Parassitologia* 40: 245–246.

Dehne, E.J. 1955. Fifty years of malaria control in the panama area. *The American Journal of Tropical Medicine and Hygiene* 4: 800–811.

Eneh, L.K., H. Saijo, A.K. Borg-Karlson, J.M. Lindh, and G.K. Rajarao. 2016. Cedrol, a malaria mosquito oviposition attractant is produced by fungi isolated from rhizomes of the grass cyperus rotundus. *Malaria Journal* 15: 478. https://doi.org/10.1186/s12936-016-1536-7

Fillinger, U., B. Ndenga, A. Githeko, and S.W. Lindsay. 2009. Integrated malaria vector control with microbial larvicides and insecticide-treated nets in western Kenya: A controlled trial. *Bull World Health Organization* 87(9): 655–665.

Gleave, K., N. Lissenden, M. Richardson, L. Choi, and H. Ranson. 2018. Piperonyl butoxide (PBO) combined with pyrethroids in insecticide-treated nets to prevent malaria in Africa. *Cochrane Database of Systematic Reviews*, 11: CD012776.

Gowelo, S., R.S. McCann, C.J.M. Koenraadt, W. Takken, H. van den Berg, and L. Manda-Taylor. 2020. Community factors affecting participation in larval source management for malaria control in Chikwawa District, Southern Malawi. *Malaria Journal* 19: 195. https://doi.org/10.1186/s12936-020-03268-8

Hemingway, J. 2017. The way forward for vector control. *Science* 358: 998–999.

Hemingway, J. 2018. Resistance: A problem without an easy solution. *Pesticide Biochemistry and Physiology* 151: 73–75.

Hemingway, J., H. Ranson, A. Magill, J. Kolaczinski, C. Fornadel, J. Gimnig, M. Coetzee, F. Simard, D.K. Roch, C.K. Hinzoumbe, J. Pickett, D. Schellenberg, P. Gething, M. Hoppe, and N. Hamon. 2016. Averting a malaria disaster: Will insecticide resistance derail malaria control? *Lancet* 387: 1785–1788.

Hiscox, A., M.M. Njoroge, A.K. Mutai, B. Otieno, D. Masiga, J. van Loon, U. Fillinger, and W. Takken. 2019. Developing push-pull strategies for surveillance and control of malaria vectors. *Chemical Senses* 44: E23–E23.

Homan, T., A. Hiscox, C.K. Mweresa, D. Masiga, W.R. Mukabana, P. Oria, N. Maire, A.D. Pasquale, M. Silkey, J. Alaii, T. Bousema, C. Leeuwis, T.A. Smith, and W. Takken. 2016. The effect of mass mosquito trapping on malaria transmission and disease burden (SolarMal): A stepped-wedge cluster-randomised trial. *The Lancet*, 388 (10050): 1193–1201.

James, S., F.H. Collins, P.A. Welkhoff, C. Emerson, H.C.J. Godfray, M. Gottlieb, B. Greenwood, S.W. Lindsay, C.M. Mbogo, F.O. Okumu, H. Quemada, M. Savadogo, J.A. Singh, K.H. Tountas, and Y.T. Toure. 2018. Pathway to deployment of gene drive mosquitoes as a potential biocontrol tool for elimination of malaria in sub-saharan Africa: Recommendations of a scientific working group. *American Journal of Tropical Medicine and Hygiene* 98: 1–49.

Killeen, G.F. 2020. Control of malaria vectors and management of insecticide resistance through universal coverage with next-generation insecticide-treated nets. *The Lancet* 395: 1394–1400.

Killeen, G.F., U. Fillinger, I. Kiche, L.C. Gouagna, and B.G. Knols. 2002. Eradication of *Anopheles gambiae* from Brazil: Lessons for malaria control in Africa? *Lancet Infect Dis* 2: 618–627.

Kirby, M.J., D. Ameh, C. Bottomley, C. Green, M. Jawara, P.J. Milligan, P.C. Snell, D.J. Conway, and S.W. Lindsay. 2009. Effect of two different house screening interventions on exposure to malaria vectors and on anaemia in children in The Gambia: A randomised controlled trial. *Lancet* 374: 998–1009.

Knapp, J., M. Macdonald, D. Malone, N. Hamon, and J.H. Richardson. 2015. Disruptive technology for vector control: The innovative vector control consortium and the US military join forces to explore transformative insecticide application technology for mosquito control programmes. *Malaria Journal* 14: 371–371.

Lindh, J.M., M.N. Okal, M. Herrera-Varela, A.-K. Borg-Karlson, B. Torto, S.W. Lindsay, and U. Fillinger. 2015. Discovery of an oviposition attractant for gravid malaria vectors of the *Anopheles gambiae* species complex. *Malaria Journal* 14: 119.

Lindsay, S.W., P.L. Alonso, J.R. Armstrong Schellenberg, J. Hemingway, J.H. Adiamah, F.C. Shenton, M. Jawara, and B.M. Greenwood. 1993. A malaria control trial using insecticide-treated bed nets and targeted chemoprophylaxis in a rural area of the Gambia, west Africa. 7. Impact of permethrin-impregnated bed nets on malaria vectors. *Transactions of the Royal Society Tropical Medicine and Hygiene* 87 Suppl 2: 45–51.

Lindsay, S.W., P.M. Emerson, and J.D. Charlwood. 2002. Reducing malaria by mosquito-proofing houses. *TRENDS in Parasitology* 18: 510–514.

Liu, W.H., K. Xin, C.Z. Chao, S.Z. Feng, L. Yan, R.Z. He, Z.H. Zhang, G. Gibson, and W.M. Kang. 2004. New irrigation methods sustain malaria control in sichuan province, China. *Acta Tropica* 89: 241–247.

MacDonald, G. 1957. *The Epidemiology and Control of Malaria*. London: Oxford University Press,.

Mburu, M.M., M. Juurlink, J. Spitzen, P. Moraga, A. Hiscox, T. Mzilahowa, W. Takken, and R.S. McCann. 2018. Impact of partially and fully closed eaves on house entry rates by mosquitoes. *Parasites & Vectors* 11: 383. https://doi.org/10.1186/s13071-01 8-2977-3

Menard, D., and A. Dondorp. 2017. Antimalarial drug resistance: A threat to Malaria elimination. *Cold Spring Harbor Perspectives in Medicine* 7(7): a025619.

Menger, D.J., P. Omusula, M. Holdinga, T. Homan, A.S. Carreira, P. Vandendaele, J.L. Derycke, C.K. Mweresa, W.R. Mukabana, J.J.A. Van Loon, and W. Takken. 2015. Field evaluation of a push-pull system to reduce malaria transmission. *PLoS ONE* 10(4): e0123415. https://doi.org/10.1371/journal.pone.0123415

Mmbando, A.S., E.P.A. Batista, M. Kilalangongono, M.F. Finda, E.P. Mwanga, E.W. Kaindoa, K. Kifungo, R.M. Njalambaha, H.S. Ngowo, A.E. Eiras, and F.O. Okumu. 2019. Evaluation of a push-pull system consisting of transfluthrin-treated eave ribbons and odour-baited traps for control of indoor- and outdoor-biting malaria vectors. *Malaria Journal* 18: 87. https://doi.org/10.1186/s12936-019-2714-1

Mutero, C.M., C. Mbogo, J. Mwangangi, S. Imbahale, L. Kibe, B. Orindi, M. Girma, A. Njui, W. Lwande, H. Affognon, C. Gichuki, and W.R. Mukabana. 2015. An assessment of participatory integrated vector management for malaria control in Kenya. *Environmental Health Perspectives* 123: 1145–1151.

Nabarro, D. 1999. Roll back Malaria. *Parassitologia* 41: 501–504.

Oria, P.A., C. Leeuwis, A. Hiscox, D. Masiga, W. Takken, and J. Alaii. 2015. Malaria control with solar-powered mosquito trapping systems: Socio-economic and perceived health outcomes of house lighting in Rusinga Island, Western Kenya. *American Journal of Tropical Medicine and Hygiene* 93: 115–115.

Ranson, H., and N. Lissenden. 2016. Insecticide resistance in African *Anopheles* mosquitoes: A worsening situation that needs urgent action to maintain Malaria control. *Trends in Parasitology* 32: 187–196.

Rocco, F. 2003. *The Miraculous Fever-Tree: Malaria and the Quest for a Cure That Changed the World,* 1st ed. New York: Harper Collins.

Ross, R. 1900. The relationship of Malaria and the mosquito. *The Lancet* 156: 48–50.

Ross, R. 1910. *The Prevention of Malaria*. London: Murray.

Sachs, J., and P. Malaney. 2002. The economic and social burden of malaria. *Nature* 415: 680–685.

Sarma, N., E. Patouillard, R.E. Cibulskis, and J.L. Arcand. 2019. The economic burden of Malaria: Revisiting the evidence. *American Journal of Tropical Medicine and Hygiene* 101: 1405–1415.

Schoelitsz, B., V. Mwingira, L.E.G. Mboera, H. Beijleveld, C.J.M. Koenraadt, J. Spitzen, J.J.A. van Loon, and W. Takken. 2020. Chemical mediation of oviposition by *Anopheles* mosquitoes: A push-pull system driven by volatiles associated with larval stages. *Journal of Chemical Ecology* 46: 397–409.

Sherrard-Smith, E., A.B. Hogan, A. Hamlet, O.J. Watson, C. Whittaker, P. Winskill, F. Ali, A.B. Mohammad, P. Uhomoibhi, I. Maikore, N. Ogbulafor, J. Nikau, M.D. Kont, J.D. Challenger, R. Verity, B. Lambert, M. Cairns, B. Rao, M. Baguelin, L.K. Whittles, J.A. Lees, S. Bhatia, E.S. Knock, L. Okell, H.C. Slater, A.C. Ghani, P.G.T. Walker, O.O. Okoko, and T.S. Churcher. 2020. The potential public health consequences of COVID-19 on malaria in Africa. *Nature Medicine* 26: 1411–1416.

Shretta, R., A.L.V. Avancena, and A. Hatefi. 2016. The economics of malaria control and elimination: A systematic review. *Malaria Journal* 15: 593. https://doi.org/10.1186/s12936-016-1635-5

Syafruddin, D., P.B.S. Asih, I.E. Rozi, D.H. Permana, A.P. Nur Hidayati, L. Syahrani, S. Zubaidah, D. Sidik, M.J. Bangs, C. Bøgh, F. Liu, E.C. Eugenio, J. Hendrickson, T. Burton, J.K. Baird, F. Collins, J.P. Grieco, N.F. Lobo, and N.L. Achee. 2020. Efficacy of a Spatial repellent for control of Malaria in Indonesia: A cluster-randomized controlled trial. *The American Journal of Tropical Medicine and Hygiene* 103: 344–358.

Takken, W., and B.G.J. Knols. 1999. Odor-mediated behavior of *Afrotropical* malaria mosquitoes. *Annual Review of Entomology* 44: 131–157.

Takken, W., W.B. Snellen, J.P. Verhave, B.G.J. Knols, and S. Atmosoedjono. 1990. *Environmental Measures for Malaria Control in Indonesia. A Historical Review on Species Sanitation*. Wageningen: Agricultural University.

Traore, M.M., A. Junnila, S.F. Traore, S. Doumbia, E.E. Revay, V.D. Kravchenko, Y. Schlein, K.L. Arheart, P. Gergely, R.D. Xue, A. Hausmann, R. Beck, A. Prozorov, R.A. Diarra, A.S. Kone, S. Majambere, J. Bradley, J. Vontas, J.C. Beier, and G.C. Muller. 2020. Large-scale field trial of attractive toxic sugar baits (ATSB) for the control of malaria vector mosquitoes in Mali, West Africa. *Malaria Journal* 19 (72): 2324. https://doi.org/10.1186/s12936-020-3132-0

Tusting, L.S., C. Bottomley, H. Gibson, I. Kleinschmidt, A.J. Tatem, S.W. Lindsay, and P.W. Gething. 2017. Housing improvements and Malaria risk in sub-saharan Africa: A multi-country analysis of survey data. *Plos Medicine* 14 (2): e1002234. https://doi.org/10.1371/journal.pmed.1002234

Tusting, L.S., J. Thwing, D. Sinclair, U. Fillinger, J. Gimnig, K.E. Bonner, C. Bottomley, and S.W. Lindsay. 2013. Mosquito larval source management for controlling malaria. *Cochrane Database System Review* 8: CD008923. doi: 10.1002/14651858.CD008923. pub2

Uwimana, A., E. Legrand, B.H. Stokes, J.-L.M. Ndikumana, M. Warsame, N. Umulisa, D. Ngamije, T. Munyaneza, J.-B. Mazarati, K. Munguti, P. Campagne, A. Criscuolo, F. Ariey, M. Murindahabi, P. Ringwald, D.A. Fidock, A. Mbituyumuremyi, and D. Menard. 2020. Emergence and clonal expansion of in vitro artemisinin-resistant plasmodium falciparum kelch13 R561H mutant parasites in Rwanda. *Nature Medicine,* 26: 1602–1608.

van den Berg, H., M. van Vugt, A.N. Kabaghe, M. Nkalapa, R. Kaotcha, Z. Truwah, T. Malenga, A. Kadama, S. Banda, T. Tizifa, S. Gowelo, M.M. Mburu, K.S. Phiri, W. Takken, and R.S. McCann. 2018. Community-based malaria control in southern Malawi: A description of experimental interventions of community workshops, house improvement and larval source management. *Malaria Journal* 17: 266. https://doi.org/10.1186/s12936-018-2415-1

Warrell, D.A., and H.M. Gilles. 2002. *Bruce-Chwatt's Essential Malariology*, 4th ed. Boca Raton, FL: CRC Press.

Watson, M. 1921. *The Prevention of Malaria in the Fedreated Malay States*, 2nd ed. London: John Murray.

Webb, James L.A., Jr. 2009. *Humanity's Burden: A Global History of Malaria*. New York: Cambridge University Press.

White, N.J., S. Pukrittayakamee, T.T. Hien, M.A. Faiz, O.A. Mokuolu, and A.M. Dondorp. 2014. Malaria. *Lancet* 383: 723–735.

Wilson, A.L., O. Courtenay, L.A. Kelly-Hope, T.W. Scott, W. Takken, S.J. Torr, and S.W. Lindsay. 2020. The importance of vector control for the control and elimination of vector-borne diseases. *PLoS Neglected Tropical Diseases* 14: e0007831.

Wilson, K.L., K.L. Flanagan, M.D. Prakash, and M. Plebanski. 2019. Malaria vaccines in the eradication era: Current status and future perspectives. *Expert Review of Vaccines* 18: 133–151.

Wooding, M., Y. Naude, E. Rohwer, and M. Bouwer. 2020. Controlling mosquitoes with semiochemicals: A review. *Parasites & Vectors* 13: 80. https://doi.org/10.1186/s13071-020-3960-3

Word Health Organization. 2005. *The Roll Back Malaria Programme*. Geneva, p. 52.

Word Health Organization. 2017. *Global Vector Control Response 2017–2030*. W. H. Organization [ed.]. Geneva, p. 53.

Word Health Organization. 2019. *World Malaria Report 2019*. Geneva, p. 232.

Yang, G.G., D. Kim, A. Pham, and C.J. Paul. 2018. A meta-regression analysis of the effectiveness of mosquito nets for Malaria control: The value of long-lasting insecticide nets. *International Journal of Environmental Research and Public Health* 15: 546–546.

9

LIVING WITH MOSQUITOES IN DISEASE-FREE CONTEXTS

Attitudes and perceptions of risk in English wetlands

Adriana Ford, Mary Gearey and Tim G. Acott

Mosquitoes are amongst a small coterie of insects whose mention within general conversation provokes an instant reaction. Joining ticks, horseflies and midges, mosquitoes conjure in the mind a time, a place, of interaction. Human and mosquito lives are entwined. Most people can recollect mosquito encounters—of high-pitched whines that prevent sleep, of walking through swarms on a summer's evening, of inflamed bites scratched until they bleed. Mosquitoes are intrinsic to what cultural cartographer Rebecca Solnit (2010) describes as the "living maps" of our perambulations through our lives and through places; an unbidden fellow traveller whose companionship we never quite manage to shake off, and whose presence appears at the most intimate of times.

Humans and wetlands have been interconnected across time, deep time. Though deep time is a contentious term (Irvine 2014), we can say that over the millennia, humanity's dependence on wetlands for all aspects of survival is non-contestable (Schmidt 2017). This is true even now, as wetlands across the globe provide a range of ecosystem services which humans depend on, including food provisioning in forms as diverse as agro-industrial rice production, cranberry harvesting, subsistence fishing, foraging and wildfowling. Human development is closely linked with wetland environments, and this in turn has meant that humans have sought to live alongside fellow wetland species—including mosquitoes.

This interspecies co-mingling as espoused by Haraway (2007) has not necessarily prompted empathy with other forms of being. The progression towards settled farming practices, from the Neolithic onwards, resculpted landscapes anthropomorphically. Cleared forests, for example, have become over time the sites of our present-day peatlands (Gearey et al. 2000). This is evident more clearly in the ways in which wetland ecosystems have been adapted by humans over time, particularly in the Global North, where draining wetlands to extend agricultural land becomes, over time, closely tied with nation-building and forms

DOI: 10.4324/9781003056034-9

of political economy (Gearey et al. 2020) and, by extension, colonialist projects of empire building (Howell 2018). This encroachment of human activity upon and within wetlands disrupted and altered human–mosquito relationships. Social historians (Watts 2006, Cohen 1983) cite the development of drainage channels as part of wetland co-option into agricultural artefacts as the driver of increased incidences of malaria. These drainage channels provide emergent breeding grounds for mosquitoes. More intensive forms of agriculture bring humans and mosquitoes into closer proximity to enable vector transmission of the disease.

Malaria, once known as ague, was endemic in Britain from the fifteenth century and was often associated with wetland areas as "marsh fevers," attributed to "the noxious vapours of stagnant marshes" (Dobson 1989: 3). In the first half of the twentieth century, prominent scientists at the British Mosquito Control Institute on Hayling Island, just off the south coast of England in Hampshire, facilitated research and shaped public consciousness around the "gravity of the menace" of the British mosquito (Hogarth 1928, Coates, this volume). However, with indigenous malaria eradicated in the UK in the mid-twentieth century, local British attention to mosquitoes declined. Yet in the twenty-first century, with increasing global temperatures facilitating the spread of mosquitoes and mosquito-borne diseases in other parts of Europe (Semenza and Suk 2018), combined with tabloid headlines designed to provoke fear and panic—"Horror as plague of killer mosquitos are headed to Britain as fears ramp up over insects"—mosquitoes, and their breeding grounds, may once again be viewed with anxiety (Hudson 2019, also see Swain 2012, *Daily Mail* 2019). Mosquitoes in Britain, of which there are 36 recorded native species, are monitored by public health authorities such as Public Health England (e.g. Vaux and Medlock 2015, Public Health England 2017) and local district councils (see Dover District Council 2020). Most of the native species in Britain do not transmit diseases, but some species have transmission capability (e.g. West Nile virus by Culex mosquitoes, and dengue and chikungunya by the invasive species *Aedes albopictus*). However, little is known about the perceptions towards mosquitoes in countries such as the UK, where mosquito-borne diseases are only a possible risk and not yet (or no longer) a reality. Are mosquitoes on people's consciousness as a native pest and cause for concern, or do people live in relative harmony alongside them? Might perceptions towards mosquitoes affect wetland management, restoration and creation, or are they inconsequential when viewed alongside the multiple values, or perhaps other risks or challenges, associated with wetlands?

Within a broader exploration of the values of English wetlands and the management of mosquitoes in the interdisciplinary WetlandLIFE project, an initiative of the Valuing Nature Programme of the UK Research Councils, we relied upon the Community Voice Method (CVM) for filming interviews and making documentaries (Ranger et al. 2016), focusing especially on human experiences and perceptions of mosquitoes. Fifty-six wetland users at three sites of different English wetland typologies (Somerset Levels, Bedford urban wetland parks and the Alkborough Flats), provided a snapshot into experiences and perceptions of these notorious insects in a very local context [see Box 9.1 and Figure 9.1].

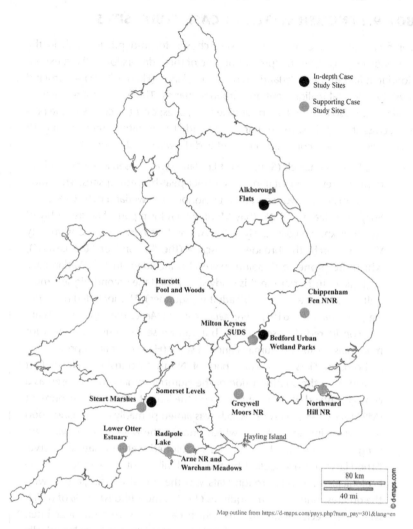

In-depth Case
Study Sites

Supporting Case
Study Sites

Alkborough
Flats

Hurcott
Pool and Woods

Chippenham
Fen NNR

Milton Keynes
SUDS

Bedford Urban
Wetland Parks

Somerset Levels

Steart Marshes

Greywell
Moors NR

Northward
Hill NR

Lower Otter
Estuary

Radipole
Lake

Hayling Island

Arne NR and
Wareham Meadows

80 km

40 mi

Map outline from https://d-maps.com/pays.php?num_pay=301&lang=en

FIGURE 9.1 WetlandLIFE case study sites. Courtesy of WetlandLIFE, UK.

The interviews of farmers, reserve managers, volunteers, walkers, bird-watchers, and other recreational wetland users and local residents, conducted throughout 2018, were designed to capture people's relationships with their local wetland environments, to interrogate the ways in which their sense of place and attendant health and well-being practices are produced and articulated within these spaces, and to suggest implications these have for wetland management. In this chapter, we present our findings from the mosquito-related dialogue, a deliberate line of exploration, which helps us to understand how people experience living with mosquitoes in disease-free contexts such as the UK. Some of these views are also captured in a short film, *Mosquito & Me – a narrative on mosquitoes in English wetlands in 2018* (Ford, 2019b).

BOX 9.1 ENGLISH WETLAND CASE STUDY SITES

Three case study sites in England were chosen for in-depth research in the WetlandLIFE project, each representing one of three drivers for wetland expansion identified in the "Wetland Vision for England" (Hulme 2008) – farmland reversion, coastal realignment and urban wetlands. The ecological research in WetlandLIFE also included a further nine study sites; over the course of the project across the 12 sites, more than 39,000 adult mosquitoes, representing 19 British species, were collected and identified (Hawkes et al. in prep).

· The Somerset Levels (South West England) was chosen as an example of farmland reversion wetlands, as former peat-harvesting sites. The study site consisted of two separate but neighbouring wetland nature reserves, Shapwick Heath and Westhay Moor, which form part of an assembly of wetlands known collectively as the Avalon Marshes. For the Community Voice research, the broader landscape (the "moors" or "the Levels"), which are prone to flooding, were also included. In the WetlandLIFE ecological study, traps in this study site yielded the second-highest mosquito abundance (over 9,000 adult mosquitoes). This included nine species, the majority (81%) were *Aedes cantans/Aedes annulipes*, which are not considered disease vectors, but can be serious nuisance-biters for mammals, including humans and livestock (Hawkes et al. in prep).

· Alkborough Flats, in a rural part of North Lincolnshire (North East England) on the southern side of the Humber Estuary, was chosen as a coastal wetland. It is the site of one of the largest managed realignment (MRA) schemes in Europe, which was aimed primarily at reducing flood risk further inland. The site, which prior to the MRA scheme was low-lying agricultural land, is now an established wetland nature reserve. "The Flats" are overlooked by the small village of Alkborough. In the ecological study, Alkborough Flats was the site of the single trap with the greatest number of mosquitoes (11,228 mosquitoes), 92% of which were the species *Aedes caspius*, which can be a severe nuisance-biter. *Anopheles claviger*, a recognized malaria vector (although not historically in Britain), was also present (Hawkes et al. in prep).

· Two country parks with wetland habitats, located close to Bedford town centre (East of England), were chosen as the location of urban wetland research. There are few natural lakes in Bedfordshire and both the study sites—Priory Country Park and Millennium Country Park—were created from the former sites of industrial extraction of gravel and clay. Both parks are managed for recreation, wildlife conservation, environmental education and community participation, as well as cultural and heritage value, and have high visitation. In the ecological study, the Bedford sites had the greatest species richness, with 13 species present, but yielded moderate to low numbers of adult mosquitoes (Hawkes et al. in prep).

This following section explores what Mick Smith (2013) has described as the relevance of post-humanist perspectives for uncovering the myriad ways that humans and the-more-than-human collaborate together. These often low-visibility "ecological communities" provide ways to counter dominant extinction narratives that view certain life forms as a pest and possibly a threat to human health. One can consider the ways in which scientific funding has been provided to try to eradicate those insects and animals seen as threats: termites, tsetse flies and tape worms amongst others. Yet removing these creatures entirely from the "web of life" (Moore 2015) may have untold long-term consequences for food chains and ecosystems. In other words "staying with the trouble," to reiterate Haraway (2016), enables us to recognize that other forms of "being together" may enable alternative sustainable futures. When we consider mosquitoes as potential disease vectors, understanding how they are currently valued and factored into wetland ecosystems may help us all manage change in the future. To understand mosquitoes as the "enemy" is to view ourselves within a framing in which nature is a battlefield and humans are the conquerors. Posthumanism, by contrast, seeks to recognize the fundamental connectivity of humans within nature, and that our animal selves have always been connected in relationships of kinship both with other animals and attendant environments. Malone (2019: 107) has described this connectivity as, "a recognition that we are animal, we are nature, and we carry the ghostly tracings of our shared past."

Human–mosquito interactions: interrogating the lived experiences of interspecies co-mingling

Whilst ecological surveillance provides information on the status, distribution and abundance of endemic mosquitoes, and identifies occurrences of invasive species (Public Health England 2017), an analysis of the "lived experience" of human–mosquito interactions, derived from the social sciences, provides insight into what the presence of mosquitoes means to people. The experiences, or encounters, people have with mosquitoes may influence their attitudes towards perceived risks, and so possibly towards the habitats with which they are associated, such as wetlands, and how these habitats should be used or managed. As a baseline for understanding how people are living with mosquitoes, one thus needs knowledge of people's experiences with mosquitoes. Do they see mosquitoes? Do they get bitten by them or experience other types of interactions with them? Have such interactions changed over time?

As anticipated when considering various wetland sites, we found the extent and frequency of human–mosquito interactions varied considerably across the sites, individuals and time. In many cases, human–mosquito interactions were not experienced at all in their local wetlands—mosquitoes were neither seen, nor felt—particularly at the urban sites in Bedford. Some respondents said they had never even thought about mosquitoes in the context of their local wetland site, until participating in this study (we made clear that the sites were not chosen because there is an exceptional mosquito problem!). Often though, mosquitoes were noticeably present, seen visibly (although people can mistake other insects for mosquitoes)—sometimes just one or two, sometimes in swarms, and usually in the summer months—and of course, sometimes the mosquitoes were felt. And it was not just the human–mosquito interactions that were relevant; farmers reported bothersome swarms, and biting, by mosquitoes, of their horses and livestock.

Perception of change may influence perception of future risk; thus, if mosquito presence appears to be increasing, that may create or add to fears for the future. We had no preconception about whether there may have been more, less or the same current density of mosquitoes compared to the past in our study sites, and most of our respondents could not identify or recollect any patterns or changes in mosquito presence and density over time. There were some exceptions though; for example an ornithologist in Bedford noted that "they've declined quite a lot; there were quite big swarms of them 20 years ago ... which they're not now; it's just the occasional one or two in comparison to what they used to be" (Int. B10), and in Somerset a farmer noted: "I think we are so close to open water and over the years, the 20 years that we've been here, living as a couple here with our family, I would say that it has progressively, year on year, got worse" (Int. S2). Some participants of the Alkborough site emphasized that they had not seen a "before and after" change in mosquitoes since the creation of the wetlands, although one farmer perceived there to be more of them, and more vicious:

> There are more. There are more. And I don't know whether it's just because there are more, but they seem to be hungrier. If you're down there on the wrong sort of day, it's bad, and also the cows suffer far more with flies than they did in the past. But it's not an insurmountable problem.
>
> *(Int. A8)*

These apparently inconsistent claims about mosquito numbers may seem perplexing. One explanation is that mosquitoes can be misidentified, giving rise to a perception of change that is not actually occurring. Another possibility is that even at the same study site, there are diverse habitats and ways of interacting with the wetlands that vary by location, time of day or duration. The heterogeneity of mosquito habitats, and therefore their populations, can create very localized experiences. Another explanation may lie in the context within which insects, and particularly mosquitoes, are viewed in individual cultural contexts. Attitudes and perceptions of risk are both culturally coded and heuristically shaped. The ways in which we frame our "sense of place" is a two-way dynamic between our lived experiences and the wider "meta-narratives" of the contemporary social representations we are embedded within, and then communicated through various forms of epistemological knowledge dissemination, whether pedagogical, scientific, legal, medical or cultural. Articulations of mosquito encounters, and perceptions of risk, then become something much more; they become articulations of a sense of place, and of the actors' own understanding of their contribution to world-making. As we explore in the sections below, understanding these often contrary articulations of perceptions of mosquitoes within English wetlands may be less about differences in species and habitat across the wetland sites, and more about which actors share sensibilities around their own senses of place within natural settings.

To explore sensitivities to place and to the mosquitoes that inhabit them, the next section reports on the ways in which study participants articulated their experiences with mosquitoes. Even if some of the participants did not encounter mosquitoes in their local wetlands, one can learn from those who do, allowing us to identify three types of impacts associated with mosquitoes: health impacts, the nuisance factor and behavioural adaptions.

Health impacts

As mosquitoes in the UK no longer transmit diseases to people, their effects on human health is virtually absent when compared to countries that are rife with mosquito-borne diseases. The only negative effects of mosquitoes in the UK stem from their bites. Many of our participants had observed that some individuals are more susceptible, and react more severely, to a mosquito bite, even if most agreed that a mosquito bite was a trifling occurrence. There were some exceptions to this generalization, the most notable being in Somerset, where a couple with children on a small farm located near a wetland environment complained about vicious mosquitoes. There, mosquitoes have led to skin reactions in one child who required medical treatment:

> One of them, from a very young age, whenever she was bitten, she has eczema as well, and it just would exacerbate her eczema, and then she would end up with very bad skin infections which most summers would result in two or three courses of antibiotics. We're just finding now that her skin problems are still continuing, even though she's at an age when really she should be growing out of it, so that's requiring some more significant treatment now.
>
> *(Int. S2)*

Another farmer at Somerset reiterated the severe reaction one might get from a mosquito bite: "my whole hand swelled up didn't it, for about three or four days. I couldn't do anything with it" (Int. S17). In the Alkborough site, one participant living just above the Flats shared an even more serious story of biting mosquitoes, albeit from 20 years ago:

> There's been rare mosquitos, when I lived in [the neighbouring village] Walcot we all got bit one year and we had terrible reactions that sort of hospitalized

a lot of my friends. It was my 18th party, and they all got bit and they swelled up really, really badly. Some had to go to A&E, some just went to the doctor's and got a prescription. Okay it was 20 years ago, but there was a really … they said there was a really bad batch so to speak that people had reacted.

(Int. A6)

Whilst other parts of Europe have seen a number of incidences of mosquito-borne diseases that adversely affect human health (Semenza and Suk 2018), there has not been a reported case of a mosquito disease infection in the UK for decades. However, tick-borne Lyme disease is a recognized growing health concern, debilitating its human host in episodic cycles over many years, serving to diminish the concern over mosquitoes. The arthropodal enemy has apparently shifted. Mosquito bites in the UK, even severe reactions to them, pale in comparison with the threats carried by ticks, which lurk in grasses and attach to our skin with neither whine nor flight to alert us to their presence. Returning once again to Smith (2013), one must also consider the web of life's connectivity to the tick's survival, which like the mosquito, depends on the blood of a host mammal or bird to provide the sustenance for its reproductive cycle. This connects us again to the ecological community in which humans are enmeshed with other species. A mosquito may be less enemy than co-respondent; to live alongside one another may be to accept how each affects the other's well-being.

The nuisance factor

Although mosquitoes may be perceived as an irritant in the UK rather than something to be immediately feared, they are still considered a nuisance by many of the respondents, and perhaps a blight to long English summers. Negative human–mosquito interactions are easy to recall particularly by marring the "rural idyll." Here, human contentment rests with a natural setting, prompting an idea of a wholesomeness and sense of well-being that can only be gained in nature—even if this is illusory. Mosquitoes, along with such sensory irritants as smelly slurry pits and obstructive electricity pylons, disrupt our imaginative framing of what the countryside should look like and what we, as humans, should experience. All of the disruptors can be classed as "nuisance factors."

Even so, many participants reported that mosquitoes are not something they have thought much about in a UK or local context. They gauge local mosquitoes in comparison with other places where they have perceived a far worse experience, particularly Scotland's west coast or tropical countries. Another internal gauge is their comparison of mosquitoes with more problematic creatures—particularly midges, and horseflies—who may combine forces to disrupt a paradisiacal weekend retreat. One respondent volunteered that:

Our worst experience of, I don't know about mosquitoes, is the West Coast of Scotland, isn't it? The midges and stuff like that, and there are a few months in the year where I feel that we shouldn't visit our relatives because you just get bitten to death, in fact you can come home and you're sort of red. In Lincolnshire, the worst thing is you're in a wooded area, you get horse flies and stuff don't you?

(Int A1)

Another participant noted more graphically that in Scotland, "the mosquitoes come attached with chainsaws" (Int. S11) (Figure 9.2 and 9.3).

The irritation and annoyance effected by mosquitoes, though not universal amongst respondents, commonly elicited such terms such as "hate" and "death." Yet, as will be discussed further, these negative reactions place mosquitoes as free agents who loom large in the imagination as foraging biters. The role of humans in creating mosquito-friendly habitats was rarely mentioned in conversations: nature as salve and nature as irritant reveals our complex positionality with our other-than-human brethren. Wickson (2010) sums up a positivist approach to human relationships with nature, declaring "Mosquitoes: just how much bio-diversity does humanity need?" Whilst humans may remain centre stage as administrators of life on the planet, there is less likely to be simple acceptance of

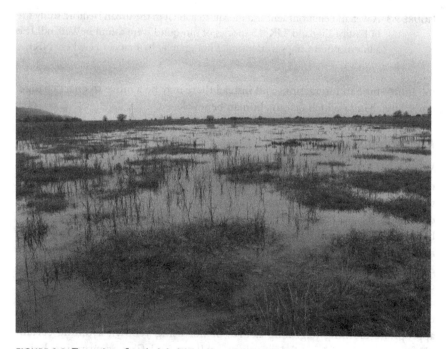

FIGURE 9.2 Estuarine flooded habitat for the *Aedes caspius* mosquito (an aggressive human biter) at Alkborough Flats, a managed realignment site in North Lincolnshire, UK. Photography by Frances Hawkes/ NRI.

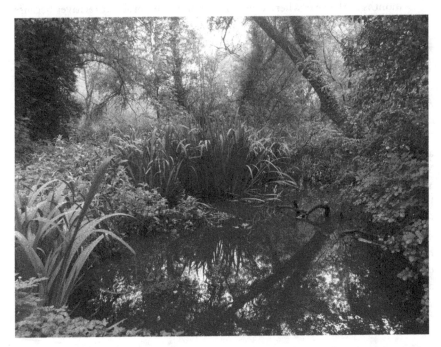

FIGURE 9.3 A wetland environment and mosquito habitat in the urban Bedford study site in East of England, UK; 13 species of mosquito were found in WetlandLIFE adult mosquito traps in Bedford. Photography by Frances Hawkes/ NRI.

mosquito–human interactions and instead there may be a move to enact change, especially change which favours human benevolence.

Behavioural adaptations

Where mosquitoes are present and a nuisance, there are three main approaches to dealing with them: ignoring them; managing their habitat and directly controlling them; or adapting one's behaviour accordingly. The last two methods, of course, are not mutually exclusive, but from the individual's perspective, behavioural adaptations are more controllable than influencing a mosquito management plan. Adaptations are dependent on the need and based on the extent or expectation of the problem, along with the ability and willingness to change. Many of our participants did not experience any mosquito interactions at all, and so required no adaptations; but for those who did notice mosquitoes, they reported taking many of the typical precautions. This included wearing appropriate clothing (e.g. long sleeves or not using yellow), avoiding certain places at certain times of day, using repellents and fires, consuming brewer's yeast (for purportedly altering the taste of blood), and even, closing one's mouth to avoid accidentally ingesting them! One extreme adaptation, given its association with more tropical environments, was draping bed nets, which was taken up by the family in Somerset referred to earlier:

> Two of my younger sisters, they [the mosquitoes] just seem to really like them; they have to sleep under mosquito nets because it's that bad some of the time, there is a lot of them down here.
>
> *(Int. S2)*

People's willingness and ability to adapt their behaviours are a vital part of learning to live with mosquitoes, and in so doing, minimizing the loss of value from the wetland environment—either by not enjoying it, or not being able to carry out such typical activities as bird-watching, strolling, farming, etc.

For our participants whose work or leisure time involved long motionless periods in the wetlands, including bat surveyors, ornithologists and wildlife photographers whose patience is repaid with an intimate knowledge of the flora and fauna or animal cosmologies, adapting to attendant mosquito environments is a pragmatic choice for using these spaces. Risk plays less of a role here than general comfort, and behavioural adaptations become a routine response to wetland conditions. These practices are sometimes multifunctional: insect repellent combined with sunscreen; longer sleeves to shield from sun and bug or the repellent actions of nettles and brambles; hats to prevent glare when peering through binoculars or camera lenses. The mosquitoes' inclusion in the matrix of wetlands means that preparations for visiting these areas become a ritual that adds to a person's sense of place: the insect repellent joins the thermos, the walking pole, the rucksack and the journal with pens. These moments of preparation attend to Shamai's (1991: 348) exploration of a sense of place as a processive collective that combines the recalled, the imagined and the actual: "A place is never merely an object, but part of a larger whole that is being felt through the "actual" experience of meaningful events." In this respect, the anticipation of a mosquito encounter is an accepted aspect of immersion into that space, even (or perhaps, especially) if the respondent finds it onerous or challenging. As Shamai explains,

> the definition of a sense of place is: feelings, attitudes, and behaviour toward a place which varies from person to person, and from one scale to another (e.g. from home to country). Sense of place consists of knowledge, belonging, attachment, and commitment to a place or part of it.
>
> *(Shamai 1991: 354)*

It is this "commitment" to a particular place that comes through clearly in our fieldwork. Our respondents' lives are embedded within these wetlands through their own volition. The attendant discomforts and "risks" of working within, living alongside, or utilizing these wetlands are connected with each person's own criteria for the negative and positive aspects of these sites, with mosquitoes occupying a shifting cost–benefit analysis as just one of many factors that must be contemplated. We realize then that human–mosquito interactions are embedded within wider personal ontologies of being-in-the-world; our perceptions are shaped both by expectation, constructed through cultural representations and social norms, and by experiencing phenomena which either support or run counter to these expectations. The Heideggerian encounter of "being-in-the-world" is simultaneously lived phenomena and part imagination and interpretation (Zahorik and Jenison 1998).

Friend or foe? Perceptions of mosquitoes

We have focused so far on the "lived experience" with the mosquito, the interactions people have with this insect and how they respond to these encounters. Yet, people's ability or willingness to live alongside mosquitoes also depends on their broader views, their interests and values, and their wider experience and understanding of mosquitoes in the world (Gearey et al. 2020). We must also recognize the importance of companionship or empathy that humans find with other animals, the "more-than-human", as an essential component of being human, and of making sense of the world. As Carol Smart suggests (2011: 36):

> The field of human-animal interactions alerts us … to be attentive to non-verbal communications and (to) forms of interaction not underscored by talk. It is a sensory world and as such is also part of everyday life.

Such sensorial experiences of a closeness with the animal world (see Ford 2019a) have been described in post-humanist philosophy as "the animal turn." Here, the hierarchy between humans and animals is flattened, focusing instead on interconnectivity and a web of life (Moore 2015) that depends on codependency. Specifically, we sought to reveal people's attitudes towards mosquitoes, linking them with broader experiences, and asking specifically whether they could be "friend" or always "foe."

Friend

Mosquitoes are normally dominated by negative connotations, as a nuisance and as killers. But from the perspective of many of the people we interviewed, "Could we or should we eliminate mosquitoes?" is a question that does not concern them since they simply do not experience mosquito interactions in their local wetlands. For those who do notice mosquitoes, they consider them mostly as nuisance rather than health threat. Of these mosquito-sensitive people, many have learned to live alongside the insects, adapting to them when using wetlands. Mosquitoes apparently occupy a fairly "neutral" role in the minds of many wetland users. Still, one wonders if mosquitoes can ever be viewed positively, as a "friend"? Our interviews revealed that, yes, the mosquito is indeed viewed positively, especially for the role that it plays in ecosystems. One conservationist with a deep passion for birds declared, "I love mosquitoes! I'll say it again, I love mosquitoes!" (Int. B8). His message was simple: mosquitoes are an insect, and insects provide food for birds; the more mosquitoes (and insects in general), the more birds. Insect populations, generally, have been in global decline, with some 40% of species threatened with extinction (Sánchez-Bayo and Wyckhuys 2019), and with the insect trend in the UK being no exception (Leather 2017). As the conservationist explained "I'm convinced that one of the biggest problems facing … our bird life, certainly farmland birds and wetland birds, is the lack of insects" (Int B8). The importance and decline of insects were mentioned by several others, including a reserve manager:

> I feel like even when I first moved here 30 years ago there were a lot more insects in the area and there were a lot more mozzies and midges, I think. I think we're losing invertebrates massively … I see them as a food source for birds and amphibians, so a sort of source of life.
>
> *(Int S9)*

Indeed, most participants across stakeholder groups acknowledged, or at least assumed, that mosquitoes play a role in the functioning of ecosystems, particularly as food for birds and bats. "It's an inconvenience but everything has its place," noted a farmer, "and maybe without the mosquitos we wouldn't have so many swallows. So it's swings and roundabouts" (Int. A8). "They're a fact of life and to be honest," said a conservation volunteer, "they are probably the biggest factor in the food chain; there are billions of them out there" (Int S11).

Another theme that emerged from the interviews was the rights of mosquitoes to exist as part of the ecosystem. "They're just part of the wildlife. They've got as much right to be here as anything else" (Int. B1). This is an ethical or moral argument that involves animal intimacies, and decentring humans as the central object of study. Anna Tsing's declamation, "human nature is an interspecies relationship," is the foundation of much of the WetlandLIFE project. Understanding and appreciating the close connectivity between humans, other animals and wetlands enabled us to appreciate how these multi-species spaces are the fabric of life on this planet. Many respondents considered mosquitoes integral to that fabric, part of the food web, or simply justifiable in their own right.

Nor are viewpoints static, inert parts of our consciousness; people constantly change their perceptions of things around them. In addition to the behavioural adaptations to mosquitoes mentioned above, there are perceptual adaptations to mosquitoes. Could we (or should we) change our perception of the mosquito from foe to friend? One Somerset resident saw this as something he might strive for: "I suppose if I was being consistent, I'd say I need to understand the sort of beings of mosquitoes and why they're there and cherish them, no doubt, but I haven't got to that stage yet! (Int. S1). Another Somerset resident adopted this approach, seeking to "learn to love the mosquito," as she says:

One night I came out here and it was incredibly warm. It was a summer evening and I bumped into a group of people, only one of whom I knew at the time, a guy called Dave. He's a chef and a fisherman and you get absolutely plagued by mosquitos in the height of summer here and it can be pretty annoying. It was one of those nights, every single inch of the air was vibrating with insects. Dave is a fisherman and was in absolute raptures about this and was pointing out the swarms and he talked about the lifecycle of larvae and he talked about the way that this was the basic food stuff of fish, so the beginning of the whole food chain and how vital it was. It was fascinating and I thought there's no point in me carrying on being irritated with the mosquitos because it's not going to make them go away. So, if I can get a bit of Dave's love for them, perhaps it'll help. So, yeah, I try to learn to love the mosquito and I did find them significantly less troublesome after that

(Int. S5)

It seems that if people understand more about mosquitoes, their biology, and their place in nature, then their attitude towards these creatures may even shift from toleration to admiration. Indeed, a reserve manager in Bedford confessed to discovering a new admiration: "I find them fascinating" (Int. B13). Or to quote one of England's early mosquito foes, A. Moore Hogarth (1928), "we may have to modify the popular view of the mosquito as an entirely useless pest; indeed, as a subject for Nature study the mosquito, especially the male mosquito, is a thing of beauty" (pp. 30–31).

Foe

Our responses to mosquitoes are greatly shaped by the dominant historical and contemporary cultural representations we live amongst. The vast majority of practices that surround navigating mosquitoes are built on narratives of destruction, most particularly the need to obliterate this foe. Timothy Winegards's work *Mosquito: A Human History of Our Deadliest Predator* (2019) highlights all too readily the contemporary, populist view of these animals as a merciless villain to be annihilated. The mosquito's label as an enemy of humankind took root in the early 1900s, after Sir Ronald Ross revealed the link between mosquitoes and malaria. Yet, beyond imported mosquito-borne diseases such as malaria carried by soldiers returning from war, Britons have lived alongside mosquitoes without the risk of contracting their diseases for over a century. Still, some Somerset residents knew local stories of malaria, or "ague," which they explicitly linked to wetlands.

I've heard stories about mosquitoes. A local farmer tells me a story there used to be some sort of fever here centuries ago, that people used to get a fever and it was from the marshes, and he said it was probably caused by all the mosquitoes. So, they've been here for a long time.

(Int. S19)

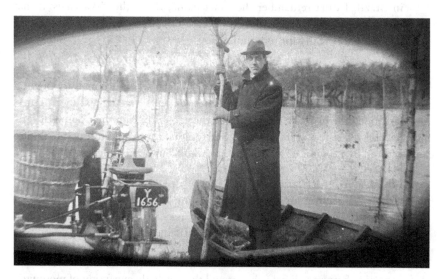

FIGURE 9.4 Dr Bracey, using a punt to visit patients in flooded moors of Somerset, circa 1913. Photograph courtesy of Hazel Hudson.

There were also rumours of a house in the Somerset moors, near Westhay Reserve, that used to treat ague—"It was an ague fever house. That's why the corner was always called Ague House Corner" (Int. S20)—along with a doctor who used to paddle across the marshes to treat those with the illness (Figure 9.4):

> the local doctor would go out in his boat to them. If it was flooded, he had a flat bottomed turf boat and he would punt out to them and treat them. They lived upstairs if it was flooded. But I can't remember … yeah, there were quite a few of them were suffering from this disease, whatever it was, that they called malaria.
>
> *(Int. S10)*

Yet despite this knowledge of indigenous malaria in Britain, there is not much explicit anxiety linked to mosquitoes or wetlands. Instead, most fear of mosquitoes stems from news about recent epidemics, global travel and climate change. Headlines about the 2015–2016 Zika outbreak, particularly in South and North America, led to heightened mosquito awareness. Although Zika's responsible mosquito, *Aedes Egypti*, does not live in the UK's cooler climate, 314 cases were confirmed across the country in those travelling from affected regions (Public Health England 2019). It is therefore not surprising that some of the respondents did mention Zika, along with the more familiar malaria, as a possible future risks for the UK:

> I think the concern around mosquitoes is if they were here in great numbers … we saw this horrible disease in places such as, parts of South America,

in Brazil, I can't remember the exact name, Zika, the Zika virus; if that was to spread to Europe and then into the UK, that could have devastating consequences really for us as humans.

(Int. B5)

And it is not just human diseases that are of concern when it comes to viewing mosquitoes as foe. For farmers, and other respondents grazing Exmoor ponies, they envisioned the primary diseases to be those confronting their domestic animals. Several references were made to Bluetongue, for example, a livestock disease vectored by midges. As a farmer near Alkborough explained,

I think as livestock farmers we're always worried about any insect, particularly if it's coming on a wind source from Europe … obviously we keep having threats of bluetongue and other associated diseases—and so, yes, there's always a big worry with any specific insect

(Int. A9)

The connection between climate change and the northerly expansion of mosquito-borne diseases, and human agency as cause of and responder to climate change, was viewed by some respondents as additional justification for confronting the climate crisis: "With climate change we know things like Zika virus have been moving … and it's why we should all take climate change seriously and we should do something about it" (Int. A12). The human role in spreading invasive mosquitoes (and the diseases that they carry) were also mentioned with reference to international transportation, and airports where "disease-ridden mosquitos would get a foothold" (Int. B2). The now heightened awareness of the role of travel in spreading disease and accelerating the COVID-19 pandemic will certainly heighten awareness, and indeed anxiety, of human agency in future mosquito threats.

Searching for Mosquitopia in English wetlands

So then, is it possible, at least in English wetlands, to learn to live side-by-side with mosquitoes without us killing them or them killing us? Or more specifically, might perceptions toward mosquitoes affect wetland management, restoration and creation? To provide an answer from an English perspective, realizing that wetlands are currently disease-free, we must declare that people living in or near these wetlands are already living in a form of Mosquitopia. Even if mosquitoes once transmitted malaria across the British Isles, with some of today's wetland users familiar with past "marsh fevers" and "ague," there are now many people who live, work or recreate in the breeding grounds of several mosquito species—coexisting with the mosquito "foe" through reluctant toleration, indifference or even admiration. A species often portrayed as villain, or nuisance, has shown itself to be an appreciated strand in the web of life, supporting a food chain that sustains other, perhaps more charismatic species appreciated by people in wetland landscapes, some of which form the very reason people visit wetlands at all.

Yet the yin of mosquitoes cannot ignore the yang of mosquitoes when developing plans to manage, restore and create wetlands. Mosquitoes here do cause severe nuisance in these wetlands even if they pose minor health threats, and so require human adaptations to fend off the wetland cohabiters. Whilst not at the forefront of people's concerns, the perceived possibility of mosquitoes carrying diseases to humans, or livestock, in the future, may modify the human–wetland–mosquito nexus. As Medlock and Vaux (2013) explain in the context of newly created wetlands (as in Alkborourgh), there is a "need for a case-by-case approach to design and management to mitigate mosquito or mosquito-borne disease issues now and in the future."

In 1928, A. Moore Hogarth wrote *British Mosquitoes and How to Eliminate Them*. If we want to avoid contributing to the "extinction narrative" but instead want to maintain a form of Mosquitopia, we need to prepare for a possible future in which mosquitoes are more prevalent, or even carrying diseases—although the actual risk in the UK is currently considered negligible. As one respondent from Bedford put it,

> I think every animal somewhere or insect has a role to play, I'm perhaps not quite sure what their role in the ecosystem is, but I would assume that we'd probably do more damage by trying to eradicate them, as opposed to, by having them.
>
> *(Int. B5)*

Through hearing the voices of those intimately connected to wetlands, we identified three key steps towards this goal. The first step, that of monitoring, is a case of "know thy enemy"; or as conservation volunteer in Somerset conveyed:

> Monitoring it helps. It helps know what species there are. It helps to know what relative numbers there are so that if there are radical changes, and those radical changes are likely to impact on other organisms, then I think we need to know and make rational decisions about that.
>
> *(Int. S6)*

The second step is to develop safe and effective management options, while recognizing that a balance must be sought. In particular, chemical methods of control may be viewed unfavourably, with more sympathetic management options (such as wetland design and management) being preferable, as an angler in Bedford, illustrated:

> I am aware that some of the chemicals that have been used to destroy mosquitoes really can do other damage so I would hope that there's research going on so if that were to be the case, then we've got a solution in waiting.
>
> *(Int B15)*

The third step is education and adaptation. Should English mosquitoes carry diseases in the future, a response might be developed by considering experiences with Lyme disease, which is managed through education and awareness of precautionary measures for avoiding and removing ticks. Indeed, many people already adapt to nuisance mosquitoes, and would extend these adaptations should the risk heighten:

> I think you'd probably adapt to it because you'd find out what the risks were and what you could do to control the risks to yourself, and you would either dress or medicate accordingly, which is what we tend to do with ticks ... you would find a way to adapt to be able to carry on doing what you wanted to do.
>
> *(Int. A1)*

Our respondents choose to live their lives embedded within these wetlands, having formed meaningful and intimate connections with these landscapes, developing senses of place and well-being, while confronting challenges that arise. Wetlands and people have formed strong relationships. Some of these places have always been wetlands; some were created over the last few thousand years during the transition from nomadic to settled farming; a few have been reclaimed more recently from coastal plains or constructed to replace other kinds of landscapes. Despite their differences and similarities, their histories recent and distant, wetlands are the setting for human–mosquito relationships. Humans and mosquitoes continue to coexist; both have, so far, resisted extinction unlike so many other creatures on this planet. The fact that mosquitoes still buzz demands a grudging respect for this most tenacious animal brethren. Communicating widely their role as pollinators, as fodder and biomass for a range of wetland creatures, whilst implementing sensitive management of their habitats where they are or may become bothersome, will play an essential part in developing a new, more intimate human–mosquito *corps à corps*.

Acknowledgements and author contribution

This research was carried out as part of WetlandLIFE project, funded and supported by the Natural Environment Research Council, the Arts and Humanities Research Council, the Economic and Social Research Council and the Department for Environment, Food and Rural Affairs under the Valuing Nature Programme (NERC grant reference number NE/NO13379/1).

Adriana Ford designed the study and collected and analyzed the data whilst working at the University of Greenwich. The chapter was written by Dr Adriana Ford and Dr Mary Gearey, with input from Dr Marcus Hall and Dr Dan Tamir. Dr Tim Acott managed the WetlandLIFE project as principal investigator, and contributed to the study design and provided the case study map. The ecological data for the case studies were provided by Dr Frances

Hawkes, of the Natural Resources Institute, University of Greenwich. We thank all of the participants of the research for sharing their time and thoughts, and for the whole WetlandLIFE team for their ideas and support throughout the project.

Interview key

A = Alkborough Flats (and surrounding area); B = Bedford urban wetland parks (Bedford Priory Country Park and Millennium Country Park); S = Somerset Levels (Westhay Moor and Shapwick Heath, and surrounding landscape). The number is the chronological interview identifier (e.g. Int. A2 = second interview conducted in Alkborough).

Data sharing and data accessibility

Please contact WetlandLIFE principal investigator Dr Tim Acott at t.g.acott@ gre.ac.uk

Bibliography

Cohen, W.B. 1983. Malaria and French imperialism. *The Journal of African History*, 24(1), 23–36.

Daily Mail. 2019. Zika mosquitoes will come to the UK because of global warming – risking a "large epidemic" of the incurable disease, MPs warn. *Daily Mail*, 3 April.

Dobson, M.J. 1989. History of Malaria in England. *Journal of the Royal Society of Medicine Supplement*, 17(Supplement 17), 82.

Dover District Council. 2020. *Mosquitoes in the Dover District*. https://www.dover.gov .uk/Environment/Environmental-Health/Pest-Control/Mosquitoes.aspx. Accessed 27 May 2020.

Ford, A. 2019a. Sport horse leisure and the phenomenology of interspecies embodiment. *Leisure Studies*, 38(3), 329–340.

Ford, A.E.S. 2019b. Mosquito and me – a narrative on mosquitoes in English wetlands in 2018. 11:30 min. https://www.youtube.com/watch?v=PPDPH0cqB-s&t=5s

Gearey, B.R., Charman, D.J. and Kent, M. 2000. Palaeoecological evidence for the prehistoric settlement of bodmin moor, Cornwall, Southwest England. Part I: The status of woodland and early human impacts. *Journal of Archaeological Science*, 27, 423–438.

Gearey, M., Church, A., and Ravenscroft, N. 2020. *English Wetlands: Spaces of Nature, Culture and Imagination*. London: Palgrave Macmillan.

Haraway, D. 2007. *When Species Meet*. Minneapolis: University of Minnesota Press.

Haraway, D. 2016. *Staying with the Trouble*. Durham, NC: Duke University Press.

Hoffman, M.A. 2016. *Malaria, Mosquitoes, and Maps: Practices and Articulations of Malaria Control in British India and WWII*. Doctoral dissertation, University of California San Diego.

Hogarth, A.M. 1928. *British Mosquitoes and How to Eliminate Them*. London: Hutchinson & Co.

Howell, J. 2018. *Malaria and Victorian Fictions of Empire*. Cambridge: Cambridge University Press.

Hudson, W. 2019. Horror as plague of killer mosquitos are headed to Britain as fears ramp up over insects. *Express*, 14 November.

Hume, C. 2008. *Wetland Vision Technical Document: Overview and Reporting of Project Philosophy and Technical Approach*. The Wetland Vision Partnership. https://www.lun evalleyfloodforum.org.uk/uploads/1/2/3/7/123753072/wetlandvision_tcm9-13295 7.pdf, accessed 05/05/21

Irvine, R. 2014. Deep time: An anthropological problem. *Social Anthropology*, 22(2), 157–172.

Leather, S.R. 2017. 'Ecological Armageddon'—more evidence for the drastic decline in insect numbers. *Annals of Applied Biology*, 172(1), 1–3.

Malone, K. 2019. Co-mingling Kin: Exploring histories of uneasy human-animal relations as sites for ecological posthumanist pedagogies. In *Animals in Environmental Education*, T. Lloro-Bidart and V. Banschbach, eds. Cham: Palgrave Macmillan, 95–115.

Medlock, J.M and Vaux, A.G.C. 2013. Colonization of UK coastal realignment sites by mosquitoes: Implications for design, management, and public health. *Journal of Vector Ecology*, 38(1), 53–62.

Moore, Jason. 2015. *Capitalism in the Web of Life*. New York: Verso.

Public Health England. 2017. Guidance. Mosquito: Nationwide surveillance. Updated August 10. https://www.gov.uk/government/publications/mosquito-surveillance/ mosquito-nationwide-surveillance

Public Health England. 2019. Guidance. Zika virus: Epidemiology and cases diagnosed in the UK. February 27. https://www.gov.uk/government/publications/zika-virus -epidemiology-and-cases-diagnosed-in-the-uk/zika-virus-epidemiology-and-cases -diagnosed-in-the-uk

Ranger, S., Kenter, J.O., Bryce, R., Cumming, G., Dapling, T., Lawes, E. and Richardson, P.B. 2016. Forming shared values in conservation management: An interpretive- deliberative-democratic approach to including community voices. *Ecosystem Services*, 21, 344–357.

Sallares, Robert and Gomzi, Susan 2001. Biomolecular archaeology of Malaria. *Ancient Biomolecules*, 3(3), 195–213.

Sánchez-Bayo, F. and Wyckhuys, K.A.G. 2019. Worldwide decline of the entomofauna: A review of its drivers. *Biological Conservation*, 232, 8–27.

Schmidt, J.J. 2017. *Water: Abundance, Scarcity, and Security in the Age of Humanity*. New York: New York University Press.

Semenza, J.C. and Suk, J.E. 2018. Vector-borne diseases and climate change: A European perspective. *FEMS Microbiology Letters*, 365, fnx244.

Shamai, S. 1991. Sense of place: An empirical measurement. *Geoforum*, 22(3), 347–358.

Smart, C. 2011. Ways of knowing: Crossing species boundaries. *Methodological Innovations Online*, 6(3), 27–38.

Smith, M. 2013. Ecological community, the sense of the world, and senseless extinction. *Environmental Humanities*, 2(1), 21–41.

Solnit, R. 2010. *Infinite City: A San Francisco Atlas*. Berkeley: University of California Press.

Swain, M. 2012. Deadly mosquito found in the UK for first time since the 1940s. *Daily Mirror*, February 9.

Tsing, A.L. 2012. Unruly edges: Mushrooms as companion species. *Environmental Humanities*, 1, 141–54.

Vaux, A.G.C. and Medlock, J.M. 2015. Current status of invasive mosquito surveillance in the UK. *Parasites & Vectors*, 8: 351. doi:10.1186/s13071-015-0936-9

Watts, S. 2006. Malaria and deaths in the English marshes. *The Lancet*, 368(9542), 1152.

Wickson, F. 2010. Mosquitoes: Just how much biodiversity does humanity need? *Nature*, 466(7310), 1041–1041.

Winegard, T.C. 2019. *The Mosquito: A Human History of Our Deadliest Predator*. New York: Dutton.

Zahorik, P. and Jenison, R.L. 1998. Presence as being-in-the-world. *Presence*, 7(1), 78–89.

10

AweWonderExcitement

Kerry Morrison and Helmut Lemke

Little one
I hold my breath
So you can't find me
He's still breathing
Bite him

This is the story of two artists who set out to shift perceptions of the mosquito from a nuisance and the spoiler of summer evenings to an arresting creature, more breath-taking than blood-taking, and a creature worthy of the appreciation of a public venturing out of doors.

This is a very northern and indeed very British story: from a country where mosquitoes have not transferred deadly diseases to humans for a long, long time.

At the beginning of their story, before the artists began their wetland mosquito quest, the artists' understanding of mosquitoes was limited to being bitten, itching, scratching and scorning the beast. However, both were experienced in creating artwork in response to the natural environment, the more-than-human, and human-and-nature interdependencies; and finding and conveying "beauty" and value in the natural world where others saw "ugly" and "pest." Yet, this venture presented a new challenge, as never before had they championed wildlife that bites, seemingly without provocation, and wildlife that is seen as a real threat to human health.

The artists are Kerry Morrison and Helmut Lemke. This is their mosquito story.

In 2017, we, as a collaborative partnership, were selected from an open call to artists to be a part of the WetlandLIFE research project, a three-year, UK research initiative within the Valuing Nature Programme[1] funded through UK Research and Innovation. Bringing together an interdisciplinary team, WetlandLIFE set

DOI: 10.4324/9781003056034-10

out to explore ecological, economic, social, and cultural values of wetlands in England, exploring ecological connections and focusing on mosquitoes and mosquito management—now and in the future, given climate change scenarios of a wetter and warmer England. The research also explored the disvalue of wetlands, specifically how these watery and buggy areas are negatively perceived and how mosquitoes in particular are perceived and reported with disdain, historically and currently.

To extend knowledge and understanding about wetlands and mosquitoes, the research team launched an open call to artists. The description read:

> Perceptions of wetlands vary considerably—from disease-ridden "swamps" that should be drained for farmland or housing, to wildlife havens generating local employment and enjoyment for thousands of visitors. Meanwhile, the mosquitoes that live in them are typically seen as a nuisance with no useful purpose—few people champion them for their aesthetic or intrinsic value, and their contribution to the resilience of wetland ecosystems remains largely unrecognized.
>
> We are looking for artists whose work can contribute to our knowledge and appreciation of wetlands and mosquitoes ... This might be done by communicating the findings of researchers about wetlands and mosquitoes to new audiences, challenging how we think about them, or changing how we feel about them—perhaps helping us connect with them in new ways.

A challenging and very tall order. Nevertheless, we grew excited about the prospect of exploring wetlands and mosquitoes, their aesthetic and intrinsic value, and how we may perceive them. We were thrilled to be selected and itching to begin on our journey of learning within the multidisciplinary research team of entomologists, social scientists, human geographers, historians, natural capital economists and artists (Figure 10.1).

The WetlandLIFE research project required the establishment of three, in-depth, case study sites connected to wetland expansion. Three wetland habitat types were selected and the research sites secured: farmland reversion at Alkborough Flats, North Lincolnshire; coastal realignment at the Somerset Levels; and urban wetlands at Priory Country Park and the Millennium Country Park, Bedford.

We were then allocated Alkborough Flats, Priory Country Park and the Millennium Country Park as our creative practice and research sites. The Somerset Levels were allocated to a third commissioned artist: creative writer, Victoria Lesley. (Sadly, part-way through the research project the ranger team at Priory Country Park were made redundant due to government cuts. This resulted in us not being able to continue with socially engaged work in Priory Park.)

As artists—not entomologists—we were starting from a position of knowing almost nothing about mosquitoes, their habits or their anatomy, and found ourselves on a dramatic learning curve, gorging on any informative publication we could

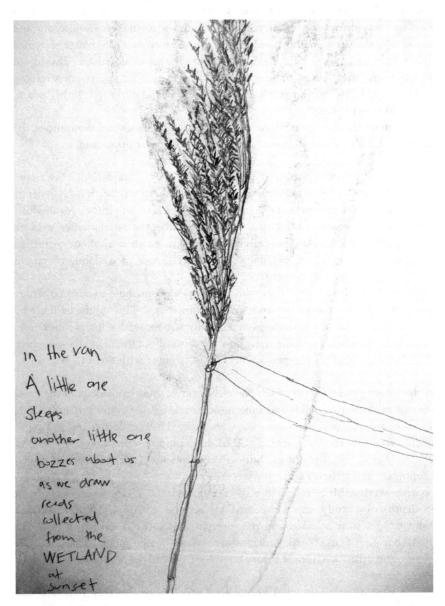

In the van
A little one
sleeps
another little one
buzzes about us
as we draw
reeds
collected
from the
WETLAND
at
sunset

FIGURE 10.1 "In the van a little one sleeps." Drawing graphite and ink on paper by Kerry Morrison.

find about mosquitoes. The entomologists in the team helped us with our hunger by feeding us germane publications. From the outset, we found a synergy between our entomologist partners and ourselves; palpable in conversations was a passion and shared love for the vilified in nature. They invited us on a site visit to one of the reconnaissance research sites, the Kent Marshes, which enabled us to experience how a mosquito expert reads the landscape, which is notably different to how many artists read landscapes. Both artists and entomologists move through the landscape with focused intent and although they eye the same subjects, the mosquito and the terrain, their interpretation varies by discipline. The entomologist hones in on specifics of habitat: where mosquitoes are likely to breed, feed and overwinter. The artist lets their ears and eyes bask in the aesthetic whilst envisaging an array of interventions and expositions. This detail of difference reveals how our professional disciplines guide our research and interpretations of landscape and emphasizes the strengths of a multidisciplinary team. If we wish to capture and make greater sense of a natural setting, more than one perspective is required. Our journey of learning also took us into the laboratory where we experienced cutting-edge mosquito research. We observed acoustic research tracking mating patterns and sounds. We experienced how mosquitoes are bred and supported in an artificial setting, which included the human feeding of adult females (Figures 10.2– Figures 10.3)

These background experiences were crucial to our understanding of the subject, the mosquito, and our understanding of a scientist's connection to their research and its subject. Through this initial step, our perception of the mosquito shifted: from a nuisance that is a potential threat to human health, to an insect that is integral to a functioning ecosystem, which includes many other species dependent upon the mosquito eggs, larvae and adults as food sources. More than that, we were amazed to discover that mosquitoes follow an intricate mating ritual, which involves males singing and dancing in murmurations to attract females. Only when a male and female harmonize with the beats of their wings do they mate. We had come to realize that the mosquito is a highly developed and successful insect that imbues awe.

We were in AWE
A = appreciation W = wonder E = excitement
We were inspired.

With a deeper understanding of mosquitoes and our new-found awe and wonder of this creature, we then designed our field research, which we framed around the question of how contemporary art practice can reorient the value of these landscapes and its vilified insect inhabitants. We aimed to (re)present a wetland nature aesthetic that intrigues and allures new audiences, and conserves and protects the seemingly ugly—which we know has ecological value and provides ecosystem services.[2] Aesthetics is often equated to beauty. Yet, when it comes to the health of an ecosystem, its beauty—or ugliness—would seem irrelevant. Irrespective of aesthetics, ecosystems can provide multifarious health and well-being benefits. Yet, the value of nature and the cultural services it provides may

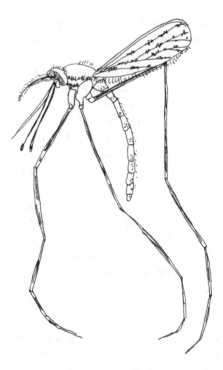

FIGURE 10.2 "Itching for Understanding" mosquito. Drawing by Kerry Morrison.

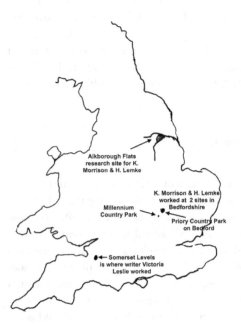

FIGURE 10.3 Map illustrating Wetland Life Research Sites. Drawing by Helmut Lemke.

be heavily dependent on aesthetics. So we asked: how do we shift the perception of a disease-ridden "swamp" to a landscape permeated with value and therefore with beauty? Having examined mosquitoes in more detail, we had discovered their tangible beauty: the iridescent streaks at 10× magnification, the harmonic buzzing when amplified, the murmuration choreography of mating males. In exploring the physical landscape of two urban wetlands and a farmland reverted to wetland, we aimed to discover which other layers of beauty emanated from these habitats Figures 10.4, 10.5 and 10.6.

Inspired with awe and sparkling with new mosquito insights, we set about our artistic investigations—art practice research—at Alkborough Flats, Priory Park and Millennium Park with the aim to:

- Immerse ourselves in the landscape.
- Explore the patterns that connect the mosquito to our enjoyment of wetland habitats.
- Converse with people we met about "this" wetland and its wildlife inclusive of mosquitoes.
- Illuminate what is beautiful about mosquitoes.
- Highlight the role and benefits of mosquitoes within the delicate web of interdependence in wetland ecosystems.
- Create new artwork to challenge how we think about mosquitoes and wetlands, thereby raising awareness and understanding towards the hopes that we can shift how we feel about mosquitoes emotionally, aesthetically, ecologically and socially.
- Create new conversations about the values and meanings of wetlands and mosquitoes for repositioning the vilified mosquito.

Our on-site interventions began through a process of art whereby art is a verb: the action of doing. Art as verb, as action, moves away from the idea of art as noun and object on display, as we most often experience in art galleries. Instead, art happens beyond traditional art venues and moves into everyday places or specific locations whereby the art can connect to everyday life (human and non-human) and the lived experiences of that location. This social practice, which is also conversational, engages people and addresses issues directly relevant to their lives. This is not a new concept, but one that has been evolving since the late 1960s with the rise of Happenings, community art and the feminist art movement. In the UK, artist (and co-founder of the Artist Placement Group) John Latham argued that artists with an understanding of art as process, who work across disciplines, are skilled in "imaginative and durational thinking, that can produce a transformation in the viewer's consciousness of the world" (Latham, in Kester, 2004, p. 62).[3] In creating art as process, out in wetlands, we were creating a more social art that invites interaction: art that is ecologically and socially engaged. Our social and ecological approach creates a situation where people can talk, be listened to, and reason and learn together. It enables a situation where

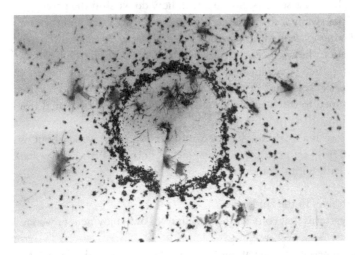

FIGURE 10.4 Mosquito eggs, Greenwich University. Alternatively, through the artists' lens: *objet trouvé* mosquito filter drawing. By Kerry Morrison and Helmut Lemke.

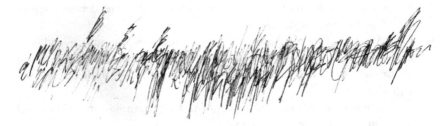

FIGURE 10.5 Alkborough Flats "Reeds and Wind." Ink on paper. Drawing by Helmut Lemke.

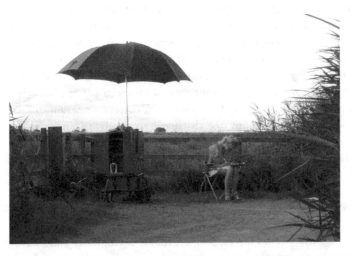

FIGURE 10.6 "Kerry and the Art Cart." Drawing on Alkborough Flats, 2018. Photograph by Kerry Morrison and Helmut Lemke.

we can pass on the knowledge we have gained about mosquitoes and wetlands as a result of being part of the WetlandLIFE interdisciplinary research team. Furthermore, our understanding of the world of wetlands increases and becomes informed by voices that exist outside of academia and the art world. This way of working is exhilarating and humbling. It is ever fresh and enlightening, and often yields the unexpected (Figures 10.7, 10.8 and 10.9).

We therefore created a mobile unit as our studio on wheels, the repository for our equipment and resources, our shelter, our desk, our hub, our wetland art cart.

Through creating a visual spectacle—a performative happening[4]—we made visible what we do as artists: data collection, sound recording, drawing, photographing, mapping, creative writing. Our approach, which is both performative and socially engaging, raised curiosity, sparking conversations with visitors about wetland life and valuing nature, inclusive of mosquitoes. With our art cart, we immersed ourselves in each of the three wetland landscapes, deepening our connectedness to wetland habitats and wildlife, learning about other's connectedness to "this" wetland and expanding our understanding of wetland aesthetics: the smells, the sounds, the views, the tactility. We observed movements and stillness, human life, more than human life, patterns created by nature, patterns that connect us (Figures 10.10 and 10.11).

We engaged in on-site conversations with stakeholders, visitors and locals. We documented and recorded sights, sounds, movements, patterns and conversations. Our process of performative patterns, action and dialogue resulted in new, shared experiences and unfolding narratives. We imaged ways of integrating these experiences and narratives with the wider WetlandLIFE research. The artist's rendition alone cannot convey the whole wetland ecosystem. The artist can frame the chaotic and soggy and sometimes seemingly hostile in ways that reimagine the subject and re-present a challenging landscape or species wrapped up in the presentation of the artwork. However, if we want to have a holistic or a panoramic view of wetlands, inclusive of mosquitoes, an interdisciplinary approach is required and research needs to be integrated. Within WetlandLIFE we were part of a multidisciplinary team. The team approach was interdisciplinary, whereby we extended thinking beyond our single disciplinary boundary to share and gather methodologies, findings and knowledge. Together, combined knowledge, combined experiences, and combining research, creates a holistic view of wetlands and their Nested Ecosystem Services,[5] inclusive of non-material value. Mindful that the WetlandLIFE project had been commissioned by UK Research and Innovation with typical outputs being academic papers and therefore not readily accessible to non-academics, we wanted to return to the wetlands to convey this much bigger, much richer, much deeper interdisciplinary picture of wetland life to visitors and stakeholders. We aimed to create a mechanism, through art, that could bring together the WetlandLIFE research into one interactive and public hub. We wanted to create a bridge, or a conduit, between the academic, the art and the everyday. Our desire was to

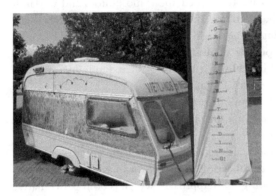

FIGURE 10.7 WoW Wetlands on Wheels. On site, Millennium Park, Bedford. Photograph by Kerry Morrison and Helmut Lemke.

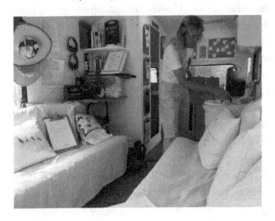

FIGURE 10.8 Kerry inside WoW just before visitors arrive. Photograph by Kerry Morrison and Helmut Lemke.

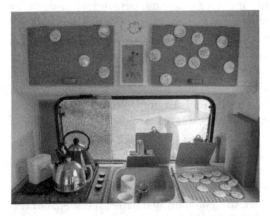

FIGURE 10.9 The kitchen, left intact so that refreshments could be offered to visitors in WetlandLIFE mosquito food-chain mugs. Photograph by Kerry Morrison and Helmut Lemke.

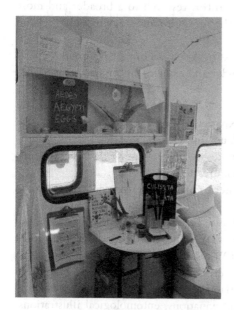

FIGURE 10.10 Display cabinet for small and fragile artefacts and curiosities, including the *objet trouvé* mosquito filter drawing. Photograph by Kerry Morrison and Helmut Lemke.

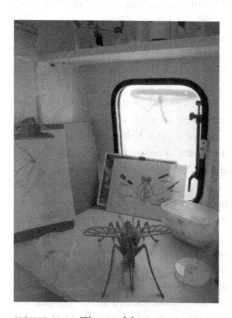

FIGURE 10.11 The wet laboratory: a mini research lab with mosquito and wetland insect specimens, microscope, mosquito research papers, entomological diagrams of mosquitoes and the sound of mosquitoes buzzing. Photograph by Kerry Morrison and Helmut Lemke.

make accessible the breadth of WetlandLIFE research to a broader and more diverse audience, thereby devilifying the mosquito and demystifying wetland ecosystems.

We imagined WoW—Wetlands on Wheels—as an immersive micro experience to facilitate the appreciation, wonder and excitement, or awe, of wetlands and mosquitoes.

WoW: a touring site-specific micro studio/lab/gallery of WetlandLIFE research. WoW: an immersive micro experience. WoW: a participatory space for conversations and exchange about wetlands and wetland research that offers visitors new ways of seeing and connecting to mosquitoes and wetland ecosystems. WoW: a repurposed vintage caravan (Figures 10.12 and 10.13).

Every part of the exterior and the interior of WoW conveyed elements of the WetlandLIFE research.

Almost all team members (Tim Acott, Frances Hawkes, Anil Graves, Joe Morris, Peter Coates, Mary Geary, Victoria Leslie, Jolyon Medlock and Lionel Feugere) participated in the creation of WoW, sharing elements of their research for the WoW experience. Tea-towels were printed with the Nested Ecosystem Service diagram; a screen displayed wetland photographs; the walls were covered with economic valuation diagrams and equations, entomological illustrations, historic newspaper cuttings about mosquitoes, maps and poetry.

Integral to our artwork is participation and creating opportunities for people to engage. Through headphones, visitors to WoW could listen to underwater wetland sounds, mosquitoes buzzing and harmonizing, and excerpts from a short story by Victoria Lesley.

In July of 2019, WoW toured to Millennium Park. Our presence, and the presence of others, within the exposition animated WoW and transformed it into a live and interactive experience. WoW came alive and was filled with, and surrounded by, wetland life exchanges.

Every day, for 14 days, we interacted with WoW visitors and also offered "Itching for Understanding" workshops led by us with sound recording and nature drawing; Dr Frances Hawkes, a mosquito behavioural entomologist who took visitors on mosquito safaris; and Professor Joe Morris and Dr Sharanya Basu Roy, Ecosystem Service and Natural Capital economists, who offered a wetland ecosystem valuation walk and a natural capital talk with tea and biscuits. These workshops gave the visiting public insights into creative approaches and wetland academic research happening in their park (Figures 10.14, 10.15 and 10.16).

WoW was far more than a static spectacle and repository of research; it was a place of interaction, engagement, activity, learning and conversations facilitated through social engagement and workshop activities. Encounters ranged from brief exchanges to in-depth conversations. As visitors learned about mosquitoes, we learned about their connectedness to "this" wetland. A regular visitor who came to see us daily at Millennium Park once worked at this site before it was a wetland. He has witnessed the landscape change over the decades, from a brick

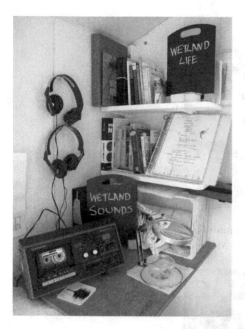

FIGURE 10.12 Sound station and reference library. Photograph by Kerry Morrison and Helmut Lemke.

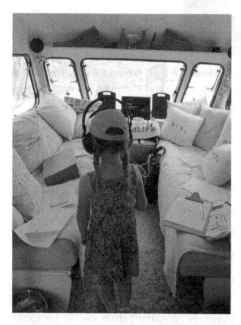

FIGURE 10.13 Mesmerized by mosquito sounds. Photograph by Kerry Morrison and Helmut Lemke.

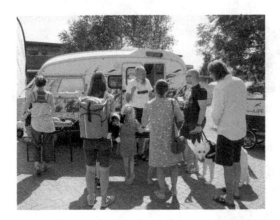

FIGURE 10.14 Helmut talking to WoW visitors at Millennium Park, Bedford, summer 2019. Photograph by Kerry Morrison and Helmut Lemke.

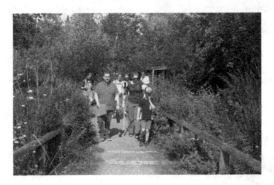

FIGURE 10.15 Mosquito safari around the Millennium Park, Bedford, led by Dr Frances Hawkes. Photograph by Kerry Morrison and Helmut Lemke.

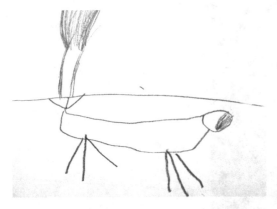

FIGURE 10.16 *Mosquito Larvae 'wriggler'*. Drawn by a young person on the mosquito safari and gifted to Kerry and Helmut.

factory, to a post-industrial wasteland site, to wetland reclamation. With awe and wonder he watched nature and wildlife taking root and flourishing where there were once furnaces, brick-dust, clay and pits. Now retired, his daily constitutional, whatever the weather, is a walk through the wetland nature reserve. He'd never given much thought to the mosquitoes before we arrived: they were just there. But learning about their behaviour and experiencing the mosquito safari with Dr Hawkes shifted his perception about mosquitoes. Before we left Millennium Park he told us he would champion the mosquito and tell people how important they are for wetlands. He was not a lone convert; others who engaged, also commented that their perceptions of mosquitoes and attitude towards them had shifted. No longer would they see mosquitoes as pests, but as integral parts of the landscape and ecosystem. For some, there was no getting away from the fact that the mosquito is a biting, bloodsucking nuisance. However, learning about their behaviour enlightened them on how to avoid being bitten, whilst still enjoying the wetland. One visitor admitted that she avoids wetlands and only comes to Millennium Park because they have a café. Learning about mosquito behaviour offered her windows of opportunity to explore the wetlands, opportunities that she was now keen to take. Learning in a novel way that mosquitoes are not omnipresent, learning that only females bite, learning that females only feed on blood during breeding, combined with learning about the wetland food web, shifted perceptions and increased appreciation, not only of mosquitoes, but also of wetlands (Figures 10.17).

WoW's second tour was to Alkborough Flats, North Lincolnshire. This winter exposition from January to February, 2020, ran concurrently with "Reclaiming Wetland Values: Marsh, Mud and Wonder",[6] an exhibition at the Royal Geographic Society, London, which brought together two Valuing Nature wetland research projects: WetlandLIFE and Coast Web.[7] WoW became an outpost to the exhibition in London, livestreaming wetland sights, sounds and encounters, along with our creative endeavours, which included writing and performing songs and poems, drawing, and performances out on the Flats.

Alkborough Flats is a very different wetland than Millennium Park. The latter was created for wildlife and for visitors, and includes a car-park, children's play area, café, shop and bike hire, as well as offering nature and conservation workshops and talks for children and adults. Millennium Park offers a full family excursion. In contrast, Alkborough Flats offers very few facilities. It is a farmland conversion on the Humber Estuary. It floods. The tenant farmers have adapted and now farm sheep and rare cattle breeds, as part of a small rural community. The Flats, open to the public, house three bird hides and no amenities. But, there are birds in abundance here, which attract plentiful birders from far and wide. These differences make for a very different site, with very different visitors. The heart of winter is perhaps not the ideal time to engage with wetland tourists about mosquitoes, since there are no mosquitoes around. However, winter is a magical time to spend in any wetland: a low sun shining through the amber

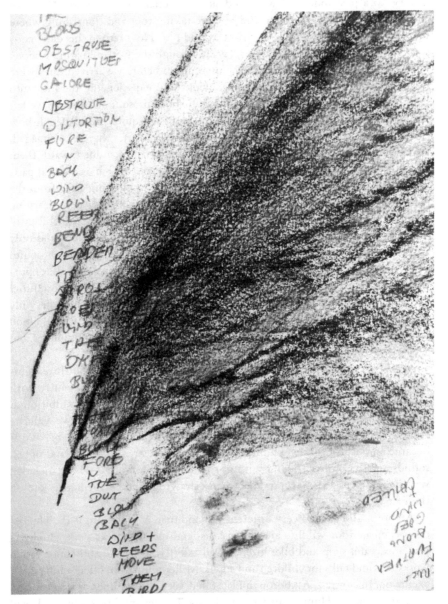

FIGURE 10.17 "Alkborough Flats." Untitled drawing. Charcoal and graphite on paper by Helmut Lemke.

reeds, a stillness of the air on a frosty morning, cold biting at your cheeks, frozen ripples at the base of reed stalks, and certainly the migrating visitors, winter waders and native marsh birds.

We pitched up next to the entrance gate and connected to London and the rest of the team through Skype. This way, The Royal Geographic Society London exhibition and audience were in Alkborough Flats, and the WoW visitors, and the Flats, were in London.

Due to the cold, much of our time was spent in WoW. When we were not in WoW we were out on the Flats, livestreaming our wetland walks and sights from the bird hides; talking to people we met; and performing in nature (Figures 10.18, 10.19 and 10.20).

When in WoW, we invited visitors to come in out of the cold wind for a cup of tea with biscuits and a chat about bird life, the beauty of wetlands, the value of wetlands and the role mosquitoes play in the complexity of wetland ecosystems. The birders we engaged with were already aware of the importance of mosquitoes. They added to our wetland experience by sharing their knowledge of birds and wildlife photography. Their dedication to capturing the perfect shot of a bird was impressive, as was their knowledge of the environment: they knew where to perch and wait for the perfect shots. The locals we met, mainly dog walkers from the village, knew less about the site's ecology and wildlife. Their connectedness to the Flats was more experiential: a great place to walk, feel the fresh air on your face and hear the wind through the reeds. Although a wetland is about ecology, it is also about how we move through and experience the more-than-human, regardless of knowing the names of species or the mechanics of nature. And, at certain times of the year, as we move through wetlands there are critters that annoy us and reduce the pleasure of our experience. What we discovered, when speaking to those who love wetlands for their aesthetics and their cultural rewards, was that the sharing of what we knew about mosquitoes shifted their perceptions. In leaning about the interdependencies of a wetland system, and the role that mosquitoes (and other insects) play, visitors' attitudes towards them relaxed.

All of this time, our presence in WoW and on Alkborough Flats was live broadcast to the exhibition in London. Museum-goers there were able to engage with us or simply observe two artists, nearing the end of their story, writing, drawing, performing, recording and conversing all things—wetlands and mosquitoes.

"Itching for Understanding—WoW" is an artwork that could not have existed without teamwork, collaboration and audience participation. It was a transdisciplinary ecological artwork, which brought together science, humanities, art and economics and in doing so created a novel space for knowledge exchange: a space that was inviting, lyrical and fun. Perhaps, when it comes to nature appreciation, value, and de-vilification, it is less about research dissemination, and more about how we disseminate research.

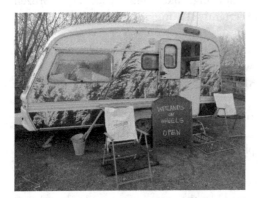

FIGURE 10.18 WoW at Alkborough Flats. January 2020. Photograph by Kerry Morrison and Helmut Lemke.

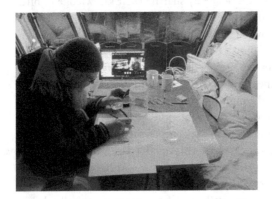

FIGURE 10.19 "Bitter cold outside, cosy warm inside." Drawing and livestreaming to London, the Royal Geographic Society exhibition: "Reclaiming Wetland Values: Marsh, Mud and Wonder". Photograph by Kerry Morrison and Helmut Lemke.

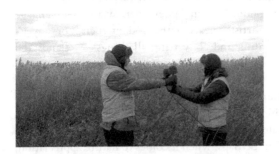

FIGURE 10.20 Reed performance. Kerry Morrison and Helmut Lemke, World Wetland Day 2020. Still video shot. Photograph by Kerry Morrison and Helmut Lemke.

Notes

1 Valuing Nature: a five-year, £6.5 million research programme funded by Natural Environment Research Council (NERC), Economic and Social Research Council (ESRC), Biotechnology and Biological Sciences Research Council (BBSRS), Arts and Humanities Research Council (AHRC) and Department for Environment, Food and Rural Affairs (DEFRA), to explore complexities of the natural environment in valuation analyses and decision-making and consider the economic, societal and cultural value of ecosystem services: https://valuing-nature.net/about

2 Acott, T. 2020. *Wetlands, Wonder and Life: Photo Essay*, https://spark.adobe.com/page /uhhjBGQc6V93z/ on 11 February 2021.

3 Kester, G. 2004. *Conversation Pieces: Community and Communication in Modern Art*. Berkeley: University of California Press.

4 The "performative happening" is a term coined by Kerry Morrison to articulate an investigative process that is part performative, part data collection and part an art event. The performative happening is a convergence of methods. It is a durational process that makes visible the research as it happens and brings the voices of others into the research process.

5 Acott, T. et al. 2020. *Ecosystem Relations and Nested Ecosystem Services*. Unpublished; in peer review.

6 "Reclaiming Wetlands: Marsh, Mud and Wonder." 2020. Exhibition at the Royal Geographic Society, 28 January–2 February. Curated by C. Freemantle and S. Reed. https://valuing-nature.net/wetlandvalues

7 CoastWeb. 2020. Natural Environment Research Council (NERC) funded Valuing Nature Project, researching health and well-being benefits derived from coastal ecosystems and salt marshes, https://www.pml.ac.uk/CoastWeb/Home

PART IV

Know thyself

11

ENACTING POLITICS *WITH* MOSQUITOES

Beyond eradication and control

Jean Segata

It was 2016. I was researching public health policy for dengue fever among mosquito workers in Brazil's coastal city of Natal. But there were more diseases there than just dengue. It was also the time of Zika and chikungunya, and that early fall, locals were also sharing pictures of dead monkeys. On WhatsApp and Facebook, news was spreading as quickly as the viruses. Many people were confused. They talked about yellow fever too, and truths about all these diseases were mixed with half-truths.[1]

Little monkeys lived in the parks, stealing the tourists' food and posing for selfies with them. The precise number of monkey deaths was unknown, and workers could not reach a consensus about precise numbers. On social media, people spoke of more than 100 deaths; Lucas, a young mosquito worker, spoke of 40; and Carlos said there are only a half dozen. Lucas warned us that the monkeys' deaths were probably caused by yellow fever, but Carlos cautiously disagreed, saying he would rather wait for new tests being carried out at the Evandro Chagas Institute in Belém do Pará, a leading research centre since the days of the Rockefeller Foundation in Brazil. Local health officials had technologies to monitor mosquitoes and ill people, but it had no means by which to map yellow fever's virus. Amid uncertainties, I asked them, "Is there yellow fever here?" Both looked at each other, and Carlos replied:

> We have no budget for yellow fever, and I don't even know if we could deal with a new epidemic. We've already had a lot of trouble with dengue, Zika and chikungunya—so yellow fever too? We must tweak the numbers. There is the tourism; there are vaccines. We have to think about everything. Let me explain: we'll develop a project to request funding to *make* the epidemic, and send it to the Ministry [of Health]. In the report we'll put in some pictures of monkeys and show their tests, and explain the troubles

DOI: 10.4324/9781003056034-11

we've been having with mosquitoes. And let's hope they approve it. So, we will *install* the epidemic, you understand? If we are then rolling in money, we'll have a yellow fever epidemic, and whatever else you want … But I don't know. The summer is over and the mosquitoes didn't help us. I hardly saw any. And now, with all this trouble in Brasília, I don't know … Maybe the epidemic will happen only next year or never. No one knows.

(Carlos, mosquito worker. Natal, February 2016)

I did not know what to say when I heard that answer. Carlos knew what he was talking about. In Natal, the battle against dengue was already permanent, having constituted a state of emergency for at least 30 years. Mosquitoes shaped all those diseases, and Carlos had made his career confronting all of them (Segata 2017, 2019). Local newspapers would refute rumours of yellow fever with claims that it was all fake news. But a few months later, dead monkeys were reported in Minas Gerais, São Paulo, Rio de Janeiro and Bahia as well. Trying to downplay the problem, the authorities said it was a kind of *jungle* yellow fever. But in the spring of 2017 people began to die across the country. Many wondered whether the disease was returning.

This chapter explores human–mosquito relations in the context of public health policies for epidemics: some of these relations are complex and go beyond the simple eradication or control of mosquito populations. Although such control programmes are being updated with new epidemiological knowledge, there are recalcitrant political frameworks that must be considered. Efforts to eradicate or control mosquito epidemics cost lives and bring suffering since people and mosquitoes alike resist top-down political machinations. Relations between humans and this insect go beyond eradication and control, producing complex political encounters and negotiations.

The first part of this chapter summarizes two different experiences from fieldwork in Natal and Porto Alegre, Brazil, highlighting the use of new digital and health technologies in monitoring and controlling mosquitoes as well as the people living with them. For more than a century, the *Aedes aegypti* mosquito was known as one of the main vectors of such diseases as yellow fever, dengue and more recently Zika and chikungunya. The mosquito's worldwide distribution puts it at the crossroads of global health science, politics and capitalism. *Aedes aegypti* is the harbinger of epidemic risk, in all its aspects. Not only do viruses travel with it, but knowledge, technology and material opportunities travel along as well: from international parameters defined by experts in the World Health Organization, to those who offer new perceptions of nature, or else represent financial interests of chemical industry shareholders at the World Bank. Local programmes for mosquito control have therefore been aligned with the interests of global health and its political connections to security. But things do not always work as imagined. The following descriptions show how fragile these local projects are and demonstrate ways such projects leak into global technologies and institutions.

The second part of this chapter explores ambivalences between new epidemiological knowledge supported by digital-biological technologies and old epidemiological knowledge represented by the framework that organizes policies of mosquito epidemics. In recent decades, epidemics have been straining global health guidelines, which have increasingly invested in predictive technologies over preventive medicine, in a broader set of so-called preparedness and response policies (Collier & Lakoff 2008, Reis-Castro & Heidrickx 2013, MacPhail 2014, Nading 2014, Caduff 2015, Lakoff 2017, Keck 2020). The maxim of this understanding can be summed up in the idea that it is no longer a question of whether a pandemic is going to happen or not. The experts predict pandemics will happen, and the question is then to know when and whether we shall be prepared for them. However, it is also necessary to realize that the focus of these policies is not new, especially in the context of mosquito epidemics. For this reason, I take up how current ethnographic situations can be compared to their historical counterparts, to show how certain "preparedness and response" mechanisms are actually militarized mosquito-centric approaches that preserve social inequality. Nonetheless, some new technologies facilitate human–mosquito interactions and help the people involved to construct a common political infrastructure.[2]

My goal in this chapter is to show that since colonial times, the project of hiding tropical epidemics has largely been a broad machination of government. This works through a tropical unconsciousness. When risks and uncertainties are enacted, new discourses, institutions and technologies are then triggered in attempts to contain them. Mosquito eradication and control programmes serve to control and repress the lives of those they mean to save. In the end, people and mosquitoes are resistant to these top-down political pressures. Both are unruly. Both are beyond control.

Natal and the digital mosquitoes

"Here, everything is digital, even mosquitoes," said Lucas about the new approach to monitoring dengue epidemics in Natal, named vigi@dengue. Using traps scattered throughout the city and having an *"at"* in its name, this digital tracking system aimed to produce a high-tech update on local public health policy (Natal 2015).

Entomological data from the traps is combined with epidemiological data provided by the local healthcare system, detailing the exact location of people either sick with dengue or suspect of being infected by the virus. Cross-checking the locations of notified patients and mosquito eggs found in the traps indicates virtual territories of risk on the city map.

Coloured circles that vary from white to red according to the "danger," highlight potential areas of risk. The epidemic risk is an imaginary value calculated by the virtual presence of mosquitoes and sick people in the same space. Red circles are designated as "combat zones," in which mosquito workers are supposed to take a series of measures required by the Ministry of Health (Brasil

2005, 2009). These measures include using pesticides to combat mosquitoes inside houses and other private properties. *Aedes aegypti* is the enemy; workers must visit all residences, check for breeding places, and eliminate them (Segata 2016a, 2016b, 2017).

Public health policymakers used to say that with technology, one can run but never hide: for them, vigi@dengue creates a sense of omnipresence and effectiveness. Indeed, technocratic fantasies about real-time monitoring have recently become a trend in epidemic surveillance systems (Caduff 2014a, 2014b, 2015, Lakoff 2015, 2017, MacPhail 2014). New digital technologies promote trust in more precise identification of risks and their control. The problem is that humans and mosquitoes do not always behave like binary codes.

The vigi@dengue was inaugurated in late 2015. Local newspapers praised the programme, heralding that the city was finally armed against the mosquito. The programme managers were already talking about delegations of politicians coming from other cities and districts interested in learning about it. Some of the mosquito workers, however, were less enthusiastic. Indeed, the project had some problems. They usually complained that "working with mosquitoes is not easy."

The first problem is that vigi@dengue's software receives inconsistent data, caused mainly by under-reporting of disease cases. Since access to medical services may be difficult in Brazil (Biehl et al. 2012, Biehl 2013), many ill people in Natal did not even bother to seek professional medical treatment, complaining about delays in care and the lack of proper care. Instead of waiting in long lines at the hospitals, they went directly to pharmacies. When someone caught dengue, Zika or chikungunya, the common treatment was simply to stay home, drink more water and treat symptoms such as temperature and pain with home remedies. Such patients went "under the radar" of the health system, and their cases were not included in the data.

A second problem is the weak correlation between infections data and mosquito data. Most of the information comes from the perspective of entomology overestimating the presence of mosquitoes. Epidemiological data considers patients' home addresses, but people can be bitten anytime and everywhere, whether at work, while commuting, or at leisure time (Segata 2017, 2019). The "enemy" does not always live in one's backyard.

A third problem is that the number of mosquitoes is estimated according to the quantity of eggs found. The number of eggs, in turn, is figured out by the surface these occupy on the trap, since mosquito eggs are too small to be numbered. As Lucas says, "you must have *a manha,*" with *manha* being slang for a kind of skill acquired in daily experience. "Mosquito eggs look like ground coffee," he said. "You only give a peek, and kick a number." Official reports constantly claim that 90% of eggs are those of *Aedes aegypti*, although this is not tested. Additionally, eggs are not checked for the presence of viruses. All such estimates are built on the assumption that the presence of mosquitoes in a certain area is sufficient to explain the incidence of the disease. The keyword in this game is probability—what philosopher Ian Hacking (2002) defined as a kind of "guide to life" which never freed itself from subjective functions of interpretation and belief. Probability is not a method, but is aimed at a goal, supported by the empowerment of numbers. Similarly, entomological data derived from the vigi@dengue's algorithm came from a mix of practice, sensitivity, popular mathematics and haste. Sometimes, the accuracy of computational calculation must count on luck (Segata 2017).

Prophets of Porto Alegre

It was Friday and everything seemed calm in the Vectors and Rodents Office of the Porto Alegre Department of Health. As we were talking about the unstable weather, the low number of mosquitoes and the uncertainty about renewing the contract with the company conducting mosquito DNA tests, the phone rang. Ligia answered, and after listening silently for a while she pulled out the computer screen to check some maps. Following a short conversation, she hung up the phone and explained that people were calling to report mosquitoes in their vicinity.

> People find mosquitoes in their house or on a nearby street and complain. But we know something about mosquitoes, and monitor everything … In the past, people were moving from door to door applying poison and killing mosquitoes wherever they could find them, but now we try to find out if they are dangerous or not … So you don't need to worry: if they don't carry a virus, they don't have a disease. Most mosquitoes are healthy. We have to learn to live with them, not all of them are bad.
>
> (Ligia, Public Policy Manager, Municipal Health
> Department. Porto Alegre, April 2017)

"Creating a new concept is part of the job," Ligia said, ending the conversation by complaining that "working with people is not easy." She argued that people assume that mosquitoes are not monitored nor does the department know which ones are infected. The popular belief was that the authorities were lying, and that nobody cares about their complaints.

Public authorities use modern technologies in Porto Alegre as well, but there they use traps to catch adult mosquitoes for DNA mapping rather than relying on eggs (Vargas 2018, Segata 2018a). More than 1,200 traps are set and geolocated, each carrying a QR code to identify it (Figure 11.1). Mosquitoes caught in them are mailed on a weekly basis to Belo Horizonte, as each mosquito sample corresponds to a specific trap. Their DNA is sequenced using PCR (polymerase chain reaction) technology, and when a virus is detected, the laboratory in Belo Horizonte warns the Department of Health in Porto Alegre. This data enables the Department of Health to locate infected areas (Figure 11.2a, Figure 11.2b).

The Department of Health operates a website called "Onde está o Aedes?" (Where is the Aedes?), which provides maps with information about the presence

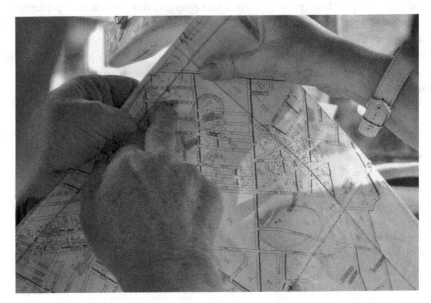

FIGURE 11.1 Mosquito workers planning an intervention in Porto Alegre, May 2018. Photograph by Jean Segata.

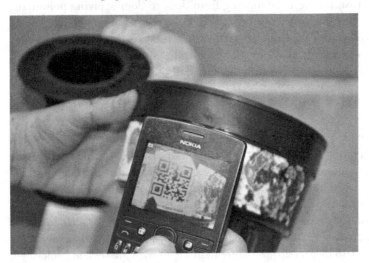

FIGURE 11.2A Inspecting a mosquito trap in Porto Alegre, May 2018. Photograph by Jean Segata.

of mosquitoes and viruses: Zika, dengue, chikungunya and, recently, yellow fever as well. In addition, the website presents tables and graphs with information about the origins of the virus in various locations: when it appeared, and whether humans were infected, or just mosquitoes. "The mosquito is our partner," Ligia told me. "People *must* learn to live with them. You can see on the map, our

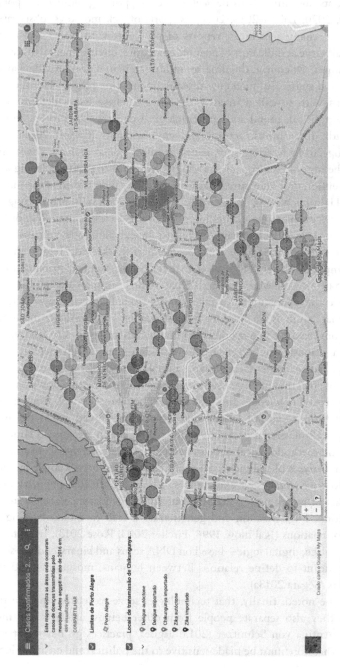

FIGURE 11.2B "Onde está o Aedes?" screenshot of the website (open access). The map pointed to the presence of local and imported dengue, Zika and chikungunya viruses in 2016. Photograph by Jean Segata.

mosquitoes are healthy and they help us fight the virus," Ligia explained: in Porto Alegre, the mosquito was even deemed a sort of prophet, by providing a set of indices that may predict epidemics.

Using mosquitoes to predict epidemics reflects a recent trend in science that relies on plants and animals to be *sentinels* for supporting biosecurity policies (Keck 2009, 2020, Lakoff 2015, 2017). Reports of sick monkeys, observations of behavioural changes in birds, reports of problems with plants and marine creatures—all serve as indicators of possible epidemics, environmental disasters or climatic changes. Of course, the illnesses of human beings also provide warning signs: avian and swine flu, mad cow disease, pneumonic plague, Leishmaniasis and problems with so-called invasive species—all these issues determine the shape of the political, moral and epistemological debates that involve animals, human health, their infrastructures and environments (Caduff 2014a, Keck 2010, Nading 2014). Keeping such issues in mind, social anthropologists have developed the idea of "multispecies ethnography" with the aim of placing at the centre of attention those creatures that were formerly maintained at the margins (Kirksey & Helmreich 2010, Tsing 2012). As a result, "animals, plants, fungi and microbes once confined in anthropological accounts to the realm of *zoe* or 'bare life'—that which is killable—have started to appear alongside humans in the realm of *bios, with legibly biographical and political lives* (Kirksey & Helmreich 2010: 545–546, emphasis mine). Thus, next to Lévi-Strauss's encyclopaedic animals are "good to think" and Marvin Harris's materialistic animals are "good to eat," we now have the opportunity to take lessons from Donna Haraway's (2007) suggestion that "animals are good for living together." Porto Alegre mosquitoes have been converted into co-workers helping health authorities to find viruses. Taking them seriously can be very useful in studying humans in society.

Despite such developments in human–animal relations, the government's new digital tools of epidemic intelligence still operate in the same top-down tradition that hierarchizes knowledge and practices. They are derived from applied science, and form a type of laboratorial experiment spread across the world (Segata 2018b). Professional decisions about public health are guided largely by theoretical and methodological choices rooted in techno-scientific assumptions than by rich analyses of individual environments, indigenous knowledge, local practices and tried-and-tested experiences. The most affected populations are often not part of public policy-making, but rather mandatory partners in their implementation. Digitalization and geneticization lead to molecularizing and squelching of relations (Rabinow 1996, Fischer 2003, Rose 2013). In Natal and Porto Alegre alike, digital logic—based on DNA scans and binary codes—shapes the devices meant to define relations between humans, mosquitoes and their environments (Segata 2018a).

It should be noted, finally, that technologies serve to separate people from people, but they also separate people from other beings, artefacts and moral regimes. As Antina von Schnitzer (2013) argues, practices go beyond specific projects and therefore must be made sensitive to the political and creative sides of technologies. I first heard about the "Onde está o Aedes?" website when I went to live in Porto Alegre in 2016. When searching for an apartment there, I was told by a real estate broker that the Moinhos de Vento neighbourhood would be a good choice. At his office, the broker turned to his laptop, and pointing to the government map said: "Look on the screen, here you're going be free of mosquitoes. It's always green." The small inconsistency, though, is that no traps are set in Moinhos de Vento. Both in Porto Alegre and Natal, traps are not placed in prosperous neighbourhoods. Authorities do indeed find mosquitoes, but exactly where they want to find them: among poor people.

Recalcitrance, uncertainties and futures

"You gotta find the enemy before it finds you," Ligia told me in an effort to justify her software, data-mining systems and PCR budget. "You must always be prepared ... As long as there are mosquitoes, there will be new biosecurity products." What she said reinforces the impression that biosecurity emerges as a global project for converting public health into a security issue. The merging of health and safety and the scaling up of the production of biosecurity goods and services has often been justified by a flexible idea of globalization: presumably, the expanding production of animal and vegetable products and their international trade—together with the global circulation of human beings—necessitate it, with modern microbiology facilitating it. This explanation, however, is not the whole story, and other explanations come to mind.

For Stephen Collier (2011), there is a tendency to transfer public health to a state of mind that almost disappeared at the end of the Cold War. This tendency to conflate safety with health was enhanced during the emergence of influenza in the early twentieth century, especially avian and swine flus, but also Ebola and more recently Zika and the COVID-19 pandemic. The global economy's vulnerability to terrorism materialized not only in the 2001 attack on the Twin Towers, but also in the bioterrorism manifested in anthrax letters dispatched the same year. Spurred on by speeches promising catastrophes, these events revived an imagery of threats ranging from nuclear bombs to mutant and antibiotic-resistant superbugs or deadly strains of a sleeping virus able to cross oceans on commercial aircraft (Caduff 2014a). Biosecurity launched a variety of messages: in Europe, the term became linked to food security and the handling of agricultural and livestock products; in Australia, biosecurity signified reducing negative effects of invasive species; and in the United States, the term addressed dangers of human contamination by biological agents, whether from zoonotic diseases or the pathogens of bioterrorism (Bingham & Hinchliffe 2008). Biosecurity policies and practices are typically woven within local contexts, although they almost always import problems and solutions from the Global North to the Global South. In the end, events described as threats on a global scale have mobilized new economies of risk, prevention and response to epidemics. Biosecurity is the buzzword that health capitalism uses to fuse health and security into a single commodity (Segata 2020).

The *Aedes aegypti* mosquito is one of the most sophisticated technologies created by tropical medicine since it causes epidemics (Benchimol 2001, 2011, Segata 2018a). For more than 100 years, this mosquito has been widely known to transmit the viruses of yellow fever and dengue, and more recently those of chikungunya and Zika. This little insect has subsequently become part of the infrastructure of science and health policies (Löwy 2006, Segata 2018a): although the diseases are quite different, they are all shaped by mosquitoes; accordingly, most public health policies surrounding these diseases rely on the monolithic method of killing mosquitoes with pesticides (Augusto et al. 1998). Mosquito-centrism is the principal symptom of our health policies. It is as persistent as the militarization of those policies.

The discovery of the mosquito's role as a disease vector went hand in hand with the beginning of US interventions in Latin America. The movement for the independence of Cuba and the construction of the Panama Canal provide two examples: in both cases, yellow fever began killing people. So, when General William Gorgas took action against the disease, the mosquito became an enemy and the war against it began: enemies and warfare, but also territories, campaigns, mapping, control, combat and struggle (Espinosa 2009, Löwy 2006, 2017, McNeill 2010, Stepan 2011). Military semantics were everywhere, and they were especially prevalent when the Rockefeller Foundation led the great campaign against yellow fever in Latin America from the 1920s to the 1950s, with the secret weapon unveiled as DDT. It sought to "kill the enemy before it killed us." Rockefeller Foundation experts established an international standard known as the "mosquito index" which measured the effectiveness of health programmes based on the link between mosquito habitats and human habits. Based on this logic, efficient mosquito control involved surveillance and joint control of humans, the insects that preyed upon them, and the territories they both shared (Löwy 1990, 1996, 1999, 2006, Segata 2017).

In the lexicon of an epidemic, the virus is an "invisible enemy," a "terrorist" that must be "fought." In arming themselves to defeat this microscopic enemy, epidemiologists must turn on the vector, for it has wings and can be neutralized with the push of a spray nozzle. The mosquito therefore becomes enemy number one, because it can be attacked. The metric tons of poison, the heaps of dead animals, the transformed environments are the war-torn landscapes of an extended mosquito battle, still not won.

This imagery is even older. Before the mosquito, theories of miasmas and contagion supported hygienist policies in Latin America and the Caribbean. In Rio de Janeiro, sanitary policies led to the destruction of *cortiços*, or dense housing developments: poor and black people were persecuted and expelled from city centres under the accusation that they were dirty and dangerous (Figure 11.3a, Figure 11.3b). Pasteurian theories led Oswaldo Cruz and his colleagues to force vaccinations on the population and invade private homes to apply pesticides (Benchimol 1992, 2001, 2003, Chalhoub 1993, 2013). Social politics reinforced microbial politics: as humans, their bodies and territories came to be controlled

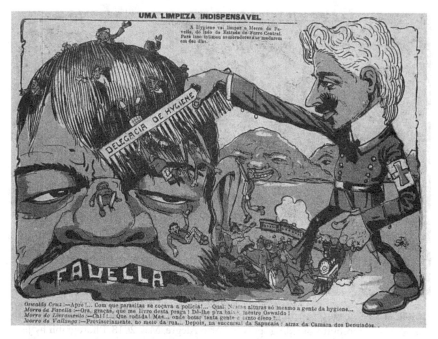

FIGURE 11.3A Caricature of Oswaldo Cruz "cleaning up" the Morro da Favela (Rio de Janeiro) published in Jornal O Malho, 8 June 1907. The criticism was that sanitary policies classified poor people and microbes as threats to the development of the nation. Unknown author.

by the state at the end of nineteenth century; microbes revealed by Pasteur would also come under state control. Hygienists and government employees established standards for what they believed to be "pure" social relations, that is, relations that would not be derailed by microbial eruptions, relations that could be predicted, and therefore rationally ordered (Paxson 2008).

The point is that despite DNA and new digital technologies, policies act in the same exclusionary manner as they did a century ago. Geolocation of breeding sites supports the maintenance and the production of distorted moralities and heightened inequalities (Segata 2016a, 2016b). In Natal, the lack of running water in poor neighbourhoods means that people must store water in buckets, where mosquitoes lay eggs. But referring only to the presence of mosquitoes takes an infrastructural issue and renders it an issue of personal responsibility amongst the poor. I found that during my fieldwork, personal responsibility for mosquitoes caused tense situations in which declarations about "the neighbour's mosquitoes" or "people with the red spot" became accusatory categories. Living in a red-designated area is an accusation of being dirty—and hence having both one's physical property and social status devalued.

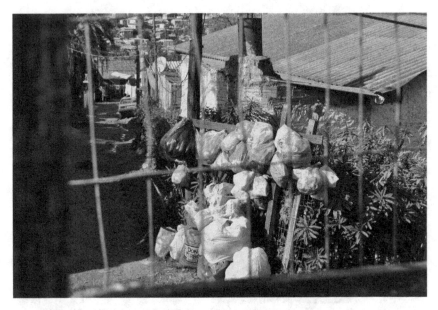

FIGURE 11.3B Current situation in low-income communities in Brazil. Area with mosquito breeding spots in Porto Alegre, May 2018. Photograph by Jean Segata.

The outcome is that the mere act of control or testing of a house for mosquitoes is conceived as a threat. As Lucas once said,

> You must go from door to door and hunt the mosquito, but people don't like it ... They become furious because they think we're accusing them of being the "owners of the mosquito." They're just living their lives, and we're just doing our mission, but people think we're persecuting them because they might be dirty and guilty. It's not true, but I don't get involved: I don't want to take a bullet—something which has happened.
>
> *(Lucas, mosquito worker. Natal, November 2015)*

In Natal, simply receiving a visit makes one into a "polluter," meaning that this person is the reason others get sick. As Lucas mentioned, conflicts are common, including violence against health agents (Segata 2017). Moreover, the virtual software makes the actual suffering invisible. The software never touches the ground and requires no physical protection, while the workers do. All the workers I lived with in Natal had already fallen ill with dengue, Zika or chikungunya. They were not given repellent, appropriate clothing, even sunscreen, and the poisons they used were also handled without gloves (Segata 2018b).

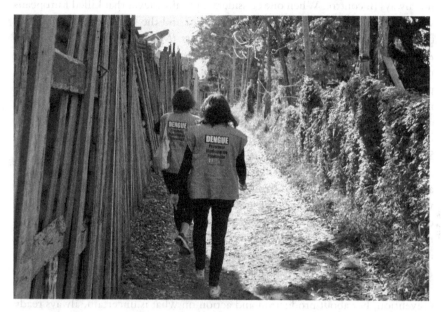

FIGURE 11.4 Doing fieldwork among mosquito workers. Porto Alegre, May–June 2018.
Photograph by Jean Segata.

In Porto Alegre, the government has implemented one of the most innovative public policies in Brazil by controlling disease through sequencing mosquito DNA. The technology is enchanting, but it contrasts dramatically with the fact that in one of the Brazilian cities with the highest per capita income, 44% of the population still do not have basic sanitation (Segata 2018b). Porto Alegre uses PCR for identifying mosquitoes, but lacks the most basic infrastructure of sealed and separated pipes for carrying drinking water and sewage. Although mosquito traps here are placed only in poor areas, some of the people who get sick live in wealthy neighbourhoods. Ashamed of getting "a poor person's disease," these dengue victims often hide being sick (Figure 11.4).

The other health workers in Porto Alegre that help locate viruses are the mosquitoes. Their terms of work are harsh: after all, some of them get caught in traps, and if they're found alive, they are usually crushed with the tip of a toothpick, intubated, and centrifuged in a laboratory to finish their careers as "genetic material" on a microscope slide. Sentient as they may be, mosquitoes nonetheless become a killable otherness. They do not receive the same respect as dogs suffering from Leishmaniasis, whose conviviality and contagion mobilize broad efforts of care and moral debate (Lewgoy et al. 2020). Mosquitoes are hardly animate creatures, and certainly not "persons" like dogs. They don't even have a face, as Lévinas (1984) might point out—and therefore they do not deserve moral consideration.

But mosquitoes are resistant. They are like the mushrooms that Anna Tsing describes in her travels: unruly (Tsing 2005, 2012). They remind us that we are not always in control. When one considers the yellow fever that killed Europeans who reached the warm sands of Latin America and the Caribbean, one realizes that mosquitoes were the first anti-colonialists (McNeill 2010). They resisted America's whitening, as well as the pesticide industry and global health imperialism. They always come back—even if it may take a while—and they make policy managers a little worried when they do not reappear immediately. Too much or too little rain may destroy their eggs, for example. Carlos complained about this when I asked him about yellow fever in Natal: "The mosquitoes were not collaborating that year," he explained. The epidemic investigation might fail. Sometimes mosquitoes are not very skilled with politics.

A lack of mosquitoes seems like a good sign, except for the mosquito workers and professional politicians. These both need the "mosquito's salary" to live, and without mosquitoes, budgets are not renewed. Beyond any dreams of control or eradication, health authorities must convince the federal government that mosquitoes still pose a threat. There is a political calculation to be made, and that is why computer models use historical information to predict future scenarios. A virtual catastrophe of an uncertain tomorrow, based on data from the past, justifies the costs and the structures of the present. The "struggle" is not about prevention, but about production and action on what is uncertain, always ready to get out of control. Uncertainty has become a subject of its own in global health policy. "Being alert and prepared" is a condition of suspending the present to create "the promise of infrastructure" (Appel et al. 2018). Such infrastructure produces expectations, allocates life—and in my case—offers false certainties in the form of digital technologies and genetic codes.

Conclusions

Beyond declarations of control and eradication, human–mosquito relations in Brazil are manifested in politics. New technologies and practices support a complex space of power. DNA and algorithms work on the same mathematical principle, and both may be expressed digitally: software or combinations of acids and proteins inscribe realities supported by confidence in computational calculation and in the universal materiality of biology. Although the world is not digital, our modern way of managing it has become so. Yet we cannot confuse genetic and computational modelling with life itself.

Digital life technologies are integral to new global infrastructures of health capitalism, manifested in information packages such as those used in Natal and Porto Alegre. At the beginning of the twentieth century, the internationalization of public health was based on technologies aimed at killing microbes; today, it is time to sell powerful global programmes aimed at managing local public policies. The goal for public health is still the same: surveillance and control of populations and territories. Now, however, the interest shifts from preventing widespread risk to "predicting enacted threats." These associated intelligences do not prevent epidemics from happening, but they do predict a future for which we must prepare. A large task of health workers is to produce data to feed to predictive technologies, rather than acting on concrete problems of the present. As Gerda Reith (2004) explains, risk helps us to colonize the future—with ongoing anti-mosquito policies depending precisely on this. The problem is that for all of this to function, "everyone must do their part," including, of course, people, but also mosquitoes, epidemiology, entomology, algorithms and viruses. As my colleague Carlos once concluded,

> "mosquitoes are a gold mine and each epidemic is a blank check. But they have to be more discreet and collaborate with us: if we show up too much, we must kill them; but if they are eradicated, the money won't come".
>
> *(Carlos, mosquito worker. Natal, November 2015)*

A lot of information has been produced by the intel of these new epidemics: maps, indexes, historical series, data sets that promise predictive ability and best response. But when monkeys started to die in Natal, mosquito workers did not know if yellow fever was coming back. The time of the disease did not coincide with the time of information, much less with that of bureaucracy. Digitalized and prophet mosquitoes are not always able to foresee new epidemics. They nonetheless help in predicting budgets that support the continuity of the few public health policies. In the right quantities, they are good partners.

Notes

1 This chapter is based on a talk presented at the Princeton University in December 2018. I am grateful to João Biehl for the invitation, and to Alex Nading and Amy Moran-Thomas for comments during the writing. I am also grateful to Jessica Leinaweaver for the support and favourable environment for teaching and research during my stay at the Center for Latin American and Caribbean Studies at Brown University, and to Andrea Mastrangelo at the Centro Nacional de Diagnóstico e Investigación en Endemoepidemias – CeNDIE of the Ministry of Health, Argentina. The research was supported with grants from CNPq (The Brazilian National Council for Scientific and Technological Development) and from CONICET (National Scientific and Technical Research Council of Argentina). An earlier version of this chapter was published in Spanish in the Colombian Journal *Tabula Rasa* (Segata 2019).

2 In this context, an important guide to my work is the intersection of ideas as "architectures of domestication" in David Andersons et al.'s (2017), also the idea of "infrastructure" as used by Susan Star (1999) and Bryan Larkin (2013) and of the "ontological politics" of Annemarie Mol (1999). Infrastructure refers to a subtle apparatus of governmentality that includes artefacts, institutions, discourses and knowledge (Star 1999). The elements that form these apparatuses cannot be reduced to a type of neutral stage where science and politics take place—before this, an infrastructure is also *political* (and *makes* politics).

Bibliography

Anderson, D., et al. 2017. Architectures of domestication: On emplacing human-animal relations in the North. *Journal of the Royal Anthropological Institute*, 23(2): 398–416.

Appel, H., Anand, N., Gupta, A. 2018. Introduction: Temporality, politics, and the promise of infrastructure. In Anand, N., Gupta, A., Appel, H., eds. *The Promise of Infrastructure*. Durham: Duke University Press, 1–41.

Augusto, L., Torrez, J.P., Costa, A., Pontez, C., Novaez, T. 1998. Programa de erradicação do *Aedes aegypti*: Inócuo e perigoso (e ainda perdulário). *Cadernos de Saúde Pública*, 14(4): 876–877.

Benchimol, J. 1992. *Pereira Passos —um Haussmann Tropical: A renovação urbana do Rio de Janeiro no início do século XX*. 2a. ed. Rio de Janeiro: Secretaria Municipal de Cultura, Turismo e Esportes.

Benchimol, J. 1999. *Dos micróbios aos mosquitos: Febre amarela e a revolução pasteuriana no Brasil*. Rio de Janeiro: EdUFRJ/Editora Fiocruz.

Benchimol, J. 2001. *Febre amarela: A doença e a vacina, uma história inacabada*. Rio de Janeiro: Editora Fiocruz.

Benchimol, J. 2003. Reforma urbana e revolta da vacina na cidade do Rio de Janeiro. In Ferreira, J., Neves, A., eds. *O Brasil republicano: Economia e sociedade, poder e política, cultura e representações*. Rio de Janeiro: Civilização Brasileira, 231–286.

Benchimol, J. 2011. *Mosquitos, doenças e ambientes em perspectiva. Anais do XXVI Simpósio Nacional de História*. São Paulo: ANPUH, 1–15.

Bingham, N.; Hinchliffe, S. 2008. Mapping the multiplicities of biosecurity. In Collier, S., Lakoff, A., eds. *Biosecurity Interventions: Global Health and Security in Question*. New York: Columbia University Press, 173–194.

Biehl, J., Amon, J.J., Socal, M.P., Petrina, A. 2012. Between the court and the clinic: Lawsuits for medicines and the right to health in Brazil. *Health and Human Rights: An International Journal*, 14(1): 1–17.

Biehl, J. 2013. The judicialization of biopolitics: Claiming the right to pharmaceuticals in Brazilian courts. *American Ethnologist*, 40(3): 419–436.

Brasil. 2005. *Ministério da Saúde, Secretaria de Vigilância em Saúde, Diretoria Técnica de Gestão. Diagnóstico rápido nos municípios para vigilância entomológica do Aedes Aegypti no Brasil - LIRAa: Metodologia para os índices Breteau e Predial*. Brasília: Ministério da Saúde.

Brasil. 2009. *Ministério da Saúde, Secretaria de Vigilância em Saúde, Departamento de Vigilância Epidemiológica. Diretrizes nacionais para a prevenção e controle de epidemias de dengue*. Brasília: Ministério da Saúde.

Caduff, C. 2014a. On the verge of death: Visions of biological vulnerability. *Annual Review of Anthropology*, 43: 105–21.

Caduff, C. 2014b. Sick weather ahead: On data-mining, crowd-sourcing and white noise. *Cambridge Anthropology*, 32(1): 32–46.

Caduff, C. 2015. *The Pandemic Perhaps: Dramatic Events in a Public Culture of Danger*. Berkeley: University of California Press.

Chalhoub, S. 1993. The politics of disease control: Yellow fever and race in Nineteenth Century Rio de Janeiro. *Journal of Latin American Studies*, 25: 441–463.

Chalhoub, S. 2013. *A cidade febril: Cortiços e epidemias na corte imperial*. São Paulo: Companhia das Letras.

Collier, S. 2011. *Post-Soviet Social: Neoliberalism, Social Modernity, Biopolitics*. Princeton: Princeton University Press.

Collier, S., Lakoff, A. 2008. The problem of securing health. Mapping the multiplicities of biosecurity. In Collier, S., Lakoff, A., eds. *Biosecurity Interventions: Global Health and Security in Question*. New York: Columbia University Press, 7–32.

Escobar, A. 2016. Bem-vindos à Cyberia: Notas para uma antropologia da cibercultura. In Segata, J., Rifiotis, T., eds. *Políticas etnográficas no campo da cibercultura*. Brasília: ABA Publicações, 21–66.

Espinosa, M. 2009. *Epidemic Invasions: Yellow Fever and the Limits of Cuban Independence, 1878–1930*. Chicago: University of Chicago Press.

Fassin, D. 2013. *Enforcing Order: An Ethnography of Urban Policing*. Malden: Polity Press.

Fischer, M. 2003. *Emergent Forms of Life and the Anthropological Voice*. Durham: Duke University Press.

Hacking, I. 2002. *L'émergence de la Probabilité*. Paris: Seuil, 2002.

Haraway, D. 2007. *When Species Meet*. Minneapolis: University of Minnesota Press.

Keck, F. 2009. Conflits d'experts: Les zoonoses, entre santé animale et santé humaine. *Ethnologie française*, XXXIX(1): 79–88.

Keck, F. 2010. *Un monde grippé*. Paris: Flammarion.

Keck, F. 2020. *Avian reservoirs: Virus hunters and birdwatchers in Chinese sentinel posts*. Durham: Duke University Press.

Kirksey, E., Helmreich, S. 2010. The emergence of multispecies ethnography. *Cultural Anthropology*, 25(4): 545–576.

Lakoff, A. 2008. From population to vital system: National security and the changing object of public health: Mapping the multiplicities of biosecurity. In Collier, S., Lakoff, A., eds. *Biosecurity interventions: Global Health and Security in Question*. New York: Columbia University Press, 33–61.

Lakoff, A. 2015. Real-time biopolitics: The actuary and the sentinel in global public health. *Economy and Society*, 44(1): 40–59.

Lakoff, A. 2017. *Unprepared: Global Health in a Time of Emergence*. Berkeley: University of California Press.

Larkin, B. 2013. The politics and poetics of infrastructure. *Annual Review of Anthropology*, 42: 327–343.

Latour, B., Woolgar, S. 1997. *A Vida de laboratório: A produção dos fatos científicos*. Rio de Janeiro: Relume Dumará.

Lévinas, E. 1984. *Éthique et Infini*. Paris: Le Livre de Poche.

Lewgoy, B., Mastrangelo, M., Beck, L. 2020. Tanatopolítica e biossegurança: Dois regimes de governo da vida para a Leishmaniose Visceral Canina no Brasil. *Horizontes Antropológicos*, 26(57): 145–176.

Löwy, I. 1990. Yellow fever in Rio de Janeiro and the Pasteur Institute Mission (1901–1905): The transfer of science to the periphery. *Medical History*, 34: 144–163.

Löwy, I. 1996. Éradication de vecteur contre vaccination: La Fondation Rockefeller et la fièvre jaune au Brésil, 1923–1939. In Waast, R., ed. *Médicenes et santé* (Les sciences hors d'Occident au XXe Siècle - Vol. 4). Paris: Orstom Édition/IRD, 91–108.

Löwy, I. 1999. Representação e intervenção em saúde pública: Vírus, mosquitos e especialistas da Fundação Rockefeller no Brasil. *História, Ciências, Saúde - Manguinhos*, 3: 647–677.

Löwy, I. 2006. *Vírus, mosquitos e modernidade: A febre amarela no Brasil entre ciência e política*. Rio de Janeiro: Editora Fiocruz.

Löwy, I. 2017. Leaking containers: Success and failure in controlling the mosquito *Aedes aegypti* in Brazil. *American Journal of Public Health*, 107(4): 517–524.

MacPhail, T. 2014. *The Viral Network: A Pathography of the H1N1 Influenza Pandemic*. Ithaca: Cornell University Press.

Mason, K. 2016. *Infectious Change: Reinventing Chinese Public Health after an Epidemic*. Stanford: Stanford University Press.

McNeill, J.R. 2010. *Mosquito Empires: Ecology and war in the Greater Caribbean, 1620–1914*. Cambridge: Cambridge University Press.

Mol, A. 1999. Ontological politics: A word and some questions. In Law, J., ed. *Actor Network Theory and after*. London: Blackwell, 74–89.

Nading, A. 2014. *Mosquito Trails: Ecology, Health and the Politics of Entanglement*. Berkeley: University of California Press.

Natal. 2015. *Vigi@dengue: nova abordagem na vigilância de dengue e outras arboviroses no município de Natal*. Natal: Secretaria Municipal de Saúde, Departamento de Vigilância em Saúde, Centro de Controle de Zoonoses (*PowerPoint presentation*).

Paxson, H. 2008. Post-Pasteurian cultures: The microbiopolitics of raw-milk cheese in the United States. *Cultural Anthropology*, 23(1): 15–47.

Rabinow, P. 1996. *Making PCR: A Story of Biotechnology*. Chicago: University of Chicago Press.

Reis-Castro, L., Heidrickx, K. 2013. Winged promises: Exploring the discourse on transgenic mosquitoes in Brazil. *Technology in Society*, 35: 118–128.

Reith, G. 2004. Uncertain times: The notion of 'risk' and the development of modernity. *Time & Society*, 13(2–3): 383–402.

Rose, N. 2013. *A política da própria vida: Biomedicina, poder e subjetividade no Século XXI*. São Paulo: Paulus.

Secretaria Municipal de Saúde. 2015. Secretaria municipal de Saúde, Departamento de Vigilância em Saúde, Centro de Controle de Zoonoses. *Vigi@dengue: Nova abordagem na vigilância de dengue e outras arboviroses no município de Natal*. Natal, (mimeo).

Segata, J. 2016a. A doença socialista e o mosquito dos pobres. *Iluminuras*, 17(42): 372–389.

Segata, J. 2016b. Os mosquitos vilões e as casas de ponta de lápis. *VI Congresso da Associação Portuguesa de Antropologia*. Coimbra.

Segata, J. 2017. O *Aedes aegypti* e o digital. *Horizontes Antropológicos*, 48(23): 19–48.

Segata, J. 2018a. Virus, algorithmics and DNA: Anthropology and new epidemics intelligence. *Symposium - Global Epidemics, Local Anthropologies? 18th IUAES World Congress*, Florianópolis.

Segata, J. 2018b. *Cuando la epidemia nos viola. Seminario Internacional Convivencia y contágio: El rol del antropólogo en las relaciones sociedad-naturaleza-enfermidad*. Argentina: IDAES, Universidad Nacional de San Martin.

Segata, J. 2019. El mosquito-oráculo y otras tecnologías. *Tabula Rasa*, 32: 103–125.

Segata, J. 2020. Covid-19, biossegurança e antropologia. *Horizontes Antropológicos* 26(57): 275–313.

Star, S. 1999. The ethnography of infrastructure. *American Behavioral Scientist*, 43(3): 377–391.

Stepan, N. 2011. *Eradication: Ridding the World of Diseases Forever?* London: Reaktion Books.

Tsing, A. 2005. *Friction: An Ethnography of Global Connection*. Princeton: Princeton University Press.

Tsing, A. 2012. Unruly Edges: Mushrooms as Companion Species: For Donna Harraway. *Environmental Humanities*, 1: 141–154.

Vargas, E. 2018. *Mosquitos, armadilhas e vírus: etnografia de uma política pública de controle ao Aedes aegypti*. Dissertação (Mestrado). Instituto de Filosofia e Ciências Humanas, Programa de Pós-Graduação em Antropologia Social. Porto Alegre: Universidade Federal do Rio Grande do Sul.

Von Schnitzer, A. 2013. Traveling Technologies: Infrastructures, ethical regimes, and the materiality of politics in South Africa. *Cultural Anthropology*, 8(4): 670–693.

12

ERADICATION AGAINST AMBIVALENCE

Alex Nading

The problem with eradication is that it is an all-or-nothing affair, and the problem with all-or-nothing affairs is that they lead to impoverished thought.

Here is what I mean. When the French structuralist Claude Levi-Strauss famously wrote that animals are "good to think," he meant that we need animals, in all their categorical diversity—the domesticated, the companionate, the hunted, the sacrificial—in order to make sense of the world (Levi-Strauss 1963, 89). What follows is *not*, Reader be assured, a structuralist argument against eradication, but it does seem worth noting that the value of human action is more accurately measured by asking what humans do *with* the world than what they do *to* the world (see e.g. Haraway 2008; Beisel 2010).

One less species walking, swimming or buzzing around the Earth is one less species to "think." With just one less species to think—no matter how unsavoury or dangerous or repulsive that creature may be—humans will be left with fewer political, social and ethical possibilities. Reflecting on my own ethnographic work around mosquitoes, I want to make the case that thought—compound, distributed, interspecies, ecological thought—has public health value. Such thought is anathema to all-or-nothing certainty (Morton 2010). Looking across a variety of mosquito-borne disease control projects, I submit that killing mosquitoes is good for public health not because of the certainty of thought it evinces in humans but because of the ambivalence it produces.

Before moving any further with that provocation, let me clarify that *species eradication* is categorically different from *disease eradication*. There is a fundamental distinction between the social and cultural categories of illness (the experience of ill health) and disease (the pathology that occasions that experience). For example, just a few years ago, the world became briefly consumed with the spread of the mosquito-borne Zika virus, but as long-term anthropological work with Zika-affected families has shown, the illness was anything but indiscriminate. Poor

DOI: 10.4324/9781003056034-12

Black women and children in Brazil fared far worse than others, both during the epidemic and in the years that followed (Diniz 2017). Zika infection causes a range of long-term complications in children born to infected mothers, and while the cost of confronting the epidemic in its acute phase was high, research with affected families in Brazil's northeast reveals how parents of children born with congenital Zika syndrome (CZS) continue to struggle to marshal resources to care for their loved ones (Williamson 2020). A similarly uneven pattern of both morbidity and social suffering emerged for COVID-19, a disease whose eradication seems too far off to contemplate just now. In the United States, data on the race or ethnicity of people with cases of coronavirus show that the rate of death among Black Americans is three times the rate among whites.[1]

Although viruses, arguably, are not species, animal vectors are. Mosquitoes, the most prominent among such vectors, are not charismatic. They occupy an unusually negative niche in the human imagination, just about everywhere. That said, mosquitoes are fascinating creatures, and the ones that transmit diseases among humans are uniquely adapted to the environments humans occupy or build, from rivers to sewers, savannahs to garbage dumps.

What kind of a thought, then, is the thought of eradication? How might it differ, for example, from the thought of extinction? In the popular imagination, the current era of extinction, known as the Sixth Extinction, is frequently understood as a tragic side effect of human–nonhuman encounters: the collateral damage of mass human migration, fossil-fuel burning and logging (Kolbert 2014). Extinction is presented as the practical consequence of human action, less as a thought than as an afterthought. As Thom Van Dooren explains, the purpose of hunting passenger pigeons was not to eradicate them from the Earth, but by 1914, the last passenger pigeon had died (Van Dooren 2014). There are interesting evolutionary biological arguments about the precise mechanism that led to that particular extinction, but it did become a touchstone in nascent conservation and environmental movements. The ethical question that energized those early movements, and which continues to drive many varieties of environmentalism today, concerns what to do about the human capacity to destroy ecosystems, species by species, and how that capacity might be curtailed in the name of sustainability and even health.

If extinction is a side effect and eradication is a purposive endeavour, then it is only the intentionality of the act of killing that seems to distinguish eradication from extinction. Alternatively, we might say that the difference has less to do with what the killer intends than with how the killer reacts. Many humans have reacted to extinction with a combination of horror and sadness—or at least a degree of wistfulness. The human agents of eradication, on the other hand, tend to look on their works with a troubling sense of triumphalism (Stepan 2011).

But neither the mourning that follows extinction nor the anticipatory triumph of eradication are innocent. As Juno Salazar Parreñas (2018, 12) describes, anti-extinction activists view their efforts to save threatened species in decidedly "moral," if mostly secular, terms. A veritable cottage industry of conservation tourism has grown up around efforts to protect endangered orangutans, whales and turtles. Tourists are drawn to exotic locales to participate in conservation because they feel compelled to take responsibility for the harm done to these creatures by extractive industries such as logging or drilling. To an extent, they recognize that the agent of extinction is not humanity writ large, but a particular historical slice of it.

Meanwhile, attempts to eradicate so-called invasive plants and animals (including some mosquito vectors) may hinge on a kind of eco-moralism. In the interest of keeping ecosystems "pristine," or of maintaining landscapes in a form that reflects a valued historical heritage, environmentalists in the United States, for example, have convinced state and federal governments to essentially criminalize the propagation of nutria, Asian carp, kudzu and fire ants. That US environmentalist anxieties about invasive species have arisen alongside right-wing anxieties about the racial and ethnic purity of European and American states is, as Hugh Raffles (2011) argues, more than a historical accident. The landscapes supposedly threatened by invasives are not, of course, "pristine." They are products of white-settler colonialism and the attempted eradication of indigenous people. As Frances Roberts-Gregory (2020) has written, drawing on her environmental research and activism in Southeast Louisiana, spaces of conservation in the United States remain explicitly and implicitly coded as white spaces.

Attempts to both stave off the tragedy of extinction and achieve the triumph of eradication are products of a white, Western and enduringly colonial attitude to the non-human world, in which experts of a certain colour and gender style themselves as the stewards of nature.[2] Such attitudes, to paraphrase Parreñas again, too often cast blame for biological crisis on the very people who interact most intimately with—who often have cultivated a capacity to *think* with—invasive or threatened species (Parreñas 2018, 13). Thinking *with* leads to a renewed appreciation not only of the uniqueness of particular creatures but also of the richness of the ecologies humans and other species create together (see Beisel and Wergin this volume).[3]

Aedes Aegypti, for example

The species of mosquito that has buzzed around much of my anthropological research, *Aedes aegypti*, is a creature whose existence and form as seen from the vantage of evolution looks rather indistinguishable from its existence and form as seen from the vantage of human history. *Ae. Aegypti* is best known as the vector for urban yellow fever, dengue and Zika viruses, but its status as an arbovirus vector *par excellence* is intimately tied to its envelopment in historical events caused and shaped by humans. Human settlement, traffic in enslaved people, wars and colonial trade and agriculture acted as evolutionary drivers in this mosquito's story.

The dengue virus probably originated in Southeast Asia as a "sylvatic" pathogen circulated among primates by *Ae. albopictus* mosquitoes. As human settlements encroached on the forest, peri-sylvatic transmission, in which humans could acquire the virus from apes but weren't particularly good at passing it to one another, became more common. Cases of dengue in humans were probably isolated, rarely resulting in widespread transmission (Gubler and Kuno 1997). Meanwhile, in eastern Africa another peri-sylvatic mosquito, *Ae. aegypti*, slowly began to change its habits, settling in villages and towns and feeding exclusively on humans. Trade in and out of Southeast Asia brought more people to ports, and as the region urbanized, *Ae. aegypti* thrived. As it turned out, the African *Ae. aegypti* was a highly competent carrier of Southeast Asian dengue—even more competent than its cousin *Ae. albopictus*. As people moved from place to place, *Ae. aegypti* moved, too. Already accustomed to laying eggs in gourds and ceramic bowls, it travelled along caravans and trade routes, stowing away on slave ships, drifting to the Indies, back to Africa, and eventually over to the Americas (Endy et al. 2010). By the mid-eighteenth century, at the height of the slave trade, dengue epidemics were occurring regularly in port cities around the world (Slosek 1986).

Through the nineteenth and early twentieth centuries, dengue remained a relatively minor epidemiological problem. World War Two was a watershed moment. The Pacific theatre was the site of road building, airstrip construction and shipping. The bombing and clear-cutting of Southeast Asian landscapes permitted mosquitoes and viral strains to spread as never before. Then, in the years after the war, there was a massive campaign against malaria, yellow fever and dengue mosquitoes, with the insecticide DDT as its centrepiece. That campaign showed some success for a certain period of time. By 1970, the wonder chemical had helped eradicate *Ae. aegypti* from most of the Western Hemisphere. It took just 20 years, however, for the mosquito to return. This return coincided with the era's structural adjustment policies. Implemented at the urging of the World Bank and the International Monetary Fund, structural adjustment policies gutted spending for health and public works. When these austerity measures intersected with intensified global transportation and trade in the late 1980s, dengue emerged as a serious health problem (Castro et al. 2010). Today, the *Ae. Aegypti* mosquito continues to develop resistance to locally applied pesticide regimes (Nading 2017).

Talk of mosquito eradication frequently appeals to the expertise of (mostly Northern, mostly white) entomologists and epidemiologists (Stepan 2011). Many of these scientific experts have cultivated their own capacity to think with mosquitoes, and they frequently share an appreciation of their diversity and even their beauty (see Hawkes, this volume). I still recall listening to one expert, an entomologist, reproduce the perfect pitch of beating mosquito wings with her own voice. Morrison and Lemke in this volume make the convincing case that non-expert publics can learn to think with the mosquitoes that surround them through participation in creative art installations.

Thinking with mosquitoes in Nicaragua

There is another group of people who have cultivated a deep sense of what it means to think with mosquitoes. I am referring to mosquito control workers in Nicaragua who, until recently, relied on organophosphate larvicides to kill *Ae. Aegypti*, but who are now switching to the biological toxin *Bacillus thuringiensis israelensis*, or *Bti*. These mosquito control workers view themselves as eliminators, not eradicators. They are in the business of killing mosquitoes, but not of ridding the Earth, or even their neighbourhoods, of them. This is a difference that makes a difference.

It turns out that it matters how you kill mosquitoes, not just in terms of the chemical you apply but also in the thought you bring to the act. It is of course possible to eliminate lots of mosquito larvae with either organophosphates or *Bti*. Doing so would not take much more thought than crushing a single adult mosquito with the palm of your hand. Mosquito control workers, however, encounter mosquitoes over and over again, in a variety of microhabitats, from upturned cookie jars to chicken troughs to bottle caps. For many of them, this repetition does not make killing rote or mindless. On the contrary, under these circumstances, the labour of killing induces a thoughtful appreciation of the complexity of the worlds shared and shaped by people, insects and microbes.

Mosquito control in Nicaragua is mostly done by low-paid community health workers (CHWs). During my fieldwork outside Managua, most of these CHWs were women who had little formal background in either science or public health (Nading 2014). Like the indigenous inhabitants of Malaysia's Sarawak described by Parreñas (2018), these women are precisely the kinds of people whose perspectives on human–insect relations are too often overlooked in policy. And like the mosquitoes themselves, it is mostly women—who are figured as responsible for managing the domestic spaces where most urban arbovirus vectors breed— who bear an inordinate share of the blame for the persistence of epidemics. If mosquitoes are not killed in high-enough numbers, and if rates of mosquito-borne disease are *too* high, this will be portrayed as a failure of women's domestic labour. Much as the conservationist ideas of nature I discussed above are frequently coded as white, the notion of hygiene in Nicaragua is frequently gendered female.

In brief, the job of the CHW in mosquito control is to think *with* mosquitoes, particularly female mosquitoes, about where to lay eggs. It is in the small, usually domestic bodies of water that harbour *Ae. aegypti* eggs where human and mosquito habitats meet. These might be in palm fronds, bromeliads, washbasins or old automobile tyres. The shared domestic or "interior" lives of humans and mosquitoes are difficult to replicate artificially (Kelly and Lezaun 2017). And it is not enough to "think like a mosquito," for a mosquito never thinks on its own. Mosquitoes move about the world by transducing physical vibrations into nervous-system signals. Their thoughts, then, are inseparable from their surroundings. They are inseparable from the thought that householders bring to

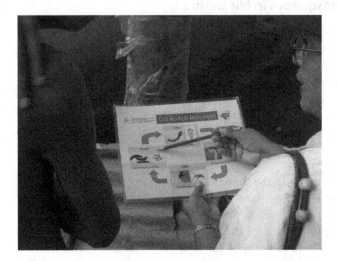

FIGURE 12.1 A Nicaraguan community health worker discussing the *Aedes aegypti* life cycle with a householder. Photograph by Alex Nading.

the arrangement of decorative flowers or the care of domestic animals. To think with mosquitoes is to think with one's kin and neighbours, human and otherwise (Figure 12.1).

One of the things CHWs report over and over again is that they find themselves unable to stop looking for mosquitoes and their breeding grounds, whether at their home, at the homes of others, or elsewhere. They have developed a version of what philosopher Timothy Morton (2010) calls "the ecological thought," the recognition of a deep interconnectedness between beings and things. For Morton, once ecological thought has been planted, it is inescapable. Such thought is neither naive nor unconscious. It entails a recognition of the vast scale of entangled life. Nor is ecological thought a fancy term for New Age fantasy. In the ecological thought, intimacy is as important as vastness and, as Kath Weston (2017) reminds us, intimacy is not always pleasant. Even when we acknowledge that the kind of intimacy between humans and mosquitoes is "full of ambiguity and darkness," it does not follow that the next step is to sever that relationship (Morton 2010, 100).

In the 1960s, the US Department of Agriculture took just this sort of step, justifying its attempts to eradicate fire ants with DDT based on a Cold War–inflected nationalism (Buhs 2004: 385). The view that the "invasive" ant was a threat to the idealized American landscape was opposed by, among others, Rachel Carson, who believed that ecological relations could not be neatly mapped onto the borders of human communities. *Ae. aegypti*, too, has been denigrated as an invasive creature by its self-styled enemies (Nading 2015). As an act that severs some relationships, eradication is simultaneously an act that preserves others. Latent in the discourse of eradication is the notion of a common good.

Who better to carry out the project of eradication, then, than the *community* health worker?

Though he advocates an environmental philosophy rooted in the inescapable relationality of life, Morton rejects the "ecology of community" as a Romantic fallacy (2010, 101; 127). Whereas Carson opposed place-based or nation-based action as inadequately attentive to the scalar dynamics of changing ecosystems, Morton is more concerned with the ways that place-based or nation-based action elides the ambiguity that undergirds all ecological relations. For Morton, community is too clean a term to encompass forms of intimacy like viral transmission or chemical exposure.

Nicaraguan CHWs speak frequently of "community" (*comunidad*). If they are Romantics, they are not rosy-eyed Romantics. *Comunidad* is not so much centred on the geographical place from which they operate (as in the local clinic, or a pandemic's "front-lines" of action) as it is the animating purpose of their mosquito control work. *Comunidad* is a form of becoming, a way of making sense of one's social, professional and environmental surroundings, not a geographical demarcation. Indeed, when presenting themselves to householders around Managua, community health workers would often say, "This *is* community."

In Nicaragua, the figure of the CHW has its origins in the country's 1979 popular Revolution, which was preceded by the 1978 Alma Ata Declaration on primary health care. The Alma Ata Declaration advocated for a horizontal approach to healthcare provision, and it saw low-level figures like CHWs as the actors best positioned to ensure a form of care that was holistic and integrated, rather than targeted and disease-focused. After Alma Ata, the presence of active CHWs in developing countries became a proxy for the political empowerment of underserved populations. After the Revolution, Nicaragua was among the most successful at putting these recommendations into practice. In the early Revolutionary period, roughly from 1979 to 1984, Nicaragua's CHWs styled themselves as *multiplicadores* (multipliers) of public health. They were influenced by a Freirean critical pedagogy, which favoured a dialogical and collaborative approach to learning about and confronting social problems (Freire 1970). Instead of styling themselves as "experts," CHWs banded together to learn *with* their neighbours about health problems and their relationship to underdevelopment. After decades of dictatorship in which most health services had been systematically denied to the majority of Nicaraguans, their hope was that demands for better care would emanate from the grassroots to the centres of political power. Evidence suggests that their advocacy led to improvements in roads, sewers, gutters and potable water systems (Nading 2014).

Among the CHWs with whom I worked between 2006 and 2011, there was a shared sense that hunting for and eliminating (rather than eradicating) mosquitoes in their domestic breeding grounds could double as a fruitful way of doing *comunidad*, of forging solidarity among human neighbours. Peri-urban Managua remains a context of entrenched poverty and low-grade violence. Under these conditions, CHWs, who hail from the same communities in which they hunt for mosquitoes, understand that doing *comunidad* has a public health value on its own. Though their work is closely audited by the Ministry of Health, CHWs are not overly concerned with bureaucratic accounting of how many insects they have killed. To put it pithily, it's the thought that counts. People are more likely to report threats to health and actively monitor the quality of their shared environments if they have regular, meaningful contact with representatives of the public health service. The act of thinking within an ecology—of witnessing and intervening in the intimate relations between humans and mosquitoes (and chickens and dogs and palms and plastic bottles)—yielded public health benefits that did not appear in dengue control records. CHWs regularly confronted householders who would blame neighbours for the presence of dengue and mosquitoes, but they also frequently would expect to relay questions and complaints back to the Ministry of Health, even about health problems beyond dengue. According to the CHWs, effecting a "quality" mosquito control visit meant taking extra time to listen to neighbours' problems and to help solve them. This was the most fulfilling part of their job. *Comunidad* connoted an ecological thought.

Though at first glance it would appear that the presence of mosquitoes was a mere pretence for discussing other health-related matters, Nicaraguan CHWs were not just instrumentalizing the mosquito's presence for a larger purpose. Getting people's attention required attending to—and getting the attention of—mosquitoes (Kelly and Lezaun 2017). The indeterminacy of the encounter (a dengue intervention? a social call? the consciousness-raising work of a Freirean pedagogue?) was the source of its value (Redfield 2016). Finding and destroying the mosquito's breeding ground was also a pathway to fostering solidarity. Mosquitoes were never fully eradicated, just as *comunidad* was never fully realized. This meant that for CHWs, the repetitive, never-quite-complete job of killing mosquitoes was not a chronic failure but a continuous form of sociality. Openness came not from the anticipated triumph of eradication but from the ambiguity and darkness of human–mosquito intimacy. As Morton (2010, 100) summarizes, "If we edit out the ambiguity and darkness, we achieve nothing but aggression." The mosquito could not be abstracted from *comunidad*. The grave threat of mosquitoes had to be confronted as a part of a larger suite of problems (Figure 12.2).

Beyond mosquito killing

The ecological thought that the CHWs call *comunidad* is not limited to mosquito-related endeavours. It resonates through other human–insect encounters. Consider, for example, human encounters with bedbugs, the pests that infest cities around the world, including in the USA, where I live and work. E. Summerson Carr (2015) studied how social workers dealt with bedbugs in a residential facility for homeless people suffering from mental illness and addiction. Carr emphasizes that these social workers do not see their job as one of

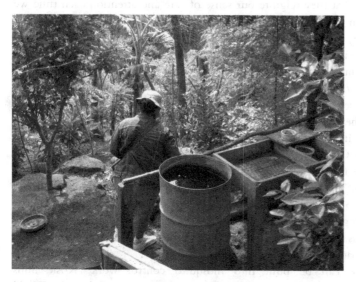

FIGURE 12.2 A community health worker "hunting" for mosquitoes in a domestic house lot. Photograph by Alex Nading.

eradication. Rather, they are constantly (if sometimes frustratingly) doing battle with bedbugs with no simple expectation of triumph. Despite repeated fumigation, the circulation of people and objects through the centre makes total elimination unlikely. For the social workers, "the bedbug infestation provides ... fertile grounds to formulate ideas about the nature, limits, and possibilities of human agency and responsibility, in ways that ultimately bolster"—rather than compromise—their "professional practice." For the social workers, doing a good job means not being "a more *intentional* actor" but rather "a more *attentive* one" (Carr 2015, 264–265). As Ann Kelly and Javier Lezaun explain with regard to mosquitoes, attention "describes ... a double movement: granting attention to and capturing the attention of" (2017, 388).

It may therefore be the partiality and ambiguity of mosquito killing, not its totality, that can translate into a sustained commitment to public health. Here, I use the term "public health" in its broadest sense, not only as a project of managing specific diseases such as malaria and dengue fever, but also as project of improving infrastructure, reducing crime and providing access to food and water, among other things. All current approaches to *Ae. aegypti* control, from systematic house-to-house larviciding, to genetic modification, to *Wolbachia* application, are incomplete successes. Evidence shows that the common thread across these approaches is not a sense of triumph but one of ambivalence (Reis-Castro 2012; Kelly and Lezaun 2014; Sims forthcoming).

Here Morton's planetary environmental philosophy can be linked to propositions like those of Peter Redfield (2016) and Maria Puig de la Bellacasa (2017), who suggest that the best we may hope for when it comes to implementing technologies is that they reignite our sense of care and attention each time we deploy them. In their clunkiness and imperfection, mosquito-killing technologies, particularly the organophosphate larvicides that my CHW friends deployed against Nicaraguan *Ae. aegypti*, do just this: they encourage care and attention towards fellow human beings as well as fellow creatures. As with dangerous mosquitoes, our relationship to the technologies that kill them is ambiguous (Morton 2010). There are many reasons to dislike these insecticides (they are poisons, after all) but they remain meaningless until they are deployed. They, too, are tools for enriching ecological thought. Even when a householder in Nicaragua refuses to let a CHW treat her water receptacles with larvicide, the chemical opens up space for what Redfield (2016) calls a "practice of community." As Redfield notes, "The one advantage of uncertainty, doubt and ambivalence is an imperative to pause and consider them" (Redfield 2016, 177). A mosquito-killing technology that kills too efficiently—even if it may produce a welcome outcome such as the reduction or eradication of disease—is not a thinkable public health approach because it eliminates ambivalence.

Ambivalence can be built into mosquito control work. Rosie Sims (forthcoming) has carried out recent ethnographic studies within the World Mosquito Program (WMP), the Australia-based project that seeks to curb *Ae. aegypti*'s ability to spread dengue by infecting mosquito populations with *Wolbachia* bacteria (Sims forthcoming). Even wildly successful *Wolbachia* infection programmes will not mean the end of dengue or Zika once and for all. In fact, the *Wolbachia* project has a limited (50-year or so) horizon of efficacy. Tellingly, the WMP does not style *Wolbachia* as a "magic bullet." Its approach is quite different from that of projects with the goal of curbing mosquito populations through, for example, genetic modification (Nading 2015). WMP organizers seem quite aware that their work will produce as much ambivalence towards mosquitoes as it eliminates. As Sims argues, the project reverses the elimination model by asking the public to consider what it might mean to live and think differently with mosquitoes. It provides no clear answer to the question of what living and thinking with mosquitoes might look like.

Eradication fails as a public health measure precisely because it forecloses the possibility of ambivalence. Ultimately, the goal of mosquito eradication does not make good policy, not because it is categorically unethical or ecologically catastrophic, but because it artificially insulates public health from the messy realities of a life lived, and a thought thought.

Notes

1 For updated data see: https://www.apmresearchlab.org/covid/deaths-by-race
2 This is far from an original point. For more on this idea, see Carter 2018; Finney 2014.
3 A similar variety of white Euro-American moralism is evident in the Global Polio Eradication Initiative, a public–private partnership that joins the WHO with non-governmental partners like the Rotary Club to promote vaccination in those parts

of the world where polio remains a problem. Critical studies of this initiative have noted that while the push to eradicate polio garnered huge support from Northern donors, enthusiasm for vaccination is less appealing in places like Karachi, Pakistan, where polio remains. One reason for this is the perceived link between eradication and neo-colonial power (Closser 2012).

Bibliography

Beisel, Uli. 2010. Jumping Hurdles with Mosquitoes? *Environment and Planning. Part D: Society and Space* 28: 46–49.

Buhs, Joshua. 2004. *The Fire Ant Wars: Nature, Science, and Public Policy in Twentieth-Century America.* Chicago: University of Chicago Press.

Carr, E. Summerson. 2015. Occupation Bedbug: Or, the Urgency and Agency of Professional Pragmatism. *Cultural Anthropology* 30(2): 257–285.

Carter, Christopher. 2018. Blood in the Soil: The Racial, Racist, and Religious Dimensions of Environmentalism. In *The Bloomsbury Handbook of Environment and Nature: The Elements,* edited by Laura Hobgood and Whitney Bauman. New York: Bloomsbury, 45–62.

Castro, Arrachu, Yasmin Khawja, and James Johnston. 2010. Social Inequalities and Dengue Transmission in Latin America. In *Plagues and Epidemics: Infected Spaces Past and Present,* edited by Ann Herring and Alan Swedlund. New York: Berg, 231–249.

Closser, Svea. 2012. "We Can't Give Up Now": Global Health Optimism and Polio Eradication in Pakistan. *Medical Anthropology* 31(5): 385–403.

De la Bellacasa, Maria Puig. 2017. *Matters of Care: Speculative Ethics in More Than Human Worlds.* Minneapolis: University of Minnesota Press.

Diniz, Deborah. 2017. *Zika: From the Brazilian Backlands to Global Threat.* Translated by Diana Grosklaus Whitty. London: Zed Books.

Endy, Timothy P., Scott Weaver, and Kathryn Hanley. 2010 Dengue Virus: Past, Present and Future. In *Frontiers in Dengue Virus Research,* edited by K. Hanley and S. Weaver. Norfolk: Caister Academic, 3–12.

Finney, Carolyn. 2014. *Black Faces, White Spaces: Reimagining the Relationship of African Americans to the Great Outdoors.* Chapel Hill: University of North Carolina Press.

Freire, Paulo. 1970. *Pedagogy of the Oppressed.* New York: Seabury Press.

Gubler, Duane, and Goro Kuno. 1997. *Dengue and Dengue Hemorrhagic Fever.* Ann Arbor: CAB International.

Haraway, Donna. 2008. *When Species Meet.* Minneapolis: University of Minnesota Press.

Kelly, Ann, and Javier Lezaun. 2014. Urban Mosquitoes, Situational Publics, and the Pursuit of Interspecies Separation in Dar es Salaam. *American Ethnologist* 41: 368–383.

Kelly, Ann, and Javier Lezaun. 2017. The Wild Indoors: Room Spaces of Scientific Inquiry. *Cultural Anthropology* 32(3): 367–398.

Kolbert, Elizabeth. 2014. *The Sixth Extinction: An Unnatural History.* New York: Henry Holt and Company.

Levi-Strauss, Claude. 1963. *Totemism.* Translated by Rodney Needham. Boston: Beacon Press.

Morton, Timothy. 2010. *The Ecological Thought.* Cambridge: Harvard University Press.

Nading, Alex. 2014. *Mosquito Trails: Ecology, Health, and the Politics of Entanglement.* Berkeley: University of California Press.

Nading, Alex. 2015. The Lively Ethics of Global Health GMOs: The Case of the Oxitec Mosquito. *BioSocieties* 10(1): 24–47.

Nading, Alex. 2017. Local Biologies, Leaky Things, and the Chemical Infrastructure of Global Health. *Medical Anthropology* 36(2): 141–156.

Parreñas, Juno Salazar. 2018. *Decolonizing Extinction: The Work of Care in Orangutan Rehabilitation.* Durham: Duke University Press.

Raffles, Hugh. 2011. Mother Nature's Melting Pot. *New York Times*, April 3, Section WK, p. 12.

Redfield, P. 2016. Fluid Technologies: The Bush Pump, the LifeStraw, and Microworlds of Humanitarian Design. *Social Studies of Science* 46(2): 159–183.

Reis-Castro, Luísa. 2012. Genetically Modified Insects as a Public Health Tool: Discussing the Different Bio-Objectification Within Genetic Strategies. *Croatian Medical Journal* 53: 635–638.

Roberts-Gregory, Frances. 2020. On Being the (Only) Black Feminist Environmental Ethnographer in Gulf Coast Louisiana. *Edge Effects*, March 31. https://edgeeffects.net /on-being-the-only-black-feminist-environmental-ethnographer-in-gulf-coast-lo uisiana/. Accessed June 23, 2020.

Sims, Rosie. Forthcoming. *Cultivating Coexistence: Global Health, Mosquitoes and the Reconfiguring of Multispecies Relations in Medellín, Colombia.* Ph.D. Dissertation, Graduate Institute of International and Development Studies. Geneva.

Slosek, Jean. 1986. *Aedes Aegypti* in the Americas: A Review of Their Interaction with the Human Population. *Social Science and Medicine* 23: 249–257.

Stepan, Nancy Leys. 2011. *Eradication: Ridding the World of Diseases Forever?* Ithaca: Cornell University Press.

Van Dooren, Thom. 2014. *Flight Ways: Life and Loss at the Edge of Extinction.* New York: Columbia University Press.

Weston, Kath. 2017. *Animate Planet: Making Visceral Sense of Living in a High-Tech Ecologically Damaged World.* Durham: Duke University Press.

Williamson, Eliza. 2020. Against Forgetting: Telling Stories after Zika. *Somatosphere* January 6. http://somatosphere.net/2020/telling-stories-zika.html/. Accessed June 23, 2020.

13

THE INNOCENT MOSQUITO?

The environmental ethics of mosquito eradication

Anna Wienhues

Who has not swatted at least one mosquito? Surely most people have crushed at least one mosquito on a hot summer evening and did not think that there could be anything morally wrong about stopping that nuisance. After all, diseases transmitted by mosquitoes are a major global health issue: malaria, dengue fever and Zika—to name a few—are diseases transmitted by mosquitoes, with substantial impact on the well-being of a large part of the world's human population. Some mosquito-borne diseases such as the West Nile virus are hosted by other animals before being spread to humans (that is, they are zoonotic diseases, like the 2020 coronavirus pandemic), thereby situating this global health problem in a web of interspecies entanglements. To address this proliferating problem, drastic means might be considered necessary, such as eradication, bringing to extinction an entire mosquito species that transmits diseases, or at least drastically diminishing their populations. Can such large-scale eradication practices be morally justified?

That is the question that I will focus on in this chapter with a specific focus on the eradication of entire vector species which is a broader aim than the elimination or control of a few populations of that species. Instead of providing arguments from within public health ethics on the problem of mosquito-borne diseases, this chapter rather looks through an environmental ethics lens to illustrate what can be said to plead the mosquito's case. The upshot in this "mosquito debate" is that we must acknowledge that in case of eradication something of moral relevance would be lost, even if we have good reasons to advocate such drastic methods: namely, mosquitoes matter. This chapter does not attempt a definitive answer or recommendation for action, but instead lays out the landscape of potential normative arguments. Importantly, the problem-framing influences what we perceive as morally salient features of a situation. If mosquito-borne diseases are considered to be borne out of a conflict of interests between humans and

DOI: 10.4324/9781003056034-13

mosquitoes, then it needs to be kept in mind that the mosquitoes are "innocent" in several senses of the term as discussed later.

Environmental ethics is a field within moral philosophy that considers questions such as whether nature has a value that is independent of its usefulness to humans; or whether animals can be considered to be holders of moral rights. It is useful to briefly engage with some arguments from this literature in order to provide a picture as inclusive as possible, covering a range of issues that are relevant to environmental moral theorizing. Moreover, this picture is not complete, since I look at the problem only from a Western analytical philosophy perspective. Introducing arguments in favour of the mosquito does not mean that there are no good counterarguments and other considerations that might outweigh the mosquito's case. As we will see, also from an environmental ethics perspective, it is not always easy to justify the strong discomfort some may feel about different mosquito eradication proposals.

Of course, a full assessment of the mosquito problem would need much more detailed analysis than can be provided here, and many more nuanced questions regarding less drastic means than complete vector species eradication need to be asked, such as disease control by insecticide treated bed nets (ITN), or regarding the different means of disease eradication, in general, and the eradication of mosquito species, in particular. The discussion will rather remain at quite an abstract level. Regarding the *elimination* of mosquito populations in a specific area, for example, one could ask whether certain practices (such as spraying large areas with biological or non-biological agents) are morally preferable or inferior to other options (such as releasing genetically altered mosquitoes into an ecosystem) in addition to questions about feasibility, even if we would reach the conclusion that eradication of disease-carrying mosquito species was all-things-considered necessary. While the elimination or reduction of mosquito populations does not have to add up to species eradication and therefore these constitute distinct aims, it is also the case that different means of eradication or elimination need to be distinguished regarding whether they have *broad* adverse effects or constitutes means of *"target killing"* the vector species in question.

Three preliminary points can be made. First, the following considerations are based on the assumption that complete eradication of certain mosquito species might be possible in the near future (despite not being possible at the moment), leaving aside the question regarding which interventions this would entail. Second, eradication is the focus here as it constitutes the most "extreme" form of disease-control from the mosquito's perspective—although most of what follows is also applicable to deliberations about population control as well. Third, although a nuanced analysis would distinguish between reducing the disease burden and eliminating it completely, we shall simply assume that there are strong normative prerogatives for both of these goals.

The following discussion is divided into five sections. The first section sketches the broader "moral landscape" of the mosquito eradication and control question to identify a few important considerations that go beyond environmental ethics, narrowly conceived. The second section shows how the lives of mosquitoes matter morally in themselves or as members of a species, while the third section discusses how the lives of mosquitoes might matter also indirectly in our moral deliberations. The fourth section is dedicated to the subject of how eradicating mosquito species constitutes a form of self-defence and whether this might constitute an appropriate framing of the disease-carrying mosquito conflict, with the last section summarizing the main points and offering some concluding remarks.

The moral landscape

The environmental ethics questions considered here are situated in the broader discourse of moral philosophy which includes other fields with important contributions to the issue of mosquito eradication, especially political philosophy and bioethics. Here there are four (not exhaustive) general issues that stand out.

For one, mosquito eradication and control require us to think about *legitimacy*. That is, who should decide about such interventions? In essence, this issue revolves around informed consent and political legitimacy. Matters of informed consent, as discussed in bioethics, account for the need of patients making voluntary decisions about their own medical treatment in clinical practice and medical research (see Manson and O'Neill 2007). Yet in this context it is more apt to speak of "group consent" (see Deplazes-Zemp 2018). Thus, field trials and other interventions on mosquitoes require the informed consent—or rather authorization via appropriate procedures—of the affected human communities in order to gain legitimacy (Meghani and Boëte 2018, Neuhaus and Caplan 2017), which leads also to the political dimension of legitimacy. Mosquito eradication projects are large-scale enterprises with effects that can transcend spatial and temporal borders to affect distant communities and future generations, involving inputs from national and international governmental and non-governmental agencies. This generates questions of political legitimacy (which is a contested area of debate) in terms of, for instance, the democratic authorization required to justify political power (see Buchanan 2002).

There is a second issue of *risk*, and the way it is embodied by different interventions which I will consider briefly in the third section. A complicated subject, risk is integral to any eradication and control proposal according to methods, aims and potential kinds of risks involved. It is precisely due to such risks that questions of legitimacy become especially salient.

A third issue that arises regards questions of *distributive justice*, since the burden of mosquito-borne diseases particularly affects the poor which, in turn, is linked to the uneven capacities of health services and relevant infrastructure (Greisman et al. 2019). There are also often special risks for pregnant women and children who catch a mosquito-borne disease. Such an unequal global distribution of the burden of disease can possibly be exacerbated by other influences such as climate change (WHO 2017). Accordingly, a global health justice lens then introduces a range of questions about such issues as the fair distribution of costs of and access to interventions, and duties to aid the most affected. Moreover, the interactions between different dimensions of injustice—economic, health-related and environmental—need to be kept in view.

Finally, and as the fourth issue, insofar as steering and monitoring people's behaviour constitute important elements of an eradication strategy, then we must be sensitive to questions about how they interfere with people's autonomy and right to privacy (Greisman et al. 2019). In light of these issues, we must acknowledge that the eradication of certain mosquito species would be of significant benefit (at least in the short term) to many people living in areas where mosquitoes are endemic. The dramatic impact mosquito-borne diseases have on the lives of many humans constitutes the main—and weighty—reason for eradication due to the fundamental interests to life and health at stake. Since several other chapters in this volume are already dedicated to the human dimensions of this ethical problem, we shall turn to other issues. As a consequence, we need to differentiate between what would be all-things-considered justified and what would be justified from the incomplete environment ethics perspective that I am presenting here.

Why mosquitoes matter

The question of whether we should eradicate disease-carrying mosquitoes is a significant challenge for many environmental ethicists who are committed to biological conservation aims. Many ethicists will not be satisfied with simply dismissing the mosquito's place in the ecosystem as a "romantic notion" (compare, for instance, Fang 2010: 434). Moreover, amongst these are also ethicists with biocentric or ecocentric commitments who argue there are many more morally relevant attributes in nature than just sentience (such as in terms of the capacity to suffer pain). So, they will not be impressed by the possibility of a pain-free "specicide" (compare, for instance, Judson and Pugh in Bates 2016, and, in more detail, Pugh 2016). In the end, any comprehensive answer to the question about whether we should eradicate disease-carrying mosquitoes will involve a complex set of moral trade-offs. In favour of the protection of the mosquitoes in question, a combination of four different (but not exhaustive) kinds of arguments could be presented based on (1) caring about each *individual* mosquito, (2) the value of each *species*, (3) what eradication says about *our moral character* and (4) whether the potential benefits outweigh the *risks* of interventions. I address each of these issues in turn, starting with the first two in this section.

The moral considerability of each individual mosquito

As biocentrists will argue, focusing on sentience alone oversimplifies the moral landscape, because all living beings matter morally in themselves. That means that the life of each individual mosquito is morally considerable and must be accounted for in our moral deliberations. As Paul Taylor phrased it, "[t]he biocentric outlook on nature ... includes a certain way of perceiving and understanding each individual organism. Each is seen to be a teleological (goal-oriented) centre of life, pursuing its own good in its own unique way" (Taylor 1986: 44–45). From this perspective each individual mosquito matters in itself independent of whether humans consider it useful, harmful or beautiful.

This theoretical commitment entails that the well-being of even such dangerous creatures as *Aedes aegypti* must be acknowledged and integrated into our moral deliberations. Although this is the necessary conclusion of any biocentric position, it is also of course a contested idea. Putting it very crudely, critics who argue that this goes too far usually maintain that *either* only humans are morally considerable (Kant 1997, 1998) *or else* that non-human beings also have moral standing, but only if they exhibit some basic capacities such as in terms of awareness or an ability to suffer pain (Singer 1975, Regan 1984). Both perspectives exclude mosquitoes from the moral realm as beings that matter in themselves as—based on present knowledge—it is unlikely that they feel pain, for instance.

In contrast, others might counter that it seems convincing to attribute moral standing to individual mosquitoes—and that they therefore deserve consideration in eradication programs—but accounting for that standing would be so demanding on our actions that we should exclude them from our moral considerations nevertheless. Besides that such considerations feed into issues we will look at in the following sections, it is important to point out that being a holder of moral status (in terms of being morally considerable) is not enough to explain the full moral context that needs to be taken into account, and so does not sufficiently explain what we should and should not do. Living beings matter in themselves, but what is ultimately morally justifiable also depends on the contextual and relational features of the situation. If a biocentrist would be committed to declaring that harm ought not be inflicted on any being with moral status under any circumstances, this would not constitute a viable position. We can refuse to pick a specific flower in a field or to kill a specific spider in our living room, but we eat plants; insects die on our windshields. And beyond contextual and relational considerations (which always matter but on which theories diverge), different theories also provide different accounts of the relative weight of the moral status of a mosquito compared to that of other beings with moral status —if they deem mosquitoes morally considerable at all. Broadly speaking, the options are between egalitarian accounts, where all beings (but not all kinds of interests) matter exactly the same (Taylor 1986), and hierarchical accounts, where mosquitoes have less moral significance than, for example, sentient animals (Agar 2001), or else non-hierarchical accounts, in which the moral significance of different living beings is incommensurable which strongly emphasizes contextual and relational considerations (Wienhues 2020).

Even if moral standing is insufficient for safeguarding all mosquitoes even in situations that do not involve substantial public health considerations, the minimum that this requires of us is to consider whether there are alternative means that are as good from a public health perspective that do not require such drastic actions that might harm such a large number of mosquitoes. Alternatives to mosquito eradication include, for example, vaccines, the reduction of mosquito breeding grounds or the improvement of healthcare and sanitary facilities which might create considerable public health benefits. If individual mosquitoes are morally considerable, then we have an additional reason for seriously considering disease-control interventions that cause less harm to mosquitoes than eradication campaigns might do.[1]

The moral value of each mosquito species

Besides the moral status and related inherent worth of an individual mosquito, we may also attach some kind of moral value to each mosquito *species* (which, in turn, is related to considerations about biodiversity) which is particularly relevant if we speak about species eradication. The instrumental value of a species refers to its current or potential usefulness for humans, for example in terms of what some call "ecosystem services."[2] Whether certain mosquito species have such instrumental value depends ultimately on empirical evidence about, for instance, their role in various ecosystems, and whether ecosystems could perform these functions if the species were removed. However, can a mosquito species also be conceived as non-instrumentally valuable?

Some think that this is the case. From such a perspective each disease-carrying mosquito species can indeed be attributed value that goes beyond its instrumental value, if it has any. Yet, there is a range of different positions that can be taken on this matter. Amongst other things, one's position on the value of species depends, on the one side, on what position on values one takes (such as debates between objective and subjective value accounts) and on the other side, on one's position regarding what constitutes a species (such as the debates about the ontological status of species).[3]

For example, a fairly common claim is that species hold some form of objective "natural historical" value (Rolston 1995, but compare Sandler 2012), which is a type of non-instrumental value.[4] Holmes Rolston III develops a bold version of the idea of natural historical value, arguing that each extinction is a kind of "superkilling" (1995: 523) because "a biological species is not just a class. A species is a living historical form … propagated in individual organisms, that flows dynamically over generations" (1985: 721). Such reasoning suggests that the human-caused loss of a species and its associated natural historical value is morally problematic and given that this constitutes an "objective" value it is independent from peoples' preferences. Here, people are not required to personally care about mosquitoes for them to be valuable in an objective natural historical sense.

Yet even Rolston, as a strong advocate of biodiversity conservation, argues that the "duty to species [not to cause their extinction] can be overridden, for example with pests or disease organisms" (2001: 410). Thus, even if a mosquito species holds natural historical value, things do not look good for our mosquitoes. Moreover, the moral value of different species may be considered to be differently morally weighty. In terms of natural historical value, one consideration might be that a lack of distinctiveness of a species implies that it is not as valuable as another, recognizing that there are more than 3,000 mosquito species with differing degrees of distinctness around the world. Because only a small number of these mosquito species actually transmits diseases to humans, the case for protecting them based on their moral value needs to be supplemented with other considerations in their favour.

Adding context

Of course, considering the value of mosquitoes as either individuals or as species is neither sufficient for reaching a moral judgement for their protection, nor is it the only route for constructing an argument that speaks against their eradication. So far, we have only considered what matters morally (that is, has moral standing or value), but these considerations have to feed into normative theories (such as theories that focus on rights, utility or moral character). In this chapter I cannot give justice to the range of aspects different normative theories can bring to the subject of mosquito eradication and, thus, I will limit myself to mentioning just a few considerations that stand out (the points three and four mentioned previously)—starting with virtue ethics.

Hubris

To many people, the concern about hubris is an intuitive criticism to visions of mosquito eradication. Environmental virtue ethics is the most obvious lens for understanding this concern, because it puts emphasis on a person's moral character. In this context, the question that poses itself is whether eradicating entire species is compatible with being and acting as the kind of person that has internalized a range of different virtues (that is, excellent character traits). Of course, even here there is a large variety of theoretical accounts, all of which propose a range of environment-specific virtues such as humility or gratitude as central attitudes towards nature. What actions such theories justify depends, on the one side, on what they consider morally valuable, as discussed before, and on the other side on the content of the relevant virtues (Sandler 2016).

Context is very important for virtue ethics approaches. However, at first view at least, it seems that different environmental virtue ethics, including varieties that do not acknowledge the moral standing of individual mosquitoes, are at least sceptical of plans to eradicate several mosquito species. On the face of it, such plans appear hubristic by misrepresenting humanity's appropriate role in nature in addition to being epistemically hubristic by overestimating humanity's ability to control nature. That is problematic insofar as hubris is understood as a vice, and insofar that such plans are incompatible with such virtues as humility in our actions and our stance toward the environment. Such concerns, of course, appear particularly pressing if one also presupposes a particular way of understanding humanity's place in nature that rejects the role of a master or a manager.

In terms of hubris and humility such an endeavour to eradicate mosquitoes appears to share similarities with other controversial human interventions in nature, such as plans to address climate change through geoengineering (Meyer and Uhle 2015) or genetic crop modification through biotechnology (Sandler 2004). Whether different accounts of environmental virtue ethics ultimately reject or justify such wide-ranging human interventions—including the eradication of disease-carrying mosquito species—involves taking into account all morally relevant contextual features, humanity's health burden being one of such crucial concerns.

Risks

A person who is not convinced by virtue-based perspectives might, however, think differently about risk-based arguments and still be inclined to favour a precautionary approach in light of the risks involved in any such intervention (even if done for purely human-focused reasons) when weighted against its potential benefits. Much recent work about ethics and disease-carrying mosquitoes are written from a public heath perspective and highlight this specific question of risk—usually linked to the importance of community engagement mentioned earlier—in light of the current development of gene drives for containing mosquito-borne diseases (Greisman et al. 2019, Patrão Neves and Druml 2017, Resnik 2014, Resnik 2017).

Gene-drive systems, as technologies of genome editing, are developed, for example, as means for eradicating mosquito species or else creating resistances to pathogens (such as a virus) in a target population of mosquitoes. For instance, Jonathan Pugh (2016), who does not consider mosquitoes to be morally considerable in themselves, does not find the "hubris objection" convincing while discussing gene-drive technologies potentially being used on disease-carrying mosquitoes as a means of eradication. Still, he argues that a better understanding of the potential effects and success of mosquito eradication will be important to make well-informed moral decisions. Indeed, Pugh is right when claiming that "epistemic humility" does not involve the dismissal of biotechnology based on it having *some* risk (Pugh 2016: 580). Yet, the potential irreversibility of gene drives, for example, is definitely a risk to take into account. Even by relying on solutions less technical than gene drives, the eradication of a species by more "conventional" means carries a risk for ecosystems and may be irreversible (when putting the controversial possibility of "de-extinction" with technological solutions aside). Accordingly, one might still be inclined to favour the precautionary principle in light of the risks involved in any intervention—even ones carried out for purely human-focused reasons—which are intertwined with a range of empirical questions.[5]

Self-defence

So far, we have seen several ethical considerations that can justify a reluctance in wanting to eradicate mosquitoes. This reluctance may be based on a mosquito's moral standing, the natural historical value of a mosquito species, concerns about our own moral character or concerns about risk. In turn, these considerations will be part of a broader assessment of mosquito eradication proposals, most inclusively by providing a pluralistic picture that engages with different normative theories. Besides the virtue ethics approach mentioned above, one could ask questions about whether mosquitoes have certain rights that must be accounted for or whether certain strategies are better than others to maximize well-being. However, there is an additional dimension to dealing with mosquitoes not yet addressed. The question is what constitutes the appropriate problem-framing of the conflict between humans and disease-carrying mosquitoes and can it be framed as a matter of self-defence?[6]

Humans stand in a multitude of different moral relationships with non-human animals, each of which comes with a different set of moral demands. For example, most mosquito species do not prey on humans, a fact which makes living alongside them on a shared planet possible as long as human impact on their habitats, say in the forms of soil degradation or air pollution, is contained.[7] The case is different, however, for our relationship with those few mosquito species that "prey" on humans by having a preference for human blood. Yet, again only a subset of these anthropophilic mosquito species also carry malaria, dengue fever, Zika and so on.

At first glance, these cases of disease-carrying mosquitoes look like straightforward cases of self-defence which usually are considered morally permissible even if killing the aggressor is the only means to defend one's own life. For instance, self-defence could be a way of justifying the extermination of the smallpox pathogen, which was declared accomplished in 1979 (WHO 2019). Mosquitoes, like insects generally, have not featured prominently in the environmental ethics literature, but a self-defence framing stands out in this context. For instance, James Sterba has argued for a "Principle of Human Defense" which allows one to act against "harmful aggression" through harming and killing individual animals as well as *whole species*, when necessary (Sterba 2005: 295). This would cover the disease-carrying mosquito case and allow for their eradication despite the fact that Sterba, as a biocentrist, is committed to attributing moral standing to each individual mosquito. By analogy, if someone innocent was attacked by a human aggressor with a knife, we would judge violent self-defence permissible, with the human aggressor remaining a person with moral standing (see also Taylor 1986).

Indeed, Sterba explicitly mentions that killing disease-carrying mosquitoes is a justifiable act of self-defence and states the following:

In the case of human aggression, however, it is sometimes possible to effectively defend oneself and other human beings by first suffering the aggression and then securing adequate compensation later. Because in the case of nonhuman aggression by the members of other species with which we are familiar, such an approach is unlikely to work, justifying more harmful preventive actions such as killing a rabid dog or *swatting a mosquito*, potentially carrying disease. There are simply more ways to effectively stop aggressive humans than there are to effectively stop aggressive nonhumans.

(Sterba 1998: 364, italics added)

Sterba makes killing a mosquito, and in extension the eradication of a whole species, a bit more palatable by pointing out that in the case of mosquito "aggression" we do not have as many options of self-defence as we do with human conflicts. If someone vandalizes my house, I can demand compensation after the fact; but this is not the case for the mosquito who can place me in the hospital for months and neither can we "discuss" our differences in a conflict-resolution scenario. Yet, this does not necessarily allow any kind of self-defending actions because the question remains whether there are methods for protecting human health that are less harmful to mosquitoes whilst being effective enough, as mentioned above. For instance, Jake Monaghan argues that while a biocentric position allows for killing in self-defence, it demands "programs which make the mosquitoes malaria-resistant, if it is at all a possibility" (2018: 134). Of course, such programmes come with their own set of issues (particularly, when involving gene drives) that have to be taken into account. Moreover, for self-defence to be applicable, humans must apply "reasonable care" (Taylor 1986: 265) in avoiding contact with disease-carrying mosquitoes. Given the wide global spread of mosquitoes and the common use of disease-control measures (such as bed nets or protective clothing) this condition seems to be met in many instances.

Nevertheless, there is still some background missing from the mosquito story, namely that the mosquito is merely instrumentalized by the disease that it carries, the disease being the real "aggressor" from which we need self-defence. The real source of the problem is the microbe that produces malaria, dengue fever and Zika, with mosquitoes merely being the "vehicle" that transmits them. Accordingly, it is more apt to understand the disease-carrying mosquito as the "innocent" vector. The way we frame a problem determines what we identify as its morally relevant features and so the emphasis can be put on different aspects of the problem.

On the one hand, it can be seen as a clear case of (collective) self-defence where a large section of humanity justifiably tries to defend itself from an aggression against its health and lives. Excluding some forms of genetic modification (which would change the problem-framing), killing may be the only way to fend off such aggression if it comes from entities that are "innocent" in the sense of having no awareness of the consequences of their actions. The mosquito is not a moral agent. On the other hand, although all mosquitoes that feed on human blood cause irritation, the dangerous "predator" that is targeted for eradication in this case is the disease (i.e. the virus or parasite) that they carry. So, one way of framing the issue would be to consider the eradication of the mosquitoes— now "innocent" by not being the ultimate source of the harm—as problematic "collateral damage" of the eradication of the diseases in question. That would be closer to a case of killing a bystander or hostage which carries a bigger moral burden. In a sense, the mosquito is "taken hostage" by the virus or the parasite that uses the mosquito's body as a resource. If that is an appropriate representation of the problem at hand, then it deviates in certain respects from the straightforward case of self-defence.

This illustrates, for one, that there are different senses in which the mosquito may be portrayed as "innocent." For instance, there is the unaware mosquito scenario and in that sense the mosquito constitutes an innocent threat. Yet, the mosquito also constitutes an innocent threat if it is instrumentalized by the virus which also does not constitute a moral agent. This is the hostage scenario, with an unaware virus. It follows that there are at least two ways in which the mosquito might constitute an innocent threat, and many might think that the second scenario intuitively requires more to be at stake to justify doing harm to the mosquito in fending off the disease. Although some might believe that self-defence against innocent threats is justified, others regard it as inappropriate to be conceived as self-defence, since the threat is innocent.[8] In that case, the problem would need to be framed as a matter of negative side-effects in the form of eradicating a species necessary for achieving the goal of a healthier world for people. That would mean that the human–mosquito conflict could not be framed as a matter of defence.

It therefore matters if the envisaged mosquito "specicide" is the outcome of a genuine self-defence scenario, or whether the mosquitoes are just bearing the burden of humanity's wish to make the Earth safer for itself, which includes a broad set of practices that affect the life and well-being of non-humans. Because there are alternatives to specicide when it comes to controlling mosquito-borne diseases, one must keep in mind that the eradication of the "innocent" mosquito cannot be disentangled from the broader web of potential moral failings. One needs to consider whether mosquito eradication proposals potentially constitute a means of obscuring other social and economic factors that can contribute to the prevalence of mosquito-borne diseases, such as the considerations of justice mentioned in the first section.[9] For instance, a focus on mosquito eradication might obscure that there are pressing social justice concerns such as about necessary access to health services that need to be addressed urgently. The swatting of a single mosquito that landed on my arm therefore needs to be distinguished from a practice of species eradication that is connected to a range of other moral and political decisions that depend on broader ethical considerations regarding humans and non-humans alike.

Of course, this discussion of "innocence" depends on the mosquito itself having moral standing, as discussed previously. Such considerations mean that a disease-carrying mosquito is not equivalent to a virus-infected computer, for example. Any perspective that denies moral standing to mosquitoes will perceive the mosquito problem as less complex than presented here. Beyond the question of "innocence," another dimension of the mosquito problem considers the question of how far this scenario constitutes a matter of *self*-defence.

So far, we have simply framed defence as a collective self-defence in which "humanity" defends itself. In practice, there are considerable regional differences that are in the process of transformation due to climate change, with not all regions and communities being equally affected by mosquito-borne diseases. Some regions and some individuals are not affected at all while others must deal with several mosquito-borne diseases at once. More accurately would then be to frame it as a matter of self-defence of certain affected communities, if that is the course of action that they choose to pursue. Or, it could be framed as a third-party defence, because in practice such large-scale eradication programmes are instigated by national and international organizations in aid for the affected communities. As such the defence of others would generate additional issues to take into consideration in comparison to a straightforward case of self-defence (for instance, is there a duty to defend the affected party and, if so, by whom?). This question of agency therefore links, in turn, to broader questions of global health justice, such as regarding potential duties to finance mosquito interventions and technology transfer and reintroduces challenges of political legitimacy and informed consent.[10]

The upshot

As we have seen, whether the eradication of a mosquito species can be considered morally defensible depends on a range of normative and empirical questions. I have outlined how some of these considerations can be brought in the mosquito's favour. These may be based, inter alia, on the moral standing of individual mosquitoes, the moral value of a whole mosquito species, and concerns about hubris and risk.

Yet these considerations neither exhaust all that can be said from an environmental ethics perspective nor are they meant to deny the strong moral prerogative to reduce the health burden of mosquito-borne disease. That we have reached the point of even asking the question about whether mosquitoes should be eradicated, indicates that we must carefully consider its context to make sure that nothing of moral relevance is overlooked. For one, we need to ask whether, and in what form, the self-defence scenario is an appropriate problem-framing. Next, we must consider whether there are any alternative means which might be all-things-considered morally preferable. If alternatives to eradication are viable—and since the eradication of disease-carrying mosquitoes may be impossible—then part of the debate should be about whether there are moral demands, such as in terms of global justice, to fund alternative efforts to reduce diseases carried by mosquitoes and other vectors. It would also be valuable to take a step back to think about how the mosquito question is the product of moral failures that have perpetuated the global problem of mosquito-borne diseases. Such considerations lead us also to political questions, such as vested interests in different technologies, which will influence which set of options are available.

Even if our answer is ultimately affirmative—that we do need to eradicate certain mosquito species to the best of our abilities—doing so still requires awareness that something of moral value will be lost (e.g. in terms of the species) and that something of moral status has potentially been harmed (that is, individual mosquitoes). The upshot is that taking all these moral considerations seriously will leave us with an awareness that the eradication of these species cannot be taken lightly. Any environmental ethics theory that dismisses such a loss oversimplifies the complex and conflictual moral decision-making at play, even when we have very good reasons to defend and protect our own health.

Notes

1 Of course, depending on how we define harm and the well-being of individual mosquitoes, it is not necessarily the case that all potential forms of eradication or control interventions would cause any harm to individuals. What constitutes harm to insects is an area of debate, but most generally, it seems that methods that kill adult mosquitoes are likely to involve harm to individuals while preventing them from coming to life in the first place does not.

2 But note that "ecosystem services" can also be understood more broadly, involving more than instrumental values only.

3 Most plausible to me, the non-instrumental moral value of species is not identical to the moral status of individuals as discussed in the last section (Sandler 2012), but that still leaves a range of options.

4 Non-instrumental value is often labelled as "intrinsic value" but for a nuanced differentiation between various uses of "intrinsic value" see O'Neill 1992.

5 Besides questions about which kinds of risk for humans (e.g. adverse ecological effects) and their likelihood we deem acceptable or not, gene-drive technology is also entangled in a host of other normative questions that I cannot do justice to here. See Preston and Wickson (2019) for a comprehensive overview. For instance, such technological interventions raise also questions about naturalness, the ontology of species and new responsibilities in light of changing relationships between humans and non-human beings. For example, accounts that consider "naturalness"—which is a contested concept (see Siipi 2008)—to confer a non-instrumental moral value might deem synthetic gene drives particularly problematic by introducing an "artificial" element into nature.

6 Ultimately, that is a matter of choice. Alternatives need to be considered and the appropriateness of the self-defence analogy can be challenged.

7 It has been argued that keeping environmental degradation to a minimum is even a matter of doing justice to non-human living beings. Yet, while the destruction of mosquito habitats is a matter of (distributive) justice, the conflict between disease-carrying mosquitoes and humans is not (Wienhues 2020).

8 For an overview of defence against animals see Kagan 2019. See also Monaghan (2018) for a biocentric argument that justifies self-defence against innocent threats.

9 Such concerns particularly apply to the employment of biotechnological means such as gene drives. See Preston and Wickson (2019).

10 An additional matter of third-party defence is the question of the affected domestic animals. Based on the idea that we are standing with domesticated animals in a

different relationship than with animals such as the mosquito (see Palmer 2010), it could be argued, for example, that the defence of domestic animals from mosquito-borne diseases is necessitated by a duty of care for these animals (of course, while putting aside questions about the moral legitimacy of animal husbandry in the first place).

Bibliography

Agar, Nicholas. 2001. *Life's Intrinsic Value: Science, Ethics, and Nature.* New York: Columbia University Press.

Bates, Claire. 2016. Would It Be Wrong to Eradicate Mosquitoes? *BBC New Magazine,* 28 January, Online edition.

Buchanan, Allen. 2002. Political Legitimacy and Democracy. *Ethics* 112(4): 689–719.

Deplazes-Zemp, Anna. 2018. Group Consent. In *The Routledge Handbook of the Ethics of Consent,* edited by Peter Schaber and Andreas Müller, 105–116. London: Routledge.

Fang, Janet. 2010. A World Without Mosquitoes. *Nature* 466 (News Feature): 432–434.

Greisman, Laura, Barbara Koenig and Michele Barry. 2019. Control of Mosquito-Borne Illnesses: A Challenge to Public Health Ethics. In *The Oxford Handbook of Public Health Ethics,* edited by Anna C. Mastroianni, Jeffrey P. Kahn and Nancy E. Kass, 458–471. Oxford: Oxford University Press.

Kagan, Shelly. 2019. *How to Count Animals, More or Less.* Oxford: Oxford University Press.

Kant, Immanuel. 1997 (1784–5). *Lectures on Ethics (The Cambridge Edition of the Works of Immanuel Kant).* Edited by P. Heath and J. B. Schneewind. Cambridge: Cambridge University Press.

Kant, Immanuel. 1998 (1785). *Groundwork of the Metaphysics of Morals (Grundlegung Zur Metaphysik Der Sitten).* Translated by Mary J. Gregor. Cambridge: Cambridge University Press.

Manson, Neil C. and Onora ONeill. 2007. *Rethinking Informed Consent in Bioethics.* Cambridge: Cambridge University Press.

Meghani, Zahra and Christophe Boëte. 2018. Genetically Engineered Mosquitoes, Zika and Other Arboviruses, Community Engagement, Costs, and Patents: Ethical Issues. *PLOS Neglected Tropical Diseases* 12(7): e0006501.

Meyer, Kirsten and Christian Uhle. 2015. *Geoengineering and the Accusation of Hubris.* 2015–3. THERAPIESys Discussion Paper. Berlin: Humboldt-Universität zu Berlin.

Monaghan, Jake. 2018. Killing in Self-Defence and the Case of Biocentric Individualism. *Environmental Values* 27: 119–136.

Neuhaus, Carolyn and Arthur L. Caplan. 2017. Ethical Lessons from a Tale of Two Genetically Modified Insects. Correspondence in *Nature Biotechnology* 35(8): 713–716.

O'Neill, John. 1992. The Varieties of Intrinsic Value. *The Monist* 75(2): 119–137.

Palmer, Clare. 2010. *Animal Ethics in Context.* New York: Columbia University Press.

Patrão Neves, Maria and Christiane Druml. 2017. Ethical Implications of Fighting Malaria with CRISPR/Cas9. *BMJ Global Health* 2(3): e000396.

Preston, Christopher and Fern Wickson. 2019. Ethics and Governance. In *Gene Drives: A Report on Their Science, Applications, Social Aspects, Ethics and Regulations,* Report edited by Holly Dressel. Critical Scientists Switzerland (CSS) & European Network of Scientists for Social and Environmental Responsibility (ENSSER) & Vereinigung Deutscher Wissenschaftler (VDW), 215–253.

Pugh, Jonathan. 2016. Driven to Extinction? The Ethics of Eradicating Mosquitoes with Gene-Drive Technologies. *Journal of Medical Ethics* 42: 578–581.

Regan, Tom. 1984. *The Case for Animal Rights*. London: Routledge.

Resnik, David B. 2014. Ethical Issues in Field Trials of Genetically Modified Disease-Resistant Mosquitoes. *Developing World Bioethics* 14(1): 37–46.

Resnik, David B. 2017. Field Trials of Genetically Modified Mosquitoes and Public Health Ethics. *The American Journal of Bioethics* 17(9): 24–26.

Rolston III, Holmes. 1985. Duties to Endangered Species. *BioScience* 35(11): 718–726.

Rolston III, Holmes. 1995. Duties to Endangered Species. In *Encyclopedia of Environmental Biology*, edited by W. A. Nierenberg, 517–528. Cambridge, MA: Academic Press.

Rolston III, Holmes. 2001. Biodiversity. In *A Companion to Environmental Philosophy*, edited by Dale Jamieson, 402–415. Malden: Blackwell Publishing.

Sandler, Ronald. 2004. An Aretaic Objection to Agricultural Biotechnology. *Journal of Agricultural and Environmental Ethics* 17(3): 301–317.

Sandler, Ronald. 2012. *The Ethics of Species: An Introduction*. Cambridge: Cambridge University Press.

Sandler, Ronald. 2016. Environmental Virtue Ethics. In *The Oxford Handbook of Environmental Ethics*, edited by Stephen M. Gardiner and Allen Thompson, 1–14. Online Version. Oxford: Oxford University Press.

Siipi, Helena. 2008. Dimensions of Naturalness. *Ethics and the Environment* 13(1): 71–103.

Singer, Peter. 1975. *Animal Liberation*. 2nd ed. London: Thorsons.

Sterba, James P. 1998. A Biocentrist Strikes Back. *Environmental Ethics* 20(Winter): 361–376.

Sterba, James P. 2005. Global Justice for Humans or for All Living Beings and What Difference It Makes. *Journal of Ethics* 9: 283–300.

Taylor, Paul. 1986. *Respect for Nature: A Theory of Environmental Ethics*. 25th Anniversary Edition (2011). Princeton: Princeton University Press.

Wienhues, Anna. 2020. *Ecological Justice and the Extinction Crisis: Giving Living Beings Their Due*. Bristol: Bristol University Press.

Word Health Oorganization. 2017. *Ethical Issues Associated with Vector-Borne Diseases. Report of a WHO Scoping Meeting, Geneva, 23–24 February*. Geneva: World Health Organization.

Word Health Oorganization. 2019. WHO Commemorates the 40th Anniversary of Smallpox Eradication. *WHO News Release*, 13 December. https://www.who.int/news-room/detail/13-12-2019-who-commemorates-the-40th-anniversary-of-smallpox-eradication. Accessed 22/04/2020.

PART V

Improving human–mosquito relationships

14

MOSQUITO CONTROL

Success, failure and expectations in the context of arbovirus expansion and emergence

Isabelle Dusfour and Sarah C. Chaney

Mosquitoes are considered humanity's most dangerous animal due to their capability to transmit a large number of deadly viruses and parasites, causing millions of illnesses and deaths annually, along with enormous economic loss (WHO 2020, Bradshaw et al. 2016). Among the 3,500 known mosquito species, however, only a few are vectors of these pathogens.

A vector is a mosquito that is able to pick up, amplify and transmit a pathogen from one vertebrate to another through blood feeding (Marcondes 2019). Only female mosquitoes are hematophagous (blood-feeders) and are therefore responsible for all mosquito-borne disease transmission. Yet not all female mosquitoes can transmit pathogens and some are better at it than others: the ability of any given mosquito to transmit disease from one vertebrate to another depends on its behaviour, how it fits into the ecosystem of the human-built and the natural world, and its internal biology. Each of these factors can be targeted with vector control strategies to interrupt the transmission of disease.

One way of reducing mosquito populations is to alter environmental factors necessary for mosquito breeding or to apply chemicals that target flying adults (adulticiding) or immature aquatic larval stages (larviciding). However, as we will see as we explore successes and failures of mosquito control, many chemical tools seem to have reached the end of their effectiveness as a stand-alone strategy. Despite decades of chemical control efforts over the past 50 years, the world has faced the intensification of dengue outbreaks, the re-emergence of yellow fever, the spread of chikungunya and Zika and the emergence of zoonotic diseases accompanied by the geographical expansion of major vectors (Wilder-Smith et al. 2017). Vector control departments are now faced with a challenge to expand beyond immediate prevention of human disease towards a global approach that encompasses the biology, behaviour and biodiversity of mosquito species, their ecology and what makes them effective or ineffective vectors—in

DOI: 10.4324/9781003056034-14

order to formulate a realistic, multi-faceted, environmentally friendly and efficient mosquito control strategy.

This chapter reviews what has been done so far to control *Aedes aegypti*, current challenges raised by the expansion of *Aedes albopictus* and growing threats of zoonotic viruses, and what innovations are under development to reduce mosquito-borne transmission of viruses. French overseas territories and the Americas are the focus here due to the special challenges they are facing to control mosquito vectors.

Controlling *Aedes* species in urban areas: *Aedes aegypti* and *Aedes albopictus*

Aedes aegypti and *Aedes albopictus* are the main urban vectors of arboviruses, the arthropod-borne viruses of yellow fever, dengue, chikungunya and Zika that threaten more than 3 billion people living in *Aedes*-infected areas worldwide (Wilder-Smith et al. 2017). *Aedes* species are optimally adapted for transmitting viruses from human to human: they can carry multiple arboviruses, are anthropophilic (prefer humans for blood feeding), bite during the day and feed multiple times, fly only short distances and prefer to breed in small human-made containers. Additionally, *Aedes* eggs are resistant to desiccation, giving them the advantage of spreading their offspring to new territories worldwide through human travel and commercial trade (Kraemer et al. 2019, Marcondes 2019).

Even though the two dominant *Aedes* vector species look very similar, their biology, ecology, behaviour and history of colonization reveal important differences. *Ae. aegypti* originated from forests of the western part of Africa and began spreading around the world through the transatlantic slave trade in the sixteenth century (Powell et al. 2018). This forest-dwelling species adapted to urban areas by becoming more anthropophilic and breeding specifically in human-made containers such as cisterns and buckets. This urban mosquito is closely tied to human habitation in all steps of its life cycle and is found less abundantly in rural areas and rarely in natural breeding sites. *Ae. aegypti* has colonized urban areas of subtropical and tropical regions around the world and is the main vector of the yellow fever virus, along with dengue viruses, and more recently chikungunya and Zika viruses.

Aedes albopictus, the Asian tiger mosquito, originates from forests in Asia and has become the world's most invasive mosquito species, colonizing all areas of the planet over the last 30 years within its preferred temperature range. Even though its ecological niche seems similar to that of *Ae. aegypti*, this species tends to be more rural, develops in a larger variety of natural and human-made breeding sites and adapts to a wide range of temperatures due to its capacity to lay cold-resistant eggs that can survive winter temperatures during its diapause stage (Paupy et al. 2009). *Ae. albopictus* is also less selective about hosts and can be found feeding on animals as well as humans. It does not transmit dengue and yellow fever quite as efficiently as *Ae. aegypti* and has until recently been considered more of a nuisance than a public health concern. However, *Ae. albopictus* revealed its true colours during the 2006–2007 chikungunya outbreak that hit the Indian Ocean Islands, Central Africa, India and Italy. *Ae. Albopictus'* growing distribution to more temperate latitudes and its ability to transmit about 26 different arboviruses between human and animal hosts makes it a growing threat in temperate regions (Paupy et al. 2009).

In some areas, the ranges of these two species overlap, sharing resources, often laying eggs in the same breeding sites and intermingling in ways that were never possible in their native ranges. *Ae. albopictus* has largely displaced the longer-established *Ae. aegypti* in many areas in the southeastern United States, creating complex interactions of competition, cross-mating and evolutionary pressures between these two invasive species (Bargielowski et al. 2013). The ongoing expansion of these two species to new locations in urban and rural communities makes them a central concern for public health. Due to the similarities between these species, control methods are often the same regardless of the presence of one or both species in the area.

Vector control: where, when and who?

The most familiar stage of the mosquito, the winged adult, is the form that is responsible for disease transmission. However, the mosquito's life cycle involves both aquatic and aerial stages, all of which can be targeted by mosquito control methods for preventing disease. The World Health Organization (WHO) provided the first guidelines for dengue control and prevention, including vector management, in the 1990s, but the importance of *Aedes* control took a new turn with the strong support given to the Global Vector Control Response by member states during the World Health Assembly in 2017 (WHO 1997, UNICEF/UNDP/World Bank/WHO 2017). These guidelines include protocols for environmental management of natural and human-made mosquito breeding sites, chemical and biological control agents for treatment of larval and adult stages and best practices for encouraging community engagement (WHO 2012). Mosquito control activities are most successful when multiple approaches are combined and coordinated with other health, environmental and community sectors to produce an integrated approach to mosquito management.

Vector control measures targeting the aquatic larval and pupal stages focus on the removal of human-made containers where *Aedes* mosquitoes prefer to lay eggs, or these watery habitats can be treated with chemical or biological compounds (i.e. *Bacillus thuringiensis*) to arrest development or kill immature stages and consequently reduce adult population density (Achee et al. 2015). Preventive measures such as the regular removal of stagnant water (locations A–E, in Figure 14.1) or covering water storage containers are strongly recommended (control measures 1–5 in Figure 14.1). Deployment of larvivorous fish or copepods alone or in combination with other methods has shown low levels of efficacy (Lazaro et al. 2015, Han et al. 2015).

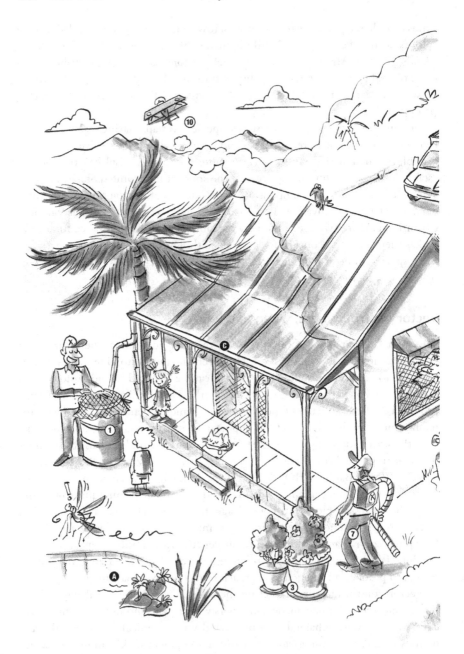

FIGURE 14.1 Suitable habitats for *Aedes* species and vector control methods. *Aedes albopictus* and *Ae. aegypti* breed in human environments. *Ae. albopictus* also develops in more natural habitats such as ponds, plants that hold water or tree holes (A). Both species are often found breeding in flower pots (B), gutters (C), water containers (D) and water collected in garbage of all sorts such as tyres, fridges and discarded containers (E). To reduce vector–human contact, several measures are used by people and public health authorities. Source reduction eliminates suitable places for females to lay eggs by properly covering

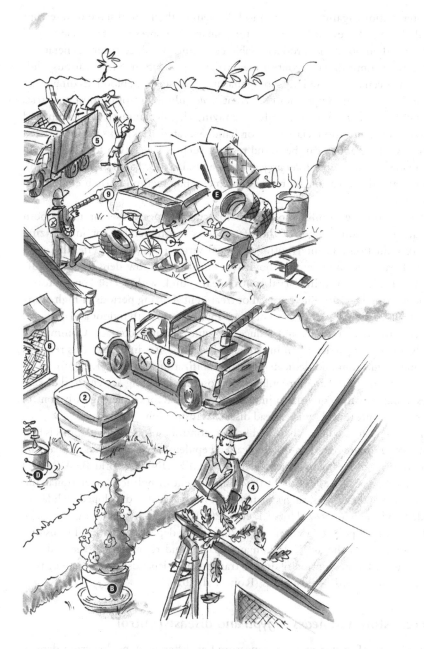

water storage (1, 2), removing stagnant water (3), cleaning household premises (4), avoiding garbage accumulation (5) and treating large ponds or reservoirs. To prevent human–vector contact, people at high risk can stay under bed nets even though *Aedes* mosquitoes are daytime biters, and screening can be installed in windows (6). Additionally, insecticide spatial spraying is performed indoors (7), outdoors (8–9) and occasionally by aircraft (10). The successful control of *Aedes* mosquitoes is based on the coordinated efforts of communities and public health authorities and by educating the youngest generation to take an active role in prevention (1). Illustration by Vincent Jacquet.

Interventions against adults aim to kill them in their aerial stage or interrupt female biting to prevent human–vector contact. Measures that target adult fertility and their ability to produce viable eggs aim to reduce future generations that may transmit disease (control measures 6–10 in Figure 14.1). Various adult behaviours can be targeted, including mating, host-seeking, blood-feeding, resting and egg-laying (oviposition). Current *Aedes* adult control in most countries around the world is based primarily on spraying chemical insecticides formulated for outdoor application via trucks or hand-operated backpacks or in targeted locations where adults can be found resting, such as vegetation for *Aedes albopictus* or indoor areas for *Aedes aegypti* (Achee et al. 2015, Faraji and Unlu 2016). Aircraft are also occasionally used as an emergency method (Britch et al. 2018, Likos et al. 2016).

An appropriate combination of vector control measures that target both immature and adult stages of the life cycle is recommended for maximizing density reduction and interrupting eventual virus transmission (Hierlihy et al. 2019). In areas with endemic arbovirus transmission, a low density of mosquitoes is achieved by routine larval control year round, with vector control teams implementing breeding site removal or treatment. During periods of high arbovirus transmission or epidemics, chemical applications, both indoor and outdoor, are used to control adults and reduce mosquito–human contact. Community involvement and participation in reducing breeding sites in urban areas requires sustained education and dedicated social mobilization (location 1, Figure 14.1). A combination of routine surveillance of mosquito breeding activity and disease cases in humans and potential animal hosts is essential for triggering early control strategies for preventing widespread disease transmission.

The decision of when, where and how to control mosquito populations is best made through integrated entomological and epidemiological surveillance as part of a comprehensive management plan (UNICEF/UNDP/World Bank/WHO 2017, Roiz et al. 2018). Without the commitment of political, operational and community stakeholders, such a plan cannot be sustainably developed, validated, funded and implemented (Horstick et al. 2010). Furthermore, local governance and operational policies are structured differently depending on local transmission patterns and the available human capacity and resources. In the end, the successful early interruption of disease transmission depends on interagency preparedness and coordinated actions (Roiz et al. 2018).

Success stories in *Aedes aegypti* and disease control

The efficacy of vector control is measured at different steps: lowering density and/or human–vector contact, epidemiological impact and its sustainability over time. There is some evidence that mosquito density can be reduced for a period of time thereby preventing epidemics, but few studies have rigorously demonstrated the long-range efficacy of vector control interventions (Wilson et al. 2015, Bowman et al. 2016). Part of the challenge is demonstrating effectiveness of a specific vector control strategy in a treatment area compared to a similar control area with no such intervention. Such experimental protocols are hard to justify during a public health emergency since the control area could be exposed to higher risk of infection and disease. This is part of the reason why clear evidence on the epidemiological impacts of vector control is scarce. However, there are three examples of sustainable success stories in interrupting yellow fever and dengue transmission.

Several reports claim stories of successfully eradicating yellow fever in the early 1900s in the Americas and the Caribbean when the yellow fever virus and its transmission by *Aedes aegypti* was first described (Soper 1963). Following reports of early successes in reducing urban yellow fever cases and the discovery of DDT (dichlorodiphenyltrichloroethane) as an effective tool in this effort, the Rockefeller Foundation embarked on a worldwide yellow fever and malaria eradication programme in the 1940s (Soper 1963). Combining vaccination with mosquito control, the Rockefeller programme paved the way for modern vector control techniques by relying on large-scale indoor residual spraying of DDT. The effects on *Ae. aegypti* populations were drastic and the species was believed to be eradicated in the Americas. For a decade no record of either the mosquito or any of the diseases it carried was published.

However, a subsequent progressive recolonization of the mosquito across the continent brought dengue fever and other arboviruses with it (Soper 1963). Pockets of urban yellow fever outbreaks were controlled with vaccination. Malathion and other organophosphorus compounds became the new adulticides of choice, combined with removing larval breeding sites and engaging community through education campaigns. During outbreaks, outdoor spraying of insecticides was favoured over indoor residual spraying.

The return of *Ae. aegypti* was accompanied by an increase in dengue outbreaks, as all four dengue serotypes colonized the Americas. One country was an exception: for 15 years from 1981 to 1997 Cuba managed to remain free of dengue and recorded very low densities of this mosquito. During this period in Cuba an intense programme of surveillance and control was enforced in two phases by combining adult and larval control. The first phase involved massive ultra-low volume (ULV) spraying of malathion by aerial and ground application both indoors and outdoors. Phase two involved nationwide breeding source removal with education programmes for the general population and law enforcement that focused on limiting suitable conditions for larval development in backyards and houses. This combination of vector control methods was accompanied by an emphasis on entomological surveillance, source reduction and larval control (Armada Gessa and Figueredo González 1986). However, in 1997 an increase in vector density, most likely due to weakening in surveillance, along with the introduction of foreign infections, caused the re-emergence of dengue on the island (Kourí et al. 1998).

Another example of success occurred in Singapore during the 1960s, when authorities combined strict larval control with law enforcement after the emergence of dengue transmission in the island city-state (Ooi et al. 2006). The programme resulted in low incidence of disease and low entomological indices for 15 years. However, since the 1980s, dengue cases have increased in the city despite low mosquito numbers. Several reasons are hypothesized to explain this disease expansion: the absence of immunity, reduced vector surveillance for case detection, introduction of foreign cases, and possibly a shift in mosquito behaviour.

Aside from these examples, worldwide *Aedes* vector control efforts have not succeeded in sustainably reducing the arbovirus burden in recent decades.

Reasons for failure: chemical and social

These experiences present many lessons to inform future surveillance and control strategies. Investigating the reasons for what has failed to sustain long-term effects is crucial to developing strategies for stopping the transmission of *Aedes*-borne diseases. The massive elimination campaigns of the 1940s in the Americas relied heavily on chemical control methods and top-down organization, neither of which are feasible or sustainable today. The authoritarian campaigns were successful for a period of time but led to neglected surveillance and vector control programmes once the vector was thought to be eradicated. *Ae. aegypti* has now recolonized all of South America, reaching all the way to its southernmost temperature limit in Argentina where it recolonized the capital, Buenos Aires, in 1991 (Zanotti et al. 2015).

With our current understanding of the long-term environmental consequences of chemical insecticides, the mass spraying of DDT and similar materials is no longer an acceptable strategy, and not only because of environmental concerns. Indeed, chemical control methods for both larvae and adults are reaching the end of their effective use for sustainable control because *Aedes* populations worldwide are becoming resistant to a wide range of compounds. Early evidence of resistance was found with DDT, followed by resistances to a range of organophosphates including the larvicide temephos (Moyes et al. 2017). Malathion remains a useful compound for mosquito control, but its toxicity to mammals restricts its use. The biological insecticide *Bacillus thuringiensis var. israelensis,* for which no resistance has yet been observed, has largely replaced temephos.

Pyrethroids, then, have become the insecticide of choice: inexpensive, harmless to wildlife, and applicable indoors as spatial and residual spray, outdoors as ultra-low volume (UVL) aerosol, and even impregnated in cloth material. These advantages are leading to a monotherapy conducive to the widespread development of resistance (Moyes et al. 2017). In addition, since 2010, pyrethroids are the only approved compounds for adult insect control in the European Union. In the absence of any alternative, some areas such as French overseas territories have arrived at a chemical control dead-end.

Aside from the widespread mosquito resistance, the method of spraying large quantities of insecticide in the environment is itself controversial because of the lack of evidence for efficacy, high cost, slow operational response, low community acceptance, and the potential impacts on non-target organisms in the environment (Esu et al. 2010, Knauer et al. 2017). Selective pressures exerted on *Aedes* populations from vector control are compounded when the same pyrethroid insecticides are used against pest mosquitoes, found in household insecticides and impregnated gardening and personal protection materials, driving pyrethroid resistance even further and possibly preventing its reversal (Macoris et al. 2018, Gray et al. 2018).

We have arrived at the point where both chemicals and the methods for applying them may be ineffective for controlling *Aedes*, with few acceptable alternatives existing. At the very least, chemical applications for emergency tools could be regained by mandating non-chemical alternatives for non-emergency situations, or by developing novel compounds that target the vectors with other modes of action and that are more selective for mosquitoes (Dusfour et al. 2019). In the absence of novel tools that are validated, recommended or available, one possibility is to increase the use of pyrethroid-impregnated materials (in window curtains, for example) and the reinstatement of indoor residual spraying with pyrethroids (Samuel et al. 2017, Banks et al. 2015). These options are less harmful for the environment as they are localized to the indoors and effective against non-resistant strains of *Ae. aegypti* which prefer to rest indoors. For *Ae. albopictus* mosquitoes that tend to rest outside households, these alternatives would not be effective. In the absence of efficient compounds against adults, the only other effective options are the application of larvicides or the alteration of larval breeding sites for large-scale mosquito population control. Typically, water collection areas or containers are drained to eliminate putative breeding sites, covered to prevent egg-laying, filled in with sand to keep moisture for gardens without stagnant water or manipulated in such a way that mosquito larvae cannot develop or grow.

Because *Aedes* females prefer to lay eggs in small human-made containers of water, households (especially those without reliable piped water) are an important source of breeding grounds for the mosquito. Community engagement, therefore, is essential for comprehensive larval control. However, such engagement has not shown long-lasting success outside of the Cuban and Singaporean examples, both of which involved strong, authoritarian enforcement. Even though education and promotion plans were integrated into strategies, top—down approaches push the population to rely on authorities and to ignore their own personal role and responsibility in source reduction (Perez-Guerra et al. 2009, Mieulet and Claeys 2014). This behaviour is exacerbated by the belief that neighbours are not doing enough and individual efforts are made in vain (Ibarra et al. 2014). The mosquito is generally and universally hated mainly because of its bite: people are often more motivated by the nuisance they cause than by diseases they transmit (Dickinson and Paskewitz 2012). Reducing *Aedes* breeding sites, however, does not always have a direct and noticeable effect on the perception of overall nuisance, since bites may continue even from a diminished population or from other mosquito species. In contexts where other, more critical health and safety concerns dominate, mosquito-borne diseases may not take priority in the lives of the community so that communication tools developed by vector control authorities may be ignored or misunderstood (Mieulet and Claeys 2014, Anderson et al. 2020). Being sensitive to local beliefs and instilling a basic understanding of disease transmission and the mosquito life cycle are also critical for mobilizing the population to act as participants in mosquito control and participate in bottom-up interventions (Ibarra et al. 2014, Paz-Soldán et al. 2011, Frank et al. 2017). Developing effective social strategies to support vector control strategies has therefore become a key recommendation and the WHO has published recommendations for guiding and supporting socially sensitive vector control teams (Bartumeus et al. 2019, Parks and Lloyd 2005).

A team of vector control specialists cannot possibly monitor all potential breeding sites when larvae can develop into adults in only two weeks under optimal temperature conditions; therefore, involving communities in control and surveillance is essential for efficiently covering or disrupting all possible breeding sites (Gubler and Clark 1996). Successful examples of community engagement also highlight the importance of regular surveillance protocols to monitor mosquito activity, disease incidence and mosquito resistance and then sustain these efforts over time (Bardach et al. 2019, Sulistyawati et al. 2019). This integrated approach has been advocated for decades but requires intensive and constant efforts from all stakeholders, even during periods when there is no disease transmission. The best results require political commitment, sustainable allocation of resources for planning and surveillance, as well as the training of public health authorities as part of an integrated and holistic approach for mosquito control. Despite decades of *Aedes* vector control experiences, widespread comprehensive and sustained strategies of mosquito control are not currently the norm in most endemic areas (Roiz et al. 2018). As a consequence, sound strategies have by and large failed to be implemented or sustained (Gubler 2005, Roiz et al. 2018, WHOPES 2010).

In the face of dramatic recent increases in dengue and other arboviruses, few success stories and little solid evidence for effective mosquito control, many questions are left open about the future prevention of vector-borne diseases (Bowman et al. 2016). For decades, the challenges and the calls for action have been stated in publications and reports—yet dengue remains a neglected disease. With a 30-fold increase in the past 50 years, dengue is finally being taken seriously (UNICEF/UNDP/World Bank/WHO 2017, WHO 2012). The re-emergence of yellow fever, the Zika outbreak and the emergence of other novel sylvatic arboviruses carry a warning to authorities and the public about an imminent threat. *Aedes*-borne arbovirus transmission is finally drawing the attention of researchers to develop new tools for surveillance and control.

The future of control against *Aedes* and disease

The global community is facing new challenges in controlling arboviruses. At the same time, modern vector control is still placed firmly in the dream of past successes, expecting old tools and old methods to be efficient against new diseases, impacting only the targeted vector, while being environmentally friendly, sustainable and acceptable by communities all over the globe. Clearly, new tools and strategies are urgently needed.

As the number of available and effective compounds continues to decrease, it is of primary importance to regain the efficacy of pyrethroids and avoid further development of resistance. Integrated vector control must include monitoring insecticide resistance and measuring current insecticide efficacy in a comprehensive plan (Dusfour et al. 2019). Available control compounds are scarce but remain crucial for emergency control during outbreaks. As mentioned earlier, the efficacy of spatial sprays is debatable but pyrethroids could be used for indoor residual spraying or impregnation of materials. To reduce the selection pressure for resistance, alternative tools must be developed, validated and deployed.

To ensure the quality and effectiveness of proposed products and tools, the WHO has established the Prequalification Team (PQT), which replaces the WHO Pesticide Evaluation Scheme (WHOPES). The PQT supports the development, evaluation and adoption of novel control methods. An independent Vector Control Advisory Group provides additional guidance to product developers, innovators and researchers, including guidelines on the acquisition of epidemiological data, study design and new vector interventions. This group also provides advice to the WHO Strategic and Technical Advisory Group for neglected tropical diseases.

Based on the failure to maintain long-term successes in past control efforts and the expanded knowledge that the research and vector control communities have accumulated over the years, a more integrated view of vector strategies and technological advances has led to a suite of novel tools and new methods to implement them. While professional teams are still mainly responsible for implementation, the general public is now involved at an early stage, becoming an obvious and necessary component to establish and sustain vector control knowledge and practices in the affected communities (Kolopack et al. 2015, Ernst et al. 2015). Research in citizen and social sciences such as anthropology are also accompanying the expanded use of social networks and integrating mobile and geospatial technologies for providing new potential for vector control (Sousa et al. 2017, Hamer et al. 2018). Better understanding of the community's perception, knowledge, practices, beliefs and reluctance/acceptance of mosquito control is crucial for developing appropriate local communication and media messages (McNaughton 2012). Education must be sustainably implemented beginning at a young age, and adapted to local beliefs, habits and infrastructure. People must mobilize not only for vector control but also for surveillance in cooperation with a coordinated public health framework.

The research and development of new tools for targeting vector species is revealing more efficient and environmentally friendly techniques. One category is based on the knowledge of the vector's biology, behaviour and ecology to trap or otherwise prevent it from coming into contact with people. For example, there are autodissemination traps, which exploit the cryptic behaviour of oviposition, when adult mosquitoes pick up a residue of larvicide that they then spread to other breeding sites (Maoz et al. 2017). Toxic baits that contain a sugar-insecticide compound target behaviours of both adult male and female sugar-feeding (Revay et al. 2014). Those tools are currently under evaluation, and even though some have proven their efficacy in reducing mosquito density, none have yet demonstrated epidemiological successes. These tools are relatively easy to implement and can be widely distributed, although their chemical composition may require authorization in areas where they are not commercially available. The fact that such tools rely on community involvement may factor into their chances of success (Faraji and Unlu 2016). Other tools such as the trapping of large numbers of adults through attractant compounds and behaviour-modifying compounds have shown promise in lab tests. However, better attractant compounds are still needed to demonstrate significant reductions in mosquito density (Degener et al. 2015, Obermayr et al. 2015).

The second category of novel control technologies relies on genetic modification (GM) of the mosquito (Qsim et al. 2017). The objective here is to produce non-fertilized eggs or non-viable offspring, thereby reducing the density of future generations. The sterile insect technique can be achieved through several methods. One method focuses on producing sterile males by irradiation (SIT); another relies on genetically modified mosquitoes to carry a lethal gene (RIDL); a third method utilizes insect incompatibilities with *Wolbachia*-modified mosquitoes (IIT) (Crawford et al. 2020, Kittayapong et al. 2019, Thomas et al. 2000). The last has the advantage of inhibiting arbovirus multiplication and interrupting its transmission (Ryan et al. 2019). In addition, the RNA interference technique is being tested for mosquito control as both SIT and insecticidal tools (Giesbrecht et al. 2020). Whether alone or in combination, SIT, RIDL and IIT mosquitoes have proven to be of some efficacy in controlling insects in field trials, but so far such techniques have shown only preliminary evidence for controlling disease (Crawford et al. 2020, Bellini et al. 2013, Carvalho et al. 2015, Kittayapong et al. 2019).

The general public and government agencies are often sceptical about genetically modified or altered mosquito technologies and more evidence for their efficacy is needed before they can become part of a public campaign to improve their acceptance (Ernst et al. 2015, Kolopack et al. 2015). Such concerns were heightened with the discovery in Brazil that genetically modified *Ae. aegypti* transferred some of their GM genes into the wild population (Evans et al. 2019). In Europe, GM mosquitoes are highly regulated and access to such technology is controlled and limited. Because mosquitoes irradiated to produce sterile offspring (SIT) are not considered genetically modified, some have been used and tested in Italy and in Reunion Island, France. Guidelines and principles for evaluating fertility-altered mosquitoes are different from one country to another (Panjwani and Wilson 2016). In any case, all methods targeting mosquito fertility entail significant costs to maintain dedicated infrastructure and personnel for long-term mosquito mass-rearing and release (Meghani and Boëte 2018). At present, none of the new tools are fully validated or widely available, leaving traditional insecticides and source reduction methods as the sole pillars for controlling mosquitoes in the context of disease epidemics.

Zoonotic and epizootic mosquito control

While urban vectors and their associated arboviruses are at the centre of control efforts in both temperate and tropical areas, a growing concern is arising around zoonotic diseases. Viruses (and other pathogens) cycle between forest-dwelling mosquitoes and wild animals. Viruses such as Zika can be transmitted to humans when the virus enters an urban cycle with *Aedes* mosquitoes or it can be aided by bridge mosquitoes like *Ae. albopictus* that move between rural and urban habitats (Pereira et al. 2020). Many of these viruses infect humans as accidental and dead-end hosts, meaning that the virus may infect a human but is insufficiently amplified in the human body to be transmitted to another mosquito (Weaver and Reisen 2010, Wilder-Smith et al. 2017). Such is the case for West Nile virus, Usutu, Eastern equine encephalitis and Serogroup California viruses, which have all attracted attention in Europe and North America in the last few years (Gill et al. 2019, Lindsey et al. 2020, Vilibic-Cavlek et al. 2019, Calzolari et al. 2020). West Nile virus is of particular concern, and has received more research since its arrival and expansion in North America in the late 1990s.

With the emergence of more viruses using humans as dead-end hosts, controlling transmission has become an important challenge. The culprit mosquito species do not all belong to the genus *Aedes*, with *Coquillettidia*, *Culex* and *Culiseta* also implicated, mosquitoes with vastly different ecologies and some already recognized as nuisance pests (Sherwood et al. 2020, Hesson et al. 2019, Martinet et al. 2019). Several of these latter mosquito species transmit viruses to humans with varying abilities. Their physiological and ecological requirements are as different as are their life cycles over the seasons. Unlike *Aedes*, few are container-breeders, for example, creating complications for integrated vector control strategies in areas they coinhabit with other vectors. Such mosquitoes do not transmit disease as readily in their urban cycles, with the effect that there is not as much research about ways to include their habits in integrated vector control plans.

Controlling these other vector mosquitoes therefore presents difficult challenges. Personal protection and prevention measures such as topical repellents are recommended along with larval control; controlling adults or releasing sterile males are not recommended against West Nile virus (Hongoh et al. 2016, Campagna, Trudel and INSPQ 2018, CDC 2019b). Reduction of West Nile vectors by larvicides or adulticides often depends on mass spraying, a decidedly old-fashioned technique. Strategies tend to be implemented in emergency mode relying on tools already in place for controlling nuisance or other vector mosquitoes (CDC 2019a, Werth 2019). With such outbreaks occurring with increasing frequency and greater severity, the means of controlling target mosquitoes or otherwise reducing disease transmission should be carried out with consideration for environmental impacts. To complicate matters, some of these species are already resistant to insecticides, leaving their efficacy unproven in both reducing mosquito numbers and transmitting diseases (Scott et al. 2015, Dunbar et al. 2018). Novel control methods need to be developed but the knowledge of these species is scarce, leaving the first-line strategy one of heightening people's awareness of using personal protections and developing efficient surveillance tools (Kading et al. 2020, Hongoh et al. 2016, Lindsey et al. 2020).

Conclusion

Since the discovery of the mosquito's capacity to transmit pathogens that cause diseases, humanity has tried to control these vectors to reduce the disease burden. The vectorial systems involve hosts, vectors and pathogens in the natural environment in a complex interplay that is constantly evolving under selective pressures. To reach a point where people and mosquitoes can achieve a sustainable and acceptable equilibrium that simultaneously preserves human health and protects the environment, one must aim to integrate all aspects of the ecology of mosquito-borne disease with the habits of the few mosquitoes that transmit those diseases. Just as the *Aedes aegypti* mosquito has fully adapted to living with humans, people must learn to adapt their own habits and urban environments to minimize their exposure to this and other dangerous mosquitoes. Targeted and integrated approaches for reducing the transmission of urban mosquito diseases have been advocated for decades but are unevenly applied due to their costs, limited human capacity, community apathy and weakness of the political will that is required to sustain these efforts during interepidemic periods. With the rising threat of mosquito-borne diseases, these approaches must be strengthened and adapted if we want to reduce pathogen transmission.

Bibliography

Achee, Nicole L., Fred Gould, T. Alex Perkins, Robert C. Reiner Jr, Amy C. Morrison, Scott A. Ritchie, Duane J. Gubler, Remy Teyssou, and Thomas W. Scott. 2015. A Critical Assessment of Vector Control for Dengue Prevention. *PLOS Neglected Tropical Diseases* 9 (5): e0003655. https://doi.org/10.1371/journal.pntd.0003655.

Anderson, Elizabeth J., Kacey C. Ernst, Francisco Fernando Martins, Cicera da Silva Martins, and Mary P. Koss. 2020. Women's Health Perceptions and Beliefs Related to Zika Virus Exposure during the 2016 Outbreak in Northern Brazil. *The American Journal of Tropical Medicine and Hygiene* 102 (3): 629–633. https://doi.org/10.4269/ajtmh.19-0311.

Armada Gessa, J.A., and R. Figueredo González. 1986. Application of Environmental Management Principles in the Program for Eradication of *Aedes* (*Stegomyia*) *aegypti* (Linneus, 1762) in the Republic of Cuba, 1984. *Bulletin of the Pan American Health Organization* 20 (2): 186–193.

Banks, Sarah DeRaedt, James Orsborne, Salvador A. Gezan, Harparkash Kaur, Annelies Wilder-Smith, Steve W. Lindsey, and James G. Logan. 2015. Permethrin-Treated Clothing as Protection against the Dengue Vector, *Aedes aegypti*: Extent and Duration of Protection. *PLOS Neglected Tropical Diseases* 9 (10): e0004109. https://doi.org/10.1 371/journal.pntd.0004109.

Bardach, Ariel Esteban, Herney Andrés García-Perdomo, Andrea Alcaraz, Elena Tapia López, Ruth Amanda Ruano Gándara, Silvina Ruvinsky, and Agustín Ciapponi. 2019. Interventions for the Control of *Aedes aegypti* in Latin America and the Caribbean: Systematic Review and Meta-Analysis. *Tropical Medicine & International Health*: 24 (5): 530–552. https://doi.org/10.1111/tmi.13217.

Bargielowski, Irka E., L. Philip Lounibos, and María Cristina Carrasquilla. 2013. Evolution of Resistance to Satyrization through Reproductive Character Displacement in Populations of Invasive Dengue Vectors. *Proceedings of the National Academy of Sciences of the United States of America* 110 (8): 2888–2892.

Bartumeus, Frederic, Guilherme B. Costa, Roger Eritja, Ann H Kelly, Marceline Finda, Javier Lezaun, Fredros Okumu, et al. 2019. Sustainable Innovation in Vector Control Requires Strong Partnerships with Communities. *PLoS Neglected Tropical Diseases* 13 (4). https://journals.plos.org/plosntds/article?id=10.1371/journal.pntd.0007204.

Bellini, R., A. Medici, A. Puggioli, F. Balestrino, and M. Carrieri. 2013. Pilot Field Trials with *Aedes albopictus* Irradiated Sterile Males in Italian Urban Areas. *Journal of Medical Entomology* 50 (2): 317–325. https://doi.org/10.1603/me12048.

Bowman, Leigh R., Sarah Donegan, and Philip J. McCall. 2016. Is Dengue Vector Control Deficient in Effectiveness or Evidence?: Systematic Review and Meta-Analysis. *PLoS Neglected Tropical Diseases* 10 (3): e0004551. https://doi.org/10.1371/j ournal.pntd.0004551.

Bradshaw, Corey J.A., Boris Leroy, Céline Bellard, David Roiz, Céline Albert, Alice Fournier, Morgane Barbet-Massin, Jean-Michel Salles, Frédéric Simard, and Franck Courchamp. 2016. Massive yet Grossly Underestimated Global Costs of Invasive Insects. *Nature Communications* 7 (1): 12986. https://doi.org/10.1038/ncomms12986.

Britch, S.C., K.J. Linthicum, R.L. Aldridge, M.S. Breidenbaugh, M.D. Latham, P.H. Connelly, and M.J.E. Rush, J.L. Remmers, J.D. Kerce, C.A. Silcox. 2018. US Navy Entomology Center of Excellence Team. Aerial ULV control of Aedes aegypti with naled (Dibrom) inside simulated rural village and urban cryptic habitats. *PLoS One* 13 (1): e0191555. doi: 10.1371/journal.pone.0191555. PMID: 29352307; PMCID: PMC5774805.

Calzolari, Mattia, Paola Angelini, Luca Bolzoni, Paolo Bonilauri, Roberto Cagarelli, Sabrina Canziani, Danilo Cereda, et al. 2020. Enhanced West Nile Virus Circulation in the Emilia-Romagna and Lombardy Regions (Northern Italy) in 2018 Detected by Entomological Surveillance. *Frontiers in Veterinary Science* 7: 243. https://doi.org/10 .3389/fvets.2020.00243.

Campagna, Céline, Richard Trudel, and INSPQ. 2018. *Évaluation de l'efficacité des larvicides contre les espèces vectrices du virus du Nil occidental: Rapport d'évaluation.* http://collections .banq.qc.ca/ark:/52327/3579857.

Carvalho, Danilo O., Andrew R. McKemey, Luiza Garziera, Renaud Lacroix, Christl A. Donnelly, Luke Alphey, Aldo Malavasi, and Margareth L. Capurro. 2015. Suppression of a Field Population of *Aedes aegypti* in Brazil by Sustained Release of Transgenic

Male Mosquitoes. *PLoS Neglected Tropical Diseases* 9 (7): e0003864. https://doi.org/10 .1371/journal.pntd.0003864.

CDC. 2019a. Information on Aerial Spraying. *Centers for Disease Control.* October 2. https ://www.cdc.gov/easternequineencephalitis/mosquitocontrol/aerial-spraying.html.

CDC. 2019b. *Prevention.* October 7. https://www.cdc.gov/lac/gen/pre.html.

Crawford, Jacob E., David W. Clarke, Victor Criswell, Mark Desnoyer, Devon Cornel, Brittany Deegan, Kyle Gong, et al. 2020. Efficient Production of Male Wolbachia -Infected *Aedes aegypti* Mosquitoes Enables Large-Scale Suppression of Wild Populations. *Nature Biotechnology* 38 (4): 482–492. https://doi.org/10.1038/s41587 -020-0471-x.

Degener, Carolin Marlen, Tatiana Mingote Ferreira de Ázara, Rosemary Aparecida Roque, Susanne Rösner, Eliseu Soares Oliveira Rocha, Erna Geessien Kroon, Cláudia Torres Codeço, et al. 2015. Mass Trapping with MosquiTRAPs Does Not Reduce *Aedes aegypti* Abundance. *Memórias Do Instituto Oswaldo Cruz* 110 (4): 517–527. https://doi.org/10.1590/0074-02760140374.

Dickinson, Katherine, and Susan Paskewitz. 2012. Willingness to Pay for Mosquito Control: How Important Is West Nile Virus Risk Compared to the Nuisance of Mosquitoes? *Vector Borne and Zoonotic Diseases* 12 (10): 886–892.

Dunbar, Mike W., Amanda Bachmann, and Adam J. Varenhorst. 2018. Reduced Insecticide Susceptibility in *Aedes vexans* (Diptera: Culicidae) Where Agricultural Pest Management Overlaps With Mosquito Abatement. *Journal of Medical Entomology* 55 (3): 747–751. https://doi.org/10.1093/jme/tjx245.

Dusfour, Isabelle, John Vontas, Jean-Philippe David, David Weetman, Dina M. Fonseca, Vincent Corbel, Kamaraju Raghavendra, et al. 2019. Management of Insecticide Resistance in the Major *Aedes* Vectors of Arboviruses: Advances and Challenges. *PLoS Neglected Tropical Diseases* 13 (10): e0007615. https://doi.org/10.1371/journal .pntd.0007615.

Ernst, Kacey C., Steven Haenchen, Katherine Dickinson, Michael S. Doyle, Kathleen Walker, Andrew J. Monaghan, and Mary H. Hayden. 2015. Awareness and Support of Release of Genetically Modified 'Sterile' Mosquitoes, Key West, Florida, USA. *Emerging Infectious Diseases* 21 (2): 320–324. https://doi.org/10.3201/eid2102.141035.

Esu, E., A. Lenhart, L. Smith, and O. Horstick. 2010. Effectiveness of Peridomestic Space Spraying with Insecticide on Dengue Transmission; Systematic Review. *Trop Med Int Health* 15 (May): 619–631. https://doi.org/10.1111/j.1365-3156.2010.02489.x.

Evans, Benjamin R., Panayiota Kotsakiozi, Andre Luis Costa-da-Silva, Rafaella Sayuri Ioshino, Luiza Garziera, Michele C. Pedrosa, Aldo Malavasi, Jair F. Virginio, Margareth L. Capurro, and Jeffrey R. Powell. 2019. Transgenic *Aedes aegypti* Mosquitoes Transfer Genes into a Natural Population. *Scientific Reports* 9 (1): 13047. https://doi.org/10.1038/s41598-019-49660-6.

Faraji, Ary, and Isik Unlu. 2016. The Eye of the Tiger, the Thrill of the Fight: Effective Larval and Adult Control Measures Against the Asian Tiger Mosquito, Aedes Albopictus (Diptera: Culicidae), in North America. *Journal of Medical Entomology* 53 (5): 1029–1047. https://doi.org/10.1093/jme/tjw096.

Frank, Amy L, Emily R Beales, Gilles de Wildt, Graciela Meza Sanchez, and Laura L Jones. 2017. "We Need People to Collaborate Together against This Disease": A Qualitative Exploration of Perceptions of Dengue Fever Control in Caregivers' of Children under 5 Years, in the Peruvian Amazon. *PLoS Neglected Tropical Diseases* 11 (9): e0005755.

Giesbrecht, David, Daniel Heschuk, Ian Wiens, David Boguski, Parker LaChance, and Steve Whyard. 2020. RNA Interference Is Enhanced by Knockdown of

Double-Stranded RNases in the Yellow Fever Mosquito *Aedes aegypti*. *Insects* 11 (6). https://doi.org/10.3390/insects11060327.

Gill, Christine M., J. David Beckham, Amanda L. Piquet, Kenneth L. Tyler, and Daniel M. Pastula. 2019. Five Emerging Neuroinvasive Arboviral Diseases: Cache Valley, Eastern Equine Encephalitis, Jamestown Canyon, Powassan, and Usutu. *Seminars in Neurology* 39 (4): 419–427. https://doi.org/10.1055/s-0039-1687839.

Gray, Lyndsey, Sergio Dzib Florez, Anuar Medina Barreiro, José Vadillo-Sánchez, Gabriela González-Olvera, Audrey Lenhart, Pablo Manrique-Saide, and Gonzalo M. Vazquez-Prokopec. 2018. Experimental Evaluation of the Impact of Household Aerosolized Insecticides on Pyrethroid Resistant *Aedes aegypti*. *Scientific Reports* 8 (August). https://doi.org/10.1038/s41598-018-30968-8.

Gubler, D.J.. 2005. The Emergence of Epidemic Dengue Fever and Dengue Hemorrhagic Fever in the Americas: A Case of Failed Public Health Policy. *Revista Panamericana de Salud Pública* 17 (4). https://doi.org/10.1590/S1020-49892005000400001.

Gubler, D.J., and G.G. Clark. 1996. Community Involvement in the Control of *Aedes aegypti*. *Acta Tropica* 61 (2): 169–179. https://doi.org/10.1016/0001-706x(95)00103-l.

Hamer, Sarah A., Rachel Curtis-Robles, and Gabriel L. Hamer. 2018. Contributions of Citizen Scientists to Arthropod Vector Data in the Age of Digital Epidemiology. *Current Opinion in Insect Science* 28: 98–104. https://doi.org/10.1016/j.cois.2018.05.005.

Han, W.W., A. Lazaro, P.J. McCall, L. George, S. Runge-Ranzinger, J. Toledo, R. Velayudhan, and O. Horstick. 2015. Efficacy and Community Effectiveness of Larvivorous Fish for Dengue Vector Control. *Tropical Medicine & International Health* 20 (9): 1239–1256. https://doi.org/10.1111/tmi.12538.

Hesson, Jenny C., Emma Lundin, Åke Lundkvist, and Jan O. Lundström. 2019. Surveillance of Mosquito Vectors in Southern Sweden for Flaviviruses and Sindbis Virus. *Infection Ecology & Epidemiology* 9 (1): 1698903. https://doi.org/10.1080/2 0008686.2019.1698903.

Hierlihy, Catherine, Lisa Waddell, Ian Young, Judy Greig, Tricia Corrin, and Mariola Mascarenhas. 2019. A Systematic Review of Individual and Community Mitigation Measures for Prevention and Control of Chikungunya Virus. *PloS One* 14 (2): e0212054. https://doi.org/10.1371/journal.pone.0212054.

Hongoh, Valerie, Céline Campagna, Mirna Panic, Onil Samuel, Pierre Gosselin, Jean-Philippe Waaub, André Ravel, Karim Samoura, and Pascal Michel. 2016. Assessing Interventions to Manage West Nile Virus Using Multi-Criteria Decision Analysis with Risk Scenarios. *PLOS ONE* 11 (8): e0160651. https://doi.org/10.1371/journal .pone.0160651.

Horstick, Olaf, Silvia Runge-Ranzinger, Michael B. Nathan, and Axel Kroeger. 2010. Dengue Vector-Control Services: How Do They Work? A Systematic Literature Review and Country Case Studies. *Transactions of the Royal Society of Tropical Medicine and Hygiene* 104 (6): 379–386. https://doi.org/10.1016/j.trstmh.2009.07.027.

Ibarra, Anna M Stewart, Valerie A Luzadis, Mercy J Borbor Cordova, Mercy Silva, Tania Ordoñez, Efraín Beltrán Ayala, and Sadie J Ryan. 2014. A Social-Ecological Analysis of Community Perceptions of Dengue Fever and *Aedes aegypti* in Machala, Ecuador. *BMC Public Health* 14 (1): 1135.

Kading, Rebekah C., Lee W. Cohnstaedt, Ken Fall, and Gabriel L. Hamer. 2020. Emergence of Arboviruses in the United States: The Boom and Bust of Funding, Innovation, and Capacity. *Tropical Medicine and Infectious Disease* 5 (2). https://doi.org /10.3390/tropicalmed5020096.

Kittayapong, Pattamaporn, Suwannapa Ninphanomchai, Wanitch Limohpasmanee, Chitti Chansang, Uruyakorn Chansang, and Piti Mongkalangoon. 2019. Combined

Sterile Insect Technique and Incompatible Insect Technique: The First Proof-of-Concept to Suppress *Aedes aegypti* Vector Populations in Semi-Rural Settings in Thailand. *PLOS Neglected Tropical Diseases* 13 (10): e0007771. https://doi.org/10.1371/journal.pntd.0007771.

Knauer, Katja, Nadzeya Homazava, Marion Junghans, and Inge Werner. 2017. The Influence of Particles on Bioavailability and Toxicity of Pesticides in Surface Water. *Integrated Environmental Assessment and Management* 13 (4): 585–600. https://doi.org/10.1002/ieam.1867.

Kolopack, Pamela A, Janet A Parsons, and James V Lavery. 2015. What Makes Community Engagement Effective?: Lessons from the Eliminate Dengue Program in Queensland Australia. *PLoS Neglected Tropical Diseases* 9 (4). https://www.ncbi.nlm.nih.gov/pmc/articles/PMC4395388/.

Kourí, Gustavo, María Guadalupe Guzmán, Luis Valdés, Isabel Carbonel, Delfina del Rosario, Susana Vazquez, José Laferté, Jorge Delgado, and María V. Cabrera. 1998. Reemergence of Dengue in Cuba: A 1997 Epidemic in Santiago de Cuba. *Emerging Infectious Diseases* 4 (1). https://doi.org/10.3201/eid0401.980111.

Kraemer, Moritz U.G., Robert C. Reiner, Oliver J. Brady, Jane P. Messina, Marius Gilbert, David M. Pigott, Dingdong Yi, et al. 2019. Past and Future Spread of the Arbovirus Vectors *Aedes aegypti* and *Aedes albopictus*. *Nature Microbiology* 4 (5): 854–863. https://doi.org/10.1038/s41564-019-0376-y.

Lazaro, A., W.W. Han, P. Manrique-Saide, L. George, R. Velayudhan, J. Toledo, S. Runge Ranzinger, and O. Horstick. 2015. Community Effectiveness of Copepods for Dengue Vector Control: Systematic Review. *Tropical Medicine & International Health* 20 (6): 685–706. https://doi.org/10.1111/tmi.12485.

Likos, Anna, Isabel Griffin, Andrea M. Bingham, Danielle Stanek, Marc Fischer, Stephen White, Janet Hamilton, et al. 2016. Local Mosquito-Borne Transmission of Zika Virus — Miami-Dade and Broward Counties, Florida, June–August 2016. *MMWR. Morbidity and Mortality Weekly Report* 65 (38): 1032–1038. https://doi.org/10.2307/24858999.

Lindsey, Nicole P., Stacey W. Martin, J. Erin Staples, and Marc Fischer. 2020. Notes from the Field: Multistate Outbreak of Eastern Equine Encephalitis Virus — United States, 2019. *MMWR. Morbidity and Mortality Weekly Report* 69 (2): 50–51. https://doi.org/10.15585/mmwr.mm6902a4.

Macoris, Maria de Lourdes, Ademir Jesus Martins, Maria Teresa Macoris Andrighetti, José Bento Pereira Lima, and Denise Valle. 2018. Pyrethroid Resistance Persists after Ten Years Without Usage against *Aedes aegypti* in Governmental Campaigns: Lessons from São Paulo State, Brazil. *PLoS Neglected Tropical Diseases* 12 (3): e0006390. https://doi.org/10.1371/journal.pntd.0006390.

Maoz, Dorit, Tara Ward, Moody Samuel, Pie Müller, Silvia Runge-Ranzinger, Joao Toledo, Ross Boyce, Raman Velayudhan, and Olaf Horstick. 2017. Community Effectiveness of Pyriproxyfen as a Dengue Vector Control Method: A Systematic Review. *PLoS Neglected Tropical Diseases* 11 (7): e0005651. https://doi.org/10.1371/journal.pntd.0005651.

Marcondes, Carlos Brisola. 2019. *Medical and Veterinary Entomology*. Atheneu. Rio de Janairo: Elsevier. https://doi.org/10.1016/C2017-0-00210-0.

Martinet, Jean-Philippe, Hubert Ferté, Anna-Bella Failloux, Francis Schaffner, and Jérôme Depaquit. 2019. Mosquitoes of North-Western Europe as Potential Vectors of Arboviruses: A Review. *Viruses* 11 (11). https://doi.org/10.3390/v11111059.

McNaughton, Darlene. 2012. The Importance of Long-Term Social Research in Enabling Participation and Developing Engagement Strategies for New Dengue

Control Technologies. *PLOS Neglected Tropical Diseases* 6 (8): e1785. https://doi.org /10.1371/journal.pntd.0001785.

Meghani, Zahra, and Christophe Boëte. 2018. Genetically Engineered Mosquitoes, Zika and Other Arboviruses, Community Engagement, Costs, and Patents: Ethical Issues. *PLoS Neglected Tropical Diseases* 12 (7): e0006501. https://doi.org/10.1371/journal.pnt d.0006501.

Mieulet, Elise, and Cécilia Claeys. 2014. The Implementation and Reception of Policies for Preventing Dengue Fever Epidemics: A Comparative Study of Martinique and French Guyana. *Health, Risk & Society* 16 (7–8): 581–599. https://doi.org/10.1080/1 3698575.2014.949224.

Moyes, Catherine L., John Vontas, Ademir J. Martins, Lee Ching Ng, Sin Ying Koou, Isabelle Dusfour, Kamaraju Raghavendra, et al. 2017. Contemporary Status of Insecticide Resistance in the Major Aedes Vectors of Arboviruses Infecting Humans. *PLoS Neglected Tropical Diseases* 11 (7): e0005625. https://doi.org/10.1371/journal.pnt d.0005625.

Obermayr, Ulla, Joachim Ruther, Ulrich R. Bernier, Andreas Rose, and Martin Geier. 2015. Evaluation of a Push-Pull Approach for *Aedes aegypti* (L.) Using a Novel Dispensing System for Spatial Repellents in the Laboratory and in a Semi-Field Environment. *PLoS ONE* 10 (6). https://doi.org/10.1371/journal.pone.0129878.

Ooi, Eng-Eong, Kee-Tai Goh, and Duane J. Gubler. 2006. Dengue Prevention and 35 Years of Vector Control in Singapore. *Emerging Infectious Diseases* 12 (6). https://doi .org/10.3201/eid1206.051210.

Panjwani, Anusha, and Anthony Wilson. 2016. What Is Stopping the Use of Genetically Modified Insects for Disease Control? *PLOS Pathogens* 12 (10): e1005830. https://doi .org/10.1371/journal.ppat.1005830.

Parks, Will, and Linda Lloyd. 2005. *Planning Social Mobilization and Communication for Dengue Fever Prevention and Control: A Step-by-Step Guide.* Geneva: World Health Organization.

Paupy, C., H. Delatte, L. Bagny, V. Corbel, and D. Fontenille. 2009. Aedes Albopictus, an Arbovirus Vector: From the Darkness to the Light. *Microbes Infect* 11 (December): 1177–1185. https://doi.org/10.1016/j.micinf.2009.05.005.

Paz-Soldan, Valerie A., Valaikanya Plasai, Amy C. Morrison, Esther J. Rios-Lopez, Shirly Guedez-Gonzales, John P. Grieco, Kirk Mundal, Theeraphap Chareonviriyaphap, and Nicole L. Achee. 2011. Initial Assessment of the Acceptability of a Push-Pull *Aedes aegypti* Control Strategy in Iquitos, Peru and Kanchanaburi, Thailand. *The American Journal of Tropical Medicine and Hygiene* 84 (2): 208–217. https://doi.org/10.4 269/ajtmh.2011.09-0615.

Pereira, T., D Roiz, R. Lourenco do Oliveira, and C. Paupy. 2020. A Systematic Review: Is *Aedes albopictus* an Efficient Bridge Vector for Zoonotic Arboviruses? Pathogens (Basel, Switzerland). *Pathogens*, July 4. https://doi.org/10.3390/pathogens9040266.

Perez-Guerra, C.L., E. Zielinski-Gutierrez, D. Vargas-Torres, and G.G. Clark. 2009. Community Beliefs and Practices about Dengue in Puerto Rico. *Revista Panamericana de Salud Publica* 25 (March): 218–226.

Powell, J.R., Gloria-Soria A., Kotsakiozi P. and Ding-Guo Gao. 2000. Recent History of *Aedes aegypti*: Vector Genomics and Epidemiology Records. *Bioscience* 68(11), 854–860. https://doi.org/10.1093/biosci/biy119

Qsim, Muhammad, Usman Ali Ashfaq, Muhammad Zubair Yousaf, Muhammad Shareef Masoud, Ijaz Rasul, Namrah Noor, and Azfar Hussain. 2017. Genetically Modified *Aedes aegypti* to Control Dengue: A Review. *Critical Reviews in Eukaryotic*

Gene Expression 27 (4): 331–340. https://doi.org/10.1615/CritRevEukaryotGeneExpr .2017019937.

Revay, Edita E., Gunter C. Müller, Whitney A. Qualls, Daniel Kline, Diana P. Naranjo, Kristopher L. Arheart, Vasiliy D. Kravchenko, et al. 2014. Control of *Aedes albopictus* with Attractive Toxic Sugar Baits (ATSB) and Potential Impact on Non-Target Organisms in St. Augustine, Florida. *Parasitology Research* 113 (1): 73–79. https://doi .org/10.1007/s00436-013-3628-4.

Roiz, David, Anne L. Wilson, Thomas W. Scott, Dina M. Fonseca, Frédéric Jourdain, Pie Müller, Raman Velayudhan, and Vincent Corbel. 2018. Integrated Aedes Management for the Control of *Aedes*-Borne Diseases. *PLOS Neglected Tropical Diseases* 12 (12): e0006845. https://doi.org/10.1371/journal.pntd.0006845.

Ryan, Peter A., Andrew P. Turley, Geoff Wilson, Tim P. Hurst, Kate Retzki, Jack Brown-Kenyon, Lauren Hodgson, et al. 2019. Establishment of WMel Wolbachia in *Aedes aegypti* Mosquitoes and Reduction of Local Dengue Transmission in Cairns and Surrounding Locations in Northern Queensland, Australia. *Gates Open Research* 3: 1547. https://doi.org/10.12688/gatesopenres.13061.2.

Samuel, Moody, Dorit Maoz, Pablo Manrique, Tara Ward, Silvia Runge-Ranzinger, Joao Toledo, Ross Boyce, and Olaf Horstick. 2017. Community Effectiveness of Indoor Spraying as a Dengue Vector Control Method: A Systematic Review. *PLoS Neglected Tropical Diseases* 11 (8): e0005837. https://doi.org/10.1371/journal.pntd.000 5837.

Scott, Jeffrey G., Melissa Hardstone Yoshimizu, and Shinji Kasai. 2015. Pyrethroid Resistance in *Culex pipiens* Mosquitoes. *Pesticide Biochemistry and Physiology* 120 (May): 68–76. https://doi.org/10.1016/j.pestbp.2014.12.018.

Sherwood, J.A., S.V. Stehman, J.J. Howard, and J. Oliver. 2020. Cases of Eastern Equine Encephalitis in Humans Associated with *Aedes canadensis, Coquillettidia perturbans* and Culiseta melanura Mosquitoes with the Virus in New York State from 1971 to 2012 by Analysis of Aggregated Published Data. *Epidemiology & Infection* 148. https://doi .org/10.1017/S0950268820000308.

Soper, Fred L. 1963. The Elimination of Urban Yellow Fever in the Americas Through the Eradication of *Aedes aegypti*. *American Journal of Public Health and the Nation's Health* 53 (1): 7–16.

Sousa, L., Mello De, D. Cedrim, A. Garcia, P. Missier, U. Anderson, O. Anderson, and A. Romanovsky. 2017. VazaDengue: An Information System for Preventing and Combating Mosquito-Borne Diseases with Social Networks. *School of Computing Science Technical Report Series*. https://eprint.ncl.ac.uk/240257.

Sulistyawati, Sulistyawati, Fardhiasih Dwi Astuti, Sitti Rahmah Umniyati, Tri Baskoro Tunggul Satoto, Lutfan Lazuardi, Maria Nilsson, Joacim Rocklov, Camilla Andersson, and Åsa Holmner. 2019. Dengue Vector Control through Community Empowerment: Lessons Learned from a Community-Based Study in Yogyakarta, Indonesia. *International Journal of Environmental Research and Public Health* 16 (6). https://doi.org/10.3390/ijerph16061013.

Thomas, D.D., C.A. Donnelly, R.J. Wood, and L.S. Alphey. 2000. Insect Population Control Using a Dominant, Repressible, Lethal Genetic System. *Science (New York, N.Y.)* 287 (5462): 2474–2476. https://doi.org/10.1126/science.287.5462.2474.

UNICEF/UNDP/World Bank/WHO. 2017. Global Vector Control Response 2017–2030. Special Programme for Research and Training in Tropical. https://apps.who .int/iris/handle/10665/259002.

Vilibic-Cavlek, Tatjana, Vladimir Savic, Tamas Petrovic, Ivan Toplak, Ljubo Barbic, Dusan Petric, Irena Tabain, et al. 2019. Emerging Trends in the Epidemiology of West

Nile and Usutu Virus Infections in Southern Europe. *Frontiers in Veterinary Science* 6: 437. https://doi.org/10.3389/fvets.2019.00437.

Weaver, Scott C., and William K. Reisen. 2010. Present and Future Arboviral Threats. *Antiviral Research* 85 (2): 328–345. https://doi.org/10.1016/j.antiviral.2009.10.008.

Werth, Julia. 2019. As Massachusetts and Rhode Island Begin Aerial Spraying, Mosquitoes in Southeast Connecticut Test Positive for Eastern Equine Encephalitis. *The Connecticut Examiner (blog).* September 10. https://ctexaminer.com/2019/09/10/as-massachusetts-and-rhode-island-begin-aerial-spraying-mosquitoes-in-southeast-connecticut-test-positive-for-eastern-equine-encephalitis/.

WHOPES. 2010. *WHO Pesticide Evaluation Scheme: 50 Years of Global Leadership. WHO/HTM/NTD/WHOPES/2010.2.* Geneva: WHO. http://www.who.int/whopes/resources/978924159927/en/.

Wilder-Smith, Annelies, Duane J. Gubler, Scott C. Weaver, Thomas P. Monath, David L. Heymann, and Thomas W. Scott. 2017. Epidemic Arboviral Diseases: Priorities for Research and Public Health. *The Lancet Infectious Diseases* 17 (3): e101–106. https://doi.org/10.1016/S1473-3099(16)30518-7.

Wilson, Anne L., Marleen Boelaert, Immo Kleinschmidt, Margaret Pinder, Thomas W. Scott, Lucy S. Tusting, and Steve W. Lindsay. 2015. Evidence-Based Vector Control? Improving the Quality of Vector Control Trials. *Trends in Parasitology* 31 (8): 380–390. https://doi.org/10.1016/j.pt.2015.04.015.

World Health Organization. 1997. *Dengue Haemorrhagic Fever : Diagnosis, Treatment, Prevention and Control.* World Health Organization. https://apps.who.int/iris/handle/10665/41988.

World Health Organization. 2012. *Global Strategy for Dengue Prevention and Control, 2012–2020.* Geneva: World Health Organization. http://apps.who.int/iris/bitstream/10665/75303/1/9789241504034_eng.pdf.

World Health Organization. 2020. *WHO.* World Health Organization. http://www.who.int/neglected_diseases/vector_ecology/mosquito-borne-diseases/en/.

Zanotti, Gabriela, María Sol De Majo, Iris Alem, Nicolás Schweigmann, Raúl E Campos, and Sylvia Fischer. 2015. New Records of *Aedes aegypti* at the Southern Limit of Its Distribution in Buenos Aires Province, Argentina. *Journal of Vector Ecology* 40 (2): 408–411.

15

DESIGNER MOSQUITOES?

Prospects and precautions of genome-edited insects for public health

Ramya M. Rajagopalan

> Some of the most fascinating of the new methods [for controlling insect pests] are those that seek to turn the strength of a species against itself—to use the drive of an insect's life forces to destroy it.
>
> —Rachel Carson, *Silent Spring*, 1962

Among the many influences theorized across human societies as the animating "life force" giving rise to the splendid diversity of Earth's biomes, perhaps none has been so fetishized by the public and scientific consciousness as the biochemical macromolecule known as deoxyribonucleic acid or DNA: made up of sequences of the nucleotides A, T, G and C, code for genes and genomes throughout the plant, animal and microbial kingdoms. DNA metaphors, like the "book of life" and "the age old language of the living cell," have been critiqued for their over-simplification of life processes (Keller 1995). Nevertheless, the idea of DNA as the animating molecule of life has been fashioned into a ubiquitous icon of heredity, unfairly burdened with the responsibility of an outsized and deterministic influence on the entirety of the intergenerational processes that support life on earth. This "mystique" of DNA as the control centre of all life (Nelkin and Lindee, 2004) is increasingly contested. New research in fields such as epigenetics show that DNA is but one factor among a host of complex biological, social and environmental interactions to which living things are subjected and which shape them at every stage of development, within and across generations. But the chemical and informational simplicity of DNA, and its ubiquity across lifeforms, have become a convenient conceptual platform from which to fantasize about the possibility of manipulating and modifying DNA, and of shaping life into new forms that are subservient to human desires.

The dream of altering or rewriting DNA has been made concrete in the twenty-first century through a set of techniques known as "gene editing" or

DOI: 10.4324/9781003056034-15

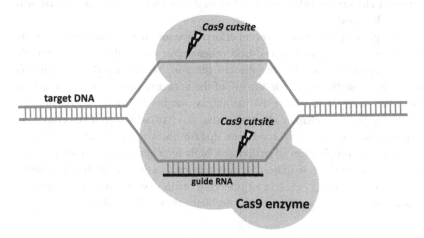

FIGURE 15.1 Schematic of CRISPR–Cas9 mediated gene editing. Source: Adapted from Jinek et al. 2012.

"genome editing," which have transformed scientific research. Gene editing repurposes the bacterial surveillance system known as CRISPR-Cas9, which microbes use as a kind of immune mechanism to identify and defend against invading pathogens like viruses. The catalytic engine of this molecular machine is the enzyme Cas9. Short sequences of ribonucleic acid (RNA) guide Cas9 in locating complementary target sequences in the genome, where Cas9 separates and cuts the two strands of DNA, initiating the rewriting of the target DNA sequence (Figure 15.1). This seemingly simple sequence of steps comprises a powerful molecular technology. Indeed, CRISPR-Cas9–mediated gene editing is just the latest in a long line of genetic engineering tools developed by molecular biologists who have sought to read, write, cut, paste and rewrite DNA to meet human needs.

Since the 1960s, scientists have used genetic engineering to successfully mass-produce vital protein-based drugs like insulin, blight-resistant crops and catalytically active enzymes that form laundry detergent and cheese. Yet many early genetic-modification tools were imprecise, time-consuming and expensive, restricting their possible applications. CRISPR-Cas9 represents a new—if controversial—kind of genetic engineering that can theoretically be used to cut, paste or edit *any* piece of DNA, in *any* organism on the planet, relatively easily and cheaply. This technology is potentially world-changing.

Envisioning it as a kind of genetic surgery, enthusiasts see limitless possibilities for gene editing, from curing disease, to improving crops, eliminating insect and fungal pests, and transforming living things into what humans wish them to be. Alongside hopes of transforming health care, agriculture and species conservation, the spectre of CRISPR-Cas9 has also sparked intense debate. This gene-editing technology may allow humans to make irrevocable, permanent changes to other species, but its downstream consequences are still poorly understood.

Within global public health, recent efforts have sought to harness gene editing to accelerate the "end of malaria" and other vector-borne diseases. By genetically modifying disease-carrying insects, the aim, borrowing Rachel Carson's framing, is to use the very "life forces" of the vector to destroy itself, or at least to block its ability to transmit the pathogens that have long decimated human populations. As this chapter discusses, the ways in which genetic engineering figures in controlling vector-borne disease illuminates the social, political and economic complexities of utilizing a high-tech approach, challenging our assumptions about the role of human intervention in a delicate global ecosystem. As with any technology, genetic engineering technologies can embody specific political and moral orientations to the problems they seek to address.

The elusive nature of vector control

Efforts to manipulate the genetic composition of mosquitoes follow on a long history of often frustrated attempts to rid human societies of mosquito-borne disease. For centuries mosquitoes have been viewed as pests, insects whose tiny size belies the throbbing, itchy sting of their blood-sucking bite. But they also serve as unwitting vectors for parasites, like those of the genus *Plasmodium*, which cause malaria, a debilitating disease that devastates hard-hit communities in South and Southeast Asia, sub-Saharan Africa, and northern South America. Annually, hundreds of thousands of children and adults lose their lives or their livelihoods to malaria (WHO 2020). Among the 112 genera and over 3,500 species of mosquitoes which have been identified, the females of just a handful of species in three genera bite humans to nourish developing eggs, sometimes transmitting disease-causing viruses and parasites. These *Anopheles*, *Aedes* and *Culex* mosquitoes have been the focus of efforts to use genetic approaches for vector control.

In the 1940s, the development of the potent insecticide known as dichlorodiphenyltrichloroethane (DDT) fueled over three decades of vector control and eradication campaigns aimed at alleviating the public health burdens posed by mosquitoes (Stepan 2011). The World Health Organization (WHO) initiated the Global Malaria Eradication Programme in the 1950s in an effort to eliminate malaria in Europe, Asia and the Americas, in part by spraying millions of tonnes of DDT. However, DDT is quite toxic and persistent in the environment, and humanity's growing reliance on it was destroying fragile ecosystems (Carson 1962). Further, mosquitoes rapidly began to develop resistance to DDT and to later pyrethroid-based insecticides that replaced it, even when exposed to previously lethal concentrations.

As eradication attempts faltered and were suspended in the 1960s, mosquito vectors returned and brought with them a resurgence of disease. Some nations and localities temporarily or permanently quashed vector-borne diseases, as the United States did for mosquito-borne malaria, while others struggled with rebound malaria. Surviving a bout of malaria could also be protective; when DDT dramatically reduced local mosquito populations and thus the incidence of malaria infections over several years, children no longer encountered the parasite early enough in their development to acquire short-term immunity. Some rebounds were therefore even more deadly than the original epidemics (Cohen et al. 2012).

Into the lively, bloody politics animating failed mosquito eradication campaigns, then, the new DNA editing technologies are being tested as a means of exerting genetic control over insect pests. These high-tech efforts are unfolding in the 2000s in the context of a renewed malaria elimination agenda crafted by the WHO's Global Malaria Programme, in concert with governments and philanthropies. Under their auspices, research groups around the world have pivoted to developing novel chemistries for next-generation insecticides, and more controversially, re-engineering the very DNA of mosquitoes. Twenty-first-century biotechnology might enhance the arsenal of vector-borne disease control, but not without social, political and ecological ramifications. It also unleashes the power to alter the direction of evolutionary change in target species (Noble et al. 2018). Community members, civil society groups, journalists, scientists, policy-makers, regulators and ethicists, have all raised cautions about deploying genetically edited mosquitoes into the wild.

Gene drives: high-tech mosquito control?

Several types of genetically modified mosquitoes are currently under development. The British-based company Oxitec has field-tested millions of laboratory-made, transgenic *Aedes aegypti* mosquitoes in Brazil and the Cayman Islands, in an effort to control dengue, Zika, chikungunya and yellow fever. They have yet to publish epidemiological results from these open field experiments, which could take years. Oxitec engineered male mosquitoes with a gene that kills female offspring; when the modified males are released and mate with wild females, only males survive to adulthood, leading to population collapse. This approach has sparked heated debates about safety, risks and the environmental and health consequences of releasing large numbers of genetically modified mosquitoes, with strong opposition voiced by environmental and civil society groups. Oxitec has also sought to conduct field trials in the United States. In 2016, municipal governments in the Florida Keys held a non-binding referendum asking residents if they would assent to a release of Oxitec's mosquitoes in their neighbourhoods. There was significant opposition to a release (Bloss et al. 2017). Nevertheless in 2020, the US Environmental Protection Agency and mosquito control district boards in the Keys approved the release of Oxitec's mosquitoes, scheduled for 2021.

Another approach known as "gene drive" aims to control malaria-transmitting *Anopheles* mosquitoes. Gene drives short-circuit the usual patterns of genetic inheritance to ensure that a particular version of a gene is inherited more often

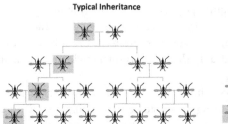

Typical Inheritance

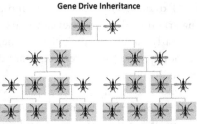

Gene Drive Inheritance

A fraction of the progeny at each generation receive the engineered version of the gene (roughly half, as indicated by the shaded boxes)

Virtually all of the progeny at each generation receive the engineered version of the gene (as indicated by the shaded boxes)

FIGURE 15.2 Gene drives override typical patterns of inheritance. Source: Adapted from E. Otwell and M. Tefler, in Saey 2015.

than by chance. Most genes are represented twice in animal genomes; each chromosomal copy or "allele" has a roughly equal (50%) chance of being passed down to a given offspring. A gene drive skews these probabilities in favour of one allele over the other. In a CRISPR-Cas9–based gene drive, gene-editing capabilities are embedded within the target organism itself, permitting the non-engineered allele to be rewritten with the same sequence as the engineered allele (Gantz and Bier 2015a, b). This allows any stretch of engineered DNA chosen by humans to be propagated from generation to generation to both chromosomal copies in virtually all descendants of a mosquito breeding population, as illustrated in Figure 15.2.

Practical applications of gene drives are enormous, but ethically fraught. Gene drives could theoretically be engineered into any target species, to rapidly spread a desired trait to every individual in a wild population. This would give humans the ability to permanently alter any wild species, with just a few genetic tweaks in the lab. Advocates of gene drive, such as some scientists and their funders, are excited by its prospects, framing it as a transformative public health tool that could finally crush the scourge of malaria. They see CRISPR-Cas9 gene-editing technology as a marked improvement over brute-force approaches of blanket insecticide spraying, thereby restricting human-induced changes to only a few species within a diverse geographic area or ecosystem. As philanthropist Bill Gates has written, "The promise of gene editing is that, instead of killing a bunch of mosquitoes indiscriminately, we could eliminate only the dangerous ones in a particular area. That would buy us time to cure all the people there of malaria" (Gates 2019).

Gene drives tantalize with their potential precision, targeting only certain genes in certain species, interrupting the devastating feature of mosquito vectors, which is their role as intermediate hosts for organisms pathogenic to humans. In the public health campaign against malaria, gene drives are being fashioned into "biomedical weapons" (Packard 2007) against two *Anopheles* vector species, *stephensi* and *gambiae*. The Bill and Melinda Gates Foundation and the Tata Trusts of India have both committed millions to fund research on gene-drive technology for malaria control, using suppression and replacement gene drives in West Africa, and a replacement gene drive in South Asia, respectively. Both types of gene drive are still in the research and development phase.

Suppression gene drives: eliminate mosquitoes by preventing reproduction

Target Malaria, a not-for-profit research consortium supported in part by the Gates Foundation, is designing suppression gene drive technology in *Anopheles gambiae*. The mosquitoes are under development in labs at Imperial College in the UK, as well as in Italy and the United States. Target Malaria is working with stakeholders, regulatory bodies and communities in Burkina Faso, Mali, Uganda and Ghana, to explore the feasibility of field release trials. Their approach exploits an "Achilles' heel" in the mosquito genome creating gene-drive-modified mosquitoes with self-destructive genetic mutations. The mutations would disrupt reproduction, heavily favouring male over female offspring, and rendering any female offspring sterile. If released in the wild, the lab-made male mosquitoes would mate with female mosquitoes and spread the sterilizing mutation to the entire population, resulting over time in a population of mostly males. As with the Oxitec mosquitoes, with fewer and fewer mating partners, the population would eventually crash, effectively wiping it out (Kyrou et al. 2018). Thus, the suppression gene drive could locally eliminate a target species.

Replacement gene drives: eliminate disease by vaccinating the mosquito

Rather than wiping out target mosquitoes, the second type of gene drive, known as a *replacement* (or *modification*) drive, seeks to break their disease transmission capabilities, rendering them harmless. These gene drive mosquitoes are under development at the Tata Institute for Genetics and Society and the University of California at Irvine Malaria Initiative, supported by funding from the Tata Trusts in India and the Gates Foundation, respectively. Engagement efforts are underway to explore the feasibility of field release trials for *Anopheles stephensi* in India and *Anopheles gambiae* in São Tomé and Principe. In this approach, engineered mosquitoes would encode small proteins designed to destroy invading *Plasmodium* parasites, thus "immunizing the mosquito" against the parasite (Aguilera 2020). If released in the wild, modified mosquitoes would mate and spread the parasite-defence genes, halting malaria-causing *Plasmodium* in their tracks before they ever reach humans. Over several generations, these replacement drives are projected to substitute a disease-spreading mosquito population with one that is incapable of transmitting malaria to humans (Gantz et al. 2015).

Gene drives: reimagining human–mosquito relations

While suppression gene drives aim to disrupt mosquito reproduction, replacement gene drives aim to disrupt infectious disease transmission. Importantly, both exploit the natural life-cycle behaviours of mosquitoes, their intricate mating rituals and reproductive movements, to effect human-desired, population-level alterations. Gene drives would harness, in Rachel Carson's words, the very "life forces" of the mosquito to destroy itself or its ability to transmit pathogens to humans. Gene drives therefore represent a new kind of public health tool by conscripting mosquitoes as central actors in the solution to the human health problems they themselves pose.

But suppression and replacement drives carry out their purposes in very different ways, each representing a contrasting vision, and a different set of political and moral orientations to the question of how human–mosquito relationships ought to look going forward. Suppression gene drives posit that a better world is one absent of vector-transmitting mosquitoes, aligning closely with the vision of earlier eradication campaigns. This anthropocentric and arguably reductive view serves to amplify the rhetoric of an age-old war between humans and mosquitoes, their significance to humans and ecosystems defined entirely by the fact that they transmit human disease. This position spotlights the pernicious role of mosquitoes in igniting pandemics that can devastate humans and their governments, economies, and health and welfare systems. It sidelines appreciation of mosquitoes' exquisite biology, the singular evolution of each unique species among a proliferation of thousands, and their remarkable ability to adapt to a variety of ecological niches and climates. Suppression drives reflect a moral orientation to efficiently control—and ideally eliminate—the handful of mosquito species that spread human diseases, so that we may peacefully coexist with the many other harmless mosquito species.

By contrast, replacement gene drives fundamentally reorient our views away from the assumption that mosquitoes are merely subservient to human needs. By rendering mosquitoes harmless, replacement gene drives serve to reimagine mosquitoes as vital parts of ecological systems that are not simply harbingers of disease. If historical campaigns waged against these winged creatures have taught us anything, it is that human efforts to completely wipe out disease-harbouring mosquitoes are likely to fail. Replacement gene drives could foster a new dynamic in human–mosquito relations, encouraging the view that humans and mosquitoes *can* coexist peacefully and amicably with each other, provided their antagonistic activities are deactivated. Here there is a move beyond the contours of a war metaphor being played out in mosquito eradication campaigns, which rely on a rhetoric of extermination and extinction, to one positioning mosquitoes as vital elements in a humanized world.

Social and ethical concerns around using gene drives for vector control

At first glance, a replacement gene drive sketches the possibility of a benign outcome dramatically reducing or even eliminating malaria, at least locally, without exterminating the mosquito vector. Genetic-control enthusiasts point to what they see as declining efficacies of existing malaria control strategies, such as insecticides and bed nets, due in part to growing resistance among wild mosquito populations. Yet many scientists acknowledge that gene-drive techniques will be insufficient to wipe out malaria, though they may complement existing control strategies in reducing malaria transmission (NASEM 2016). The current director of WHO's Global Malaria Programme, Pedro Alonso, cautions that eradication might be an unrealistic goal even if genetic technologies can be deployed successfully (WHO 2019).

Owing to their ability to irrevocably change species' germ lines, both types of gene drives have become the focus of intense social, political and ethical scrutiny, inciting guarded responses from government leaders, regulators and others tasked with assessing their safety and risk profiles. It is useful to distinguish two, somewhat overlapping sets of concerns around gene drives. The first has to do with social, political and economic dimensions of gene drives as a vector control strategy, raising questions around inequality, wealth, power and poverty within and beyond malaria-endemic regions. The second set of concerns has to do with environmental impacts of gene drives, including ecological risks and orientations around how humans may wish to structure their current and future relationships with mosquitoes and other species in the natural world, of which we are part.

The sociopolitics of gene-drive-modified mosquitoes

Relations of power, political and economic, typically configure choices and decisions about whether and how a given technology could or should be used. Gene drives are similarly entangled in social and ethical debates that raise questions about the undue influence of power, politics and access. For example, some civil society groups have cautioned against the injection of philanthrocapital into global health concerns, which allows private charities to exert a defining influence on framing priorities and their solutions. Although gene-drive advocates have promised to provide most of the economic resources for developing and deploying gene drives, this strategy represents a substantial financial investment that, some argue, could be used to more effectively reduce malaria in other ways, as discussed below. In addition, research and development on genetically modified mosquitoes is primarily being conducted by labs of the Global North, in the USA and Europe, quite distant from the sites of their intended release in Asia, Africa and Latin America. This raises concerns about how to avoid replicating colonial paternalisms, and how to distribute decision-making authority to those who are most affected by decisions to deploy a gene drive or not. It is important to acknowledge that gene drives are forms of power mediated by individuals and organizations that have likely never had to experience a debilitating life with malaria. Furthermore, not all stakeholders may view the problem as fundamentally one that can be addressed by the techno-logics of genetic solutions.

Thus, a key consideration for assessing gene-drive-modified mosquitoes is to identify whose interests are served by them. Guidance frameworks for gene-drive development have called for the involvement of diverse stakeholders in transparent, open, equitable and accountable science and decision-making (NASEM 2016). Risks and harms stemming from these technologies are likely to accrue most to those near a release site. Assessing whether communities actually desire gene drives as part of malaria control efforts, and, if so, which design best meets local needs, will require sustained public engagement activities, knowledge sharing and dialogue about potential benefits and harms that are sensitive to local culture, language and religious practices. In many communities, landscapes are culturally significant, and traditions and beliefs about the place of human intervention are built around a long history of careful environmental stewardship. Indigenous communities have valuable local knowledge of disease transmission and ecosystem dynamics, and involving them as active and equal partners in gene-drive design and decision-making could ensure that gene drives do not amplify existing vulnerabilities (Titingfong 2020). Such efforts should ensure that conflicts of interest are minimized by involving a range of stakeholders as partners in decision-making, especially because developers and funders of gene drives are interested parties with respect to decisions about their implementation.

Defining the relevant community could be challenging, as gene-drive-engineered mosquitoes are not likely to obey political boundaries. There are cases of mosquitoes being carried by winds hundreds of kilometres from their point of origin (Huestis et al. 2019) which complicates the use of mosquitoes as public health tools (Biesel and Boete 2013). Areas lying near national or regional borders may be particularly contentious. Some have proposed that every community member be given opportunities to voice opinions, raise concerns and register their free, prior and informed consent, while others suggest that elected or appointed leaders make the final decisions. As gene-drive release areas are proposed, the prevailing political, social and regulatory contexts of each should be accounted for to inform the most suitable approaches for empowering local communities in decision-making about their collective futures.

Finally, some worry that gene drives are reductive and not as cost-effective as other anti-malarial strategies, or that they fail to generate returns commensurate with the expense of creating them. Although CRISPR-Cas9 gene-editing technology is relatively inexpensive, using it to design a gene drive is a very capital-intensive endeavour. Because malaria is concentrated in regions characterized by wide economic disparities, stemming from centuries of exploitive, often violent colonization, affected communities may give first priority to poverty reduction, educational and employment opportunities, and access to adequate health care, over deploying a technology whose efficacy and side effects remain uncertain. Observers of genetic modification approaches have pointed out that alternative means of addressing malaria might have far greater impacts on reducing morbidity and mortality of a mosquito-borne disease, by using large capital injections to shore up health infrastructure, or investing in socioeconomically precarious regions in ways that would address inequities in access to housing, education and employment. Such holistic investments would not only help alleviate malaria, a preventable and treatable disease linked to socioeconomic status, but also raise the overall standard of living, ameliorating public health far beyond the quelling of a single disease.

Assessing environmental risks of gene-drive modifications

Gene drives represent an expensive, high-tech endeavour to address what may be considered fundamentally social problems of vector-borne disease. Today's patterns of mosquito distribution are legacies of military conquest and colonization, stemming from a long history of human encroachment on natural habitats. Major malaria outbreaks have followed human reshaping of natural landscapes which fundamentally altered the distribution and flow of water across the land (Packard 2007). Water is an important feature of malaria transmission because it is in stagnant pools that females lay their eggs and expand their population. In recent times, such landscape modifications often stemmed from redirecting water for power-generating dams or irrigating crops, leading to flooding in some areas and droughts in others.

Given this history, a key challenge for gene drives is to accurately assess their risks to organismal and ecosystem health, and their potential for disrupting relationships between them. The ecological impacts of gene drives are not yet understood. The World Health Organization, the US National Academies, and various national and local regulatory bodies, have all proposed stepwise, phased testing pathways through which gene drives might proceed, beginning with laboratory studies, and moving to confined and open field trials if local communities approve. Iterative rounds of data collection and assessment at each step are critical for evaluating efficacy, safety and environmental, entomological and epidemiological impacts. Could gene drives somehow damage ecosystems or reduce biodiversity? Some have argued that gene-drive-modified organisms may be pervasive and invasive, advising caution (Noble et al. 2018). Others, particularly civil society groups, worry that gene drives may be less precise and targeted than intended, potentially transferring altered DNA sequences to non-target mosquito species, or worse, to other organisms up and down the food chain. Although it still remains unclear how exactly a gene drive would perform in the wild and whether it could successfully eliminate a mosquito species locally, there is much to be learned about how mosquitoes, individually or collectively, interact with complex ecosystems, and what their elimination might mean to the biotic and abiotic environment. Might local elimination of a mosquito species inadvertently lead to local collapse of food webs? Could another mosquito species expand into the territory of the old, occupy its niche, and become a new vector for malaria parasites? What level of knowledge must be attained about knock-on effects and risks to humans, other species, and local ecological webs, before a mosquito gene drive could be deemed safe to deploy? Which uncertainties can be tolerated, and which cannot? Are there ways to know if a gene drive is getting out of control, and if so, which measures could be implemented to halt or interrupt the escalating impacts of a renegade drive? Gene-drive researchers are using mathematical modelling to investigate possible impacts on shared environments, and develop mitigation strategies, but few methods currently exist to answer these questions satisfactorily, and better assessment tools must be developed.

And finally, how might gene-drive-modified mosquitoes impair our understanding of and relationships with parasites, malaria and mosquitoes? What might be undesirably lost in our ability to control vector-borne disease through the process of deploying gene drives? For example, gene drives could powerfully shape mosquito evolution, and in turn, shape human susceptibility to mosquitoes. Gene-drive scientists worry about the potential for mosquitoes to evolve resistance to gene drives, just as they did to DDT; such resistances arise readily in the lab. Some wild mosquitoes may find ways to escape the effects of the gene drive, retaining their ability to transmit malaria, and possibly rebounding worse than before. Indeed, any intervention in nature for eliminating or neutralizing a harmful species runs the risk of ultimately aiding its own undoing, even hastening the evolution of new resistances that evade human control. So, while replacement gene drives are designed to convert current vectors into non-vectors, they may also convert these vectors into more virulent varieties (Hayes et al. 2019). Such evolutionary side effects could have long-term implications for future efforts to control malaria. Considered another way, redesigning mosquitoes might also redesign the human experience of mosquitoes, and the malaria they transmit, and not necessarily for the better. Gene drives therefore present planetary scale implications, and the practical and ethical work required to assess and make decisions surrounding them needs to be commensurate with that scale.

Conclusion: the politics of technoscience

This chapter outlines some of the prospects and precautions of genetic technologies for the control of mosquito-borne diseases. Gene drives are enlivened biotechnologies that aim to tweak mosquito DNA to nudge their biology in directions less pernicious to humans. In so doing, they internalize the problem of vector-borne disease to the mosquito, rather than to the larger web of social, economic, and political inequalities that render such diseases fatal in some bodies and treatable in others. The questions attending gene-drive technologies require us to complicate the assumption that technologies are innocent or somehow apolitical. As theorists of technology remind us, technologies are never ethically or politically neutral. Rather, they are "forms of life" that "restructure our physical and social worlds, and so how we live" (Winner 1983). The technology of gene drive, an altered but living, respiring, mosquito, is doubly a "form of life" (Sandler 2019). Technologies express the ethical and political orientations of their designers, and the futures they wish to implement. The two gene-drive designs of suppression and replacement represent starkly different responses to the question of whether disease-carrying mosquito species should exist. The choice of a suppression gene drive expresses a view that disease-carrying mosquitoes are primarily pests and so should be targeted for elimination, whereas a replacement/modification approach sees value in preserving mosquitoes as part of local ecologies, designing a gene drive for compromising only this insect's ability to transmit human disease. In the first scenario, there might not be mosquitoes left to bite humans; in the second, mosquitoes would bite, but not transmit infectious pathogens.

A choice of two mosquito scenarios dovetails into a larger set of dilemmas that loom in the discourse of genetic engineering: to what extent is it acceptable for humanity to manipulate nature to serve its own interests? Is it ethical to edit other species at will, shaping them to have the properties we want or desire, to serve our needs, fancies or whims? Are extreme measures, such as destroying a mosquito species, justified if they help save human lives from a debilitating disease like malaria, which has a disproportionate impact on children made vulnerable by economic inequality, imbalanced power relations and climate change? Would it be unjust *not* to try to deploy gene drives to eradicate disease vectors?

And yet, gene drives for malaria control can open the door to an ethical slippery slope. Should humans collectively decide it acceptable to genetically alter one species because it serves as a key node in a major health threat, how much easier does it become to justify altering any species, whether viewed as a threat or simply a mild nuisance that may interfere with human agendas and visions? In considering ways to govern decisions about exercising such consequential power, this chapter implores us to nurture humility towards each other and towards the ecosystems of which we are a part.

Genetic technologies dazzle, hypnotically. In so doing, such technologies inflate the illusion of control. But gene drives may not be a saviour. Even if deployed, a gene drive may not be as effective or efficient as anticipated, demanding that we lower our expectations about the human power to "control" mosquitoes or malaria, much less eradicate them. Mosquitoes adroitly and rapidly adapt their relations with us, reacting to our activities, and as with DDT, may resist our efforts to control them. Thoughtful and deliberate interrogations of likely outcomes of our control methods will help us prepare for resistances that are likely to arise.

Suppression and replacement gene drives represent different political and moral orientations to the challenges posed by mosquito vectors. Each gene drive envisions a different future for malaria control and for reorienting mosquito–human relationships, with competing technopolitics at play in aiming to eliminate or else refashion insect vectors. By seeking opposite avenues for living with and alongside mosquitoes, they may differ in their political, social, ecological and health implications. Gene drives of all stripes threaten to rupture our relationships with mosquitoes, and while this rupture could be beneficial, the journey towards these benefits should also alert us to the dense and complex relations we have with mosquitoes across the political, economic and moral orders of society.

Bibliography

Aguilera, M. 2020. Biologists Create New Genetic Systems to Neutralize Gene Drives. *UC San Diego News Center*, September 18.

Biesel, U. and C. Boete. 2013. The Flying Public Health Tool: Genetically Modified Mosquitoes and Malaria Control. *Science as Culture* 22(1): 38–60.

Bloss, C. et al. 2017. Public Response to a Proposed Field Trial of Genetically Engineered Mosquitoes in the United States. *Journal of the American Medical Association* 318(7): 662–664.

Carson, Rachel. 1962. *Silent Spring*. Houghton-Mifflin.

Cohen, J.M. et al. 2012. Malaria Resurgence: A Systematic Review and Assessment of its Causes. *Malaria Journal* 11: 122.

Gantz, Valentino M. and Ethan Bier. 2015a. The Mutagenic Chain Reaction: A Method for Converting Heterozygous to Homozygous Mutations. *Science* 348: 442–444.

Gantz, Valentino M. and Ethan Bier. 2015b. The Dawn of Active Genetics. *Bioessays* 38: 50–63.

Gantz, Valentino M. et al. 2015. Highly Efficient Cas9-Mediated Gene Drive for Population Modification of the Malaria Vector Mosquito *Anopheles stephensi*. *PNAS* 112(49): E6736–6743.

Gates, B. 2019. Test-Tube Mosquitoes Might Help us Beat Malaria. *GatesNotes*, April 15, https://www.gatesnotes.com/Health/Test-tube-mosquitoes-might-help-us-beat-malaria, accessed 11.02.2021.

Hayes, K.R. et al. 2019. Identifying and Detecting Potentially Adverse Ecological Outcomes Associated with the Release of Gene-Drive Modified Organisms. *Journal of Responsible Innovation* 5(suppl 1): S139–S158.

Huestis, D.L. et al. 2019. Windborne Long-Distance Migration of Malaria Mosquitoes in the Sahel. *Nature* 574: 404–408.

Jinek, M. et al. 2012. A Programmable Dual-RNA–Guided DNA Endonuclease in Adaptive Bacterial Immunity. *Science* 337(6096): 816–821.

Keller, E. 1995. *Refiguring Life: Metaphors of Twentieth Century Biology*. New York: Columbia University Press.

Kyrou, K., A.M. Hammond, R. Galizi, N. Kranjc, A. Burt, A.K. Beaghton, T. Nolan and A. Crisanti. 2018. A CRISPR–Cas9 Gene Drive Targeting Doublesex Causes Complete Population Suppression in Caged *Anopheles gambiae* Mosquitoes. *Nature Biotechnology* 36: 1062–1066.

National Academies of Sciences, Engineering, and Medicine (NASEM). 2016. *Gene Drives on the Horizon Advancing Science, Navigating Uncertainty, and Aligning Research with Public Values*. Washington, DC: National Academies Press. https://doi.org/10.17226/23405

Nelkin, D. and S.M. Lindee. 2004. *The DNA Mystique*. Ann Arbor: Ann Arbor: University of Michigan Press.

Noble, C., B. Adlam, G.M. Church, K.M. Esvelt and M.A. Nowak. 2018. Current CRISPR Gene Drive Systems Are Likely to be Highly Invasive in Wild Populations. *eLife* 7:e33423.

Packard, Randall. 2007. *The Making of a Tropical Disease: A Short History of Malaria*. Baltimore: Johns Hopkins University Press.

Patterson, Gordon. 2009. *The Mosquito Crusades: A History of the American Anti-Mosquito Movement from the Reed Commission to the First Earth Day*. New Brunswick, NJ: Rutgers University Press.

Saey, T.H. 2015. Gene Drives Spread Their Wings. *ScienceNews*, December 2.

Sandler, R. 2019. The Ethics of Genetic Engineering and Gene Drives in Conservation. *Conservation Biology* 34(2): 378–385.

Stepan, Nancy Leys. 2011. *Eradication: Ridding the World of Diseases Forever*. Ithaca: Cornell University Press.

Titingfong, R.I. 2020. Islands as Laboratories: Indigenous Knowledge and Gene Drives in the Pacific. *Human Biology* 91(2): 57–67.

Winner, L. 1983. Technologies as Forms of Life. In *Epistemology, Methodology and the Social Sciences*, eds. Cohen and Wartofsky. Kluwer Academic Publishers.

World Health Organization. 2019. *Malaria Eradication*, Virtual Press Conference with Pedro Alonso and Michel Tanner, Transcript at https://malariaworld.org/blog/trans cript-virtual-press-conference-pedro-alonso-and-marcel-tanner-malaria-eradicatio n, accessed November 1 2020.

World Health Organization. 2020. *World Malaria Report 2020: 20 years of global progress and challenges*. Geneva: World Health Organization.

16

THE MOSQUITOME

A new frontier for sustainable vector control

Frederic Simard

Invasive *Aedes* mosquitoes such as *Aedes aegypti* and *Ae. albopictus*, that support the bulk of inter-human arbovirus transmission causing dengue, chikungunya, Zika, yellow fever and others to come, are urban mosquitoes that have largely benefited and expanded from ongoing human settlement and development, such as deforestation, urbanization and increased global trade. In tropical areas, major human malaria vectors (*Anopheles* spp.) are also typically considered as highly anthropophilic mosquitoes, showing strong feeding preference for human blood over other vertebrate hosts, hence strongly contributing to inter-human transmission of life-threatening malaria parasites. All these major disease vectors are highly dependent upon humans, not only as a reliable source of blood for their hematophagous females, but also because human transformations to natural environments and ecosystems create numerous opportunities for these mosquitoes to breed and to rest, with low exposure to most of their natural enemies that do not develop in culturally modified areas. These major disease vectors represent only a small fraction of the more than 3,500 known mosquito species, but they have significantly diverged from their wild counterparts, both in their ecology (biting behaviour, host preference, reproductive dynamics, larval ecology, etc.) and their genetics (genetic diversity, gene duplications, insecticide resistance mutations, etc.) (Neafsey et al., 2015). As a matter of fact, we humans have been the major drivers of the recent evolutionary history of this group of highly synanthropic disease-vector mosquitoes, shaping what now appears to be a set of unintentionally domesticated animals that thrive where people live.

The emergence and rapid spread of resistance to artificial chemical insecticides in all major mosquito disease vectors over the last 30 years is an emblematic, ultimate evolutionary step in the adaptation of these mosquitoes to human environments. Indeed, insecticide resistance seriously jeopardizes recent public health success in the control of malaria in Africa, as well as significantly

DOI: 10.4324/9781003056034-16

hindering any preventive or reactive interventions against the highly invasive, virus-transmitting *Aedes* mosquitoes (Hemingway et al., 2016; Moyes et al., 2017). Is this another battle we are losing against our tenacious old foes? Is this the next step in our evolutionary arms race that is tightly linking us to this or that mosquito species, when we consider the pathogens they transmit? What happens next, and when and where will it end? In this chapter, I argue that it is time for a paradigm shift from aggressive "vector control" to biologically sensitive and evolutionarily lucid management of synanthropic mosquito vector populations, aiming at shrinking ecological niches of pathogen transmission in order to prevent their emergence and spread in human populations. Applying the principles of evolutionary biology to the control of mosquito-borne pathogens may suggest novel opportunities for sustainable control of diseases that result in mosquitoes helping us combat rather than propagate the diseases they transmit.

Humans and their "Mosquitome"

Just as the "Microbiome" defines a community of bacteria, fungi, viruses and other microbes that inhabit a particular environment, be it the gut or skin of a human host, it is useful to introduce the term "Mosquitome" to describe the group of mosquitoes that thrive where people live, being composed of a handful of highly synanthropic mosquito species that have successfully adapted to humans and human-made environments. Species of the Mosquitome have come to closely depend on the presence of human beings for breeding and proliferating. Indeed, these mosquitoes have developed very specific and distinctive attributes when compared to their wild counterparts, resulting in them contributing to most of the world's burden of mosquito-borne infectious diseases. Singling out the Mosquitome, rather than all mosquitoes, might help focus public and stakeholders' attention on the accurate disease target while avoiding harm to the larger amalgam that includes other natural mosquito species of benefit to ecosystems. The scope of such a Mosquitome should include the African malarial mosquitoes, *Anopheles gambiae s.l.* complex (which includes *An. gambiae s.s.*, *An. coluzzii* and *An. arabiensis*) and *An. funestus*; the invasive Indian species, *An. stephensi*; and the highly invasive *Aedes aegypti* and *Ae. albopictus* that transmit such arboviruses as dengue, yellow fever, Zika and chikungunya. Although each mosquito species has its own evolutionary pathway, humans have played a key role in shaping the evolutionary trajectories of each and every species within the Mosquitome, serving to fine-tune this weapon of mass destruction that it has become.

Crucially, mosquitoes need blood to reproduce; specifically, female mosquitoes need blood to mature and then to lay their eggs. Strong, anthropophilic preferences for human blood over other vertebrate blood have been shown to be a heritable, genetically encoded phenotype that has arisen and disappeared at multiple occasions in the course of mosquito evolution (Besansky, Hill & Costantini, 2004; Neafsey et al., 2015). Indeed, specializing in human ecosystems has provided the Mosquitome with one of the most widespread and reliable sources of blood on Earth. Humans are gregarious animals that live in groups making them easy to locate. Moreover, humans shape their own environments wherever they settle, often removing many natural enemies of the mosquito, be they competitors or predators, such as insects, birds, bats and fish. Changes in land use through deforestation, agriculture and urbanization provide further opportunities for mosquito breeding and resting. In fact, beyond being a nearly inexhaustible source of blood, humans also provide mosquitoes with reliable and permanent access to water surfaces crucial to developing larvae.

The major human malaria vector in Africa, *An. gambiae*, lays its eggs in temporary water pounds with no vegetation, producing larvae that are highly "heliophilic," or requiring direct exposure to sunlight to develop. Such surface-water collections are widespread during the rainy season throughout sub-Saharan Africa. And in areas where the rainy season is short, human environmental modifications for water management and irrigation, such as dams and rice fields, offer good breeding opportunities that expand mosquito presence and density in both space and time (Gimonneau et al., 2012). In equatorial areas with dense vegetation that blocks direct sunlight, deforestation and urbanization can expand suitable environments for *An. gambiae* that seek breeding habitats. As a result of these mosquito habitat preferences, there is a strong correlation observed between the presence of people, villages, roads and agricultural areas, and the presence of the *An. gambiae* complex in areas of sub-Saharan Africa (Costantini et al., 2009; Simard et al., 2009). In this respect, it has been hypothesized that the *An. gambiae*'s preference for feeding on humans over other vertebrates resulted from the colonization of suitable larval development sites by ancestral populations of the mosquito in Central Africa some 5,000 years ago, when Bantu agriculturalists adopted "slash and burn" agricultural techniques to open up the forest canopy and favour the breeding of larvae in the vicinity of humans (Ayala & Coluzzi, 2005).

In the same way, recent findings based on genomic, ecological and behavioural data obtained from various populations of *Ae. aegypti* strongly suggest that its preference for human-biting originally evolved as a by-product of breeding in human water containers, such as tanks and jars, in areas where doing so was the only way to survive the long and harsh Sahelian dry season (Rose et al., 2020). Here again, humans have been a reliable source of both water and blood, becoming a host of choice for those mosquitoes that have been able to adapt and continue to adapt to this human environment. In this way, *Ae. aegypti*, the "yellow fever mosquito" of African origin, was able to take hold and become the human nemesis that it is.

It is therefore fair to claim that tight relationships and intense long-lasting interactions between humans and their Mosquitome have long been driving mosquito-borne disease evolution. A recent and emblematic example of this evolution is the rapid rise of resistance in all major human disease-vector mosquitoes to all insecticidal compounds that have been used to control them

(Hemingway et al., 2016; Moyes et al., 2017). Some of the mechanisms used by mosquitoes to resist insecticides have been thoroughly described and can be monitored in wild mosquito populations. Longitudinal studies in the field as well as molecular, physiological and genomic studies have described the origin and spread of these resistances in vector populations, unraveling their extraordinary evolutionary potential, which is driven by short generation times and high levels of fecundity. Other studies have suggested that insecticide resistance may arm the mosquito with a non-specific detoxifying enzymatic capability that enables cross-resistance to other kinds of human-linked xenobiotics and pollutants, thereby further promoting mosquito colonization of areas with high human densities (Chouaibou et al., 2008).

Humans have therefore not only facilitated the instalment of their Mosquitome across the planet, but they have been a key contributor to the movement and dispersal of this group of highly anthropophilic mosquito species. This is especially the case for both *Aedes* species which have spread across the world by human transportation. In this way, *Ae. aegypti* originated in Africa and populated the Americas and Europe during the slave trade, while adapting to breeding conditions onboard ships (Powell & Tabachnick, 2013). More recently, the Asian tiger mosquito (*Ae. albopictus*) has also benefited by increased globalization and international trade, to spread from Southeast Asia to North America and the rest of the world within decades (Hawley, 1988; Paupy et al., 2009). Their physiological and behavioural traits have facilitated unintentional transportation of their eggs and mated females across long distances (Hawley, 1988; Eritja et al., 2017). Both *Ae. albopictus* and *Ae. aegypti* produce eggs that resist desiccation for several months; both prefer day-time host-seeking and biting activities; and both have a marked preference for breeding in small temporary water collections, such as tree holes, rock pools and other artificial water holders, leading to their nickname as "container mosquitoes."

One realizes that humans have indeed shaped the evolutionary history of a handful of highly synanthropic mosquitoes that take advantage of human-modified environments to thrive and spread. In other words, we humans are a major evolutionary driver of the Mosquitome. The good news is that basic knowledge of medical entomology and mosquito physiology combined with recent advances in mosquito genomics, ecological modelling and evolutionary biology should now allow us to modify the evolution of the Mosquitome for preventing, rather than promoting, the transmission of mosquito-borne human diseases.

The Mosquitome and disease transmission

One must remember that mosquitoes are not the problem; rather, the diseases they transmit are the problem. By applying evolutionary principles, mosquitoes can become part of the solution to limit mosquito-borne diseases. To date, synanthropic mosquitoes have been considered as pests that need to be fought and ultimately eliminated for the sake of public health. And to date, only transient successes have been achieved in controlling the diseases they transmit, with many regions seeing more mosquitoes flying than ever before. Adopting the Mosquitome approach may help identify novel opportunities to tackle the challenge of sustainably controlling diseases in a changing world.

There are at least three biological tenets relevant to the status of major human disease vectors that are characteristic of the Mosquitome species (Cohuet et al., 2010): (1) a high level of contact with humans, especially by preferring to bite humans over other vertebrates; (2) genetic compatibility with the pathogen for sustaining pathogen development; and (3) unusual mosquito longevity for allowing this vector to bite susceptible hosts after the pathogen has reached the salivary glands. All these specificities result from well-adapted, co-evolutionary processes between mosquitoes and their human hosts, and between the transmitted pathogen(s) and vector-specific assemblages (see Duvallet et al., 2017 and references therein).

Existing data suggest that there is a correlation between a mosquito species' level of anthropophily (measured as the level of preference for human blood), and its longevity (measured as daily survival), with mosquitoes from the Mosquitome being champions in both categories (Figure 16.1). Greater longevity is a key parameter to vector capacity because it enables the female mosquito to survive long enough for the pathogen to develop in her body, infest her salivary glands and be transmitted through subsequent biting (Garrett-Jones, 1964; Cohuet et al., 2010). Longer lifetimes are a remarkable trait of synanthropic mosquitoes, reflecting their divergence from their wild counterparts in the course of their adapting to domestic habitats, and facilitating pathogen transmission. Thus, a key strategy for disease control is to curb the extraordinary longevity of Mosquitome species, thereby diminishing pathogen transmission intensity, while preserving mosquito biodiversity as a whole.

Longevity is correlated not only with anthropophily in mosquitoes. Indeed, as is true for all living species, longevity and fecundity are major traits of a species' fitness that appear to suffer "antagonistic pleiotropy" or genetic expressions that offer beneficial as well as detrimental effects. Conflicts in resource allocation result in an evolutionary trade-off between survival and early life fecundity that is an important basis of an organism's life-history strategy. This trade-off has long been recognized and studied in a number of organisms, from insects to plants and mammals. Long-lived organisms tend to invest less in early-life reproduction, often spreading out their offspring in time and space, compared to short-lived organisms that may rely on a single, massive reproductive event during their adult life. Most mosquitoes tend to follow the strategy of massive early reproduction, and here again Mosquitome mosquitoes stand out; as compared with non-vector species of *Culex* and *Mansonia* genera, major human malaria mosquitoes typically lay their eggs in successive batches across their lifespan, investing less in early-life fecundity (Clements, 1992). This continuous fecundity may indeed benefit such mosquitoes since the *An.*

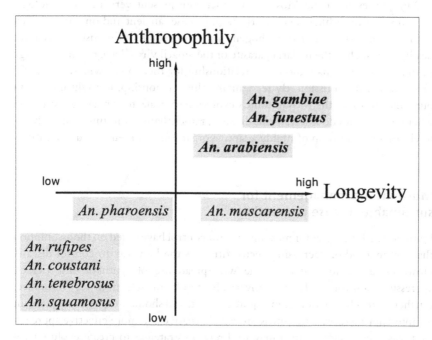

FIGURE 16.1 Schematic relationship between anthropophily and longevity in African *Anopheles* mosquito species. Anthropophily was measured as the proportion of blood meals taken on humans in natural mosquito populations in Africa (in Bruce-Chwatt et al., 1966; Gillies & de Meillon, 1968). Longevity was assessed through the average parous rate determined in natural mosquito populations (from Gillies, 1963; Hamon, 1963). Bold-font mosquito species belong to the Mosquitome and are major human malaria vectors. *Anopheles pharoensis* and *An. mascarensis* have been found naturally infected with *P. falciparum* in the field but their contribution to overall malaria transmission is anecdotal and minimal. Other mosquito species listed are zoophilic mosquito species that rarely bite humans, and are therefore not involved in human malaria transmission.

gambiae complex that inhabit harsh sub-Saharan savannahs and that rely on very intermittent surface waters, can hedge their bets to survive in this stochastic environment (Cohen, 1966). Such reproductive behaviour, also referred to as "skip oviposition," has also been described for the container-breeding *Aedes* species (Reiter, 2007). Extended lifespan, with extended periods of reproduction, is therefore an asset for both the mosquito vector to ensure survival of its progeny, and the pathogen to extend its transmission opportunities. The advantages of human-modified environments for decreasing the risk of extrinsic mortality from predation and for competitively acquiring resources, such as water, blood and nectar, further promoted the evolution of longevity within the Mosquitome.

Mosquitoes from the Mosquitome therefore present very peculiar biological traits that most likely evolved through intense, ancient and ongoing contact with humans. Many human pathogens, including some of the historically most deadly ones such as the malaria parasite or the amaril virus, have taken advantage of this intimate human–mosquito relationship for their own, widely successful inter-human transmission. By recognizing this relationship, it might now be in our hands to drive the Mosquitome's evolutionary trajectory back to a situation where mosquitoes do not transmit diseases, rather than continuing to naively try to eliminate this group of highly adaptive organisms with enormous evolutionary potential.

Mosquitome management for sustainable disease prevention

Until now, all strategies for mosquito vector control have relied on the assumption that any method of decreasing vector fitness is the best way to control disease. However, as demonstrated by the widespread use of synthetic insecticides, aggressive control tools will invariably result in selection for resistance. Furthermore, elimination of mosquitoes is not, and should not, be a requirement for interrupting disease transmission. An alternative and more effective approach to disease and vector control may well rely on strategies to create evolutionary incentives to the Mosquitome that will restore its former life history traits of epidemiological importance, especially longevity and anthropophily, to ranges typically observed in non-vector species. In other words, we must utilize evolutionary processes to drive the Mosquitome back to its natural, pre-human condition, rather than constantly attempting to counteract the effects of such processes. Countering Mosquitome longevity and anthropophily is likely the only way to achieve sustainable mosquito-borne disease prevention and vector risk-mitigation.

Opportunities exist to disentangle vector fitness from pathogen transmission (Michalakis & Renaud, 2009). Because only old female mosquitoes are actively involved in transmitting pathogens, strategies aimed at reducing their lifespans by killing them late in life, after they have reproduced but before they are able to transmit pathogens, would diminish natural selection of resistance. Biological agents such as fungi in the genus *Beauvaria* and bacteria in the genus *Wolbachia* have been considered good candidates for late-life control. By developing slowly in infected mosquitoes, the fungus allows the female to mate and lay several batches of eggs before it eventually dies from infection. For their part, strains of *Wolbachia* serve to speed up senescence in dengue-transmitting mosquitoes, shortening their lifespan and reducing the efficiency of viral transmission. Exposing the Mosquitome to this kind of innovative, late-life vector control, the theory and development of which is still being worked out, may therefore provide significant control of disease transmission, with fewer impacts on mosquito populations.

From an evolutionary perspective, a shift towards relying on late-life-acting control strategies—while reducing selection for resistance—may also promote selection of more subtle life-history adaptations in the mosquito by reallocating resources towards short-term reproduction from longer-term survival. Indeed, experimental evolution experiments conducted with the model fly *Drosophila* have shown that exposing flies to different extrinsic mortality regimes over 50–90 generations resulted in shifts towards higher fecundity and reduced lifespan even in the absence of selection (Stearns et al., 2000). Such investigations corroborate the claim that insects are able to quickly adapt their life-history strategies to changes in their environment, as by balancing fecundity and longevity to optimize reproductive outputs. Just as mosquitoes of the Mosquitome increased their lifespan when adapting to novel, low-risk human environments, the drosophila study shows that it may be possible to reverse this trend and decrease the lifespan of anthropophilic mosquitoes. Indeed, extrapolating the drosophila experiment results to mosquitoes and malaria transmission, Ferguson and colleagues (2012) demonstrated that a similar drop in mean longevity (7.7% over 90 generations in the drosophila study) would result in more than 80% reduction in malaria transmission due to the non-linear relationship between vector longevity and vector capacity. These authors propose that a similar evolutionary shift may be induced in malaria-vector mosquitoes through enforced vector-control interventions, and that this shift can act as a hidden weapon that eventually eliminates malaria transmission when the vector's lifespan drops below the parasite's development time. Other evolutionary outcomes that include selection for parasites developing faster in their vector mosquito, or increased innate vector competence in mosquito progenies, may further interfere, and so need to be monitored in the frame of scaling-up vector-control interventions.

Opportunities also exist to manipulate host preference in mosquitoes, with existing genetic variation in the Mosquitome allowing for natural selection to drive mosquitoes away from human scent when it becomes associated with higher fitness cost. Although host-preference in mosquitoes is influenced by environmental factors such as host availability, there is also a genetic basis to this preference. Ecological and ethological studies conducted in the field and lab have documented plasticity and strong shifts in host choice in response to divergent selection pressures, while genome-wide investigations have shown that the genetic basis to host preference in mosquitoes is as complex as it is evolutionarily labile (Besansky et al., 2004; Lyimo & Ferguson, 2009; Neafsey et al., 2015). Anthropophily therefore might not only be subdued, but also eliminated when the Mosquitome finds a fitness incentive for switching hosts. We should hence develop these fitness incentives in the Mosquitome for alternative host-choice by better protecting humans from aggressive bites and, at the same time, by offering other possible prey or artificial blood sources for the Mosquitome in our cities. The development of novel personal protection tools, including improved repellents and attractants to manipulate vector behaviour, next-generation mosquito nets and screens to protect homes from vector intrusion, and replenished urban biodiversity to dilute mosquito-biting pressure on humans, will be an integral part of such an endeavour.

Finally, opportunities also exist for increasing resilience of the domestic environment to mosquito breeding and spreading. Rational use and storage of water is becoming a pressing need stemming from climate change, and the way we address this urgent challenge will have a dramatic impact on the Mosquitome's ecology, and associated risks of disease transmission. Limiting surface water is key to reducing mosquito habitat suitability, and diminishing mosquito presence, density and viability. It should also be recognized that given the Mosquitome's adaptability to human-shaped environments and its extraordinary evolutionary potential, we may be doomed to share some of our space with these mosquitoes. Thus, just as we are learning how to manage our microbiome so that it can help us minimize infections and other detrimental impacts to our bodily ecosystem, we can also learn how to manage our Mosquitome so that it can help us develop more harmonious public health. Monitoring and managing our Mosquitome in a way that limits mosquito breeding in and around human dwellings will serve to limit transmission of diseases. Moreover, maintaining a resilient Mosquitome should, by occupying suitable habitats, hinder invasion by external mosquito populations with greater vector competence. Reducing vector capacity of the Mosquitome will require increasing extrinsic mortality for reducing life expectancies in resident mosquito populations. One way of decreasing mosquito longevity is by increasing natural mosquito enemies in cities and agricultural settings, which will produce novel equilibria in the Mosquitome life-history traits. Some mosquito threats in human settlements can be countered by such novel tools as mosquitoes controlling other mosquitoes. Additional mosquito-control techniques such as female-driven delivery of specific insect growth regulators, application of mosquito-specific pathogens to larval development sites, sterile-insect techniques or genetically modified mosquitoes that contain altered vector competence and/or altered vector reproduction (see also Moyes et al., 2017; Roiz et al., 2019) may all contribute to selecting for reduced longevity in the Mosquitome. The challenge now resides in our ability to carry out a gradual implementation of these complementary tools within the framework of concerted, locally designed and inclusive Mosquitome management strategies. Such a challenge will come at the cost of accepting to live with our Mosquitome. By willingly coinhabiting our Mosquitome, we may finally be achieving a Mosquitopia: that state in which mosquitoes and people can harmoniously coexist.

This scenario thus offers a paradigm shift in the way we set out to control mosquito vectors and the diseases they transmit by relying on long-term risk-mitigation of pathogen transmission, rather than short-term mosquito elimination. It is time to take care of our Mosquitome and recognize our duties in husbanding this highly specific evolutionary branch of biodiversity (Martin et al., 2015; Johnson & Munshi-South, 2017). We should strive to increase extrinsic vector mortality in cities through every means, work to (re)install mosquito biological enemies such as predators, competitors and pathogens, design effective late-life-acting control tools and chemicals that shorten mosquito lifespan while preserving lifelong fecundity, and monitor the infrastructure of our neighbourhoods and water-management systems in order to limit breeding opportunities. Recent advances in evolutionary biology and emerging frameworks of urban ecology and commensalism in anthropogenic environments should help identify opportunities for translating theory into action (Roche et al., 2018; Hulme-Beaman et al., 2016). We must also build upon recommendations from the World Health Organization for tackling research gaps and fostering intra- and inter-sectoral collaboration for implementing the Global Vector Control Response (WHO, 2017; Roiz et al., 2019).

Concluding remarks

The spring of 2020 was indeed silent. But this silence was due not to the reasons outlined in Rachel Carson's book. A sky without planes, traffic without motion and the general economic shutdown were due to a pandemic. The dramatic experience of COVID-19 highlighted the novel fate of infectious diseases in our globalized world and called for integrating preventive measures for sustainable disease mitigation. Mosquito-borne diseases are a prime public health threat for the next global emergency. They require the utmost attention. At the same time, the preservation of biodiversity has become a major societal and ecological challenge requiring immediate action, with one of the most pressing moves being an escape from our insecticide era to protect our food and health.

In this world view, I propose the Mosquitome as a concept like that of the microbiome to emphasize: (1), that when dealing with major human disease-vector mosquitoes, one deals with a very tiny fraction of the overall mosquito biodiversity and one that relies on very specific ecological attributes; (2), that this specific assemblage of mosquito species is tightly associated with and dependent upon humans; and (3), that we have long lived with these creatures and should now learn to benefit from that close association. In this view, mosquito elimination is no longer an expected or even a desirable outcome. Rather, acknowledging the Mosquitome as an integral part of our immediate environment prompts our long-term commitment to its management. Vector control programmes need to be transformed into Mosquitome management strategies to achieve sustainability in disease risk-mitigation while helping preserve biodiversity and improving ecosystem functioning, locally and globally.

Bibliography

Ayala F.J., Coluzzi M. 2005. Chromosome speciation: Humans, *Drosophila* and mosquitoes. *Proc Natl Acad Sci U S A* 102(suppl.1):6535–6542.

Besansky N., Hill C., Costantini C.. 2004. No accounting for taste: Host preference in malaria vectors. *Trends Parasitol* 20(6):249–251.

Bruce-Chwatt L.J., Garrett-Jones C., Weitz B. 1966. Ten years' study (1955–1964) of host selection by anopheline mosquitos. *Bull Wld Hlth Org* 35:405–439.

Chouaibou M., Etang J., Brévault T., Nwane P., Hinzoumbé C.K., Mimpfoundi R., Simard F. 2008. Dynamics of insecticide resistance in the malaria vector *Anopheles gambiae* s.l. from an area of extensive cotton cultivation in Northern Cameroon. *Trop Med Int Hlth* 13(4):476–486.

Clements A.N. 1992. *The Biology of Mosquitoes. Volume 1. Development, Nutrition and Reproduction.* London: Chapman & Hall.

Cohen D. 1966. Optimizing reproduction in a randomly varying environment. *J Theor Biol* 12(1):119–129.

Cohuet A., Harris C., Robert V., Fontenille D. 2010. Evolutionary forces on *Anopheles*: What makes a malaria vector? *Trends Parasitol* 26(3):130–136.

Costantini C., Ayala D., Guelbeogo W.M., Pombi M., Some C.Y., Bassole I.H.N., Ose K., Fotsing J.M., Sagon N.F., Fontenille D., Besansky N.J., Simard F. 2009. Living at the edge: Biogeographic patterns of habitat segregation conform to speciation by niche expansion in *Anopheles gambiae*. *BMC Ecology* 9: 16.

Duvallet G., Robert V., Fontenille D., eds. 2017. *Entomologie Médicale et Vétérinaire.* Marseille: Editions QUAE.

Eritja R., Palmer J.R.B., Roiz D., Sanpera-Calbet I., Bartumeus F. 2017. Direct evidence of adult *Aedes albopictus* dispersal by car. *Sci Rep* 7(1):14399. doi: 10.1038/s41598-017-12652-5.

Ferguson H.M., Maire N., Takken W., Lyimo I.N., Briet O., Lindsay S.W., Smith T.A. 2012. Selection of mosquito life-histories: A hidden weapon against malaria? *Malar J* 11(1):106.

Garrett-Jones C. 1964. Prognosis for interruption of malaria transmission through assessment of the mosquito's vectorial capacity. *Nature* 204:1173–1175.

Gillies M.T. 1963. Observations on nulliparous and parous rates in some common East African mosquitoes. *Ann Trop Med Parasitol* 57:435–442.

Gillies M.T., De Meillon B. 1968. *The Anophelinae of Africa South of the Sahara (Ethiopian Zoogeographical Region).* 2nd edition. Johannesburg: South African Institute for Medical Research, N 54, 343p.

Gimonneau G., Pombi M., Choisy M., Morand S., Dabiré R.K., Simard F. 2012. Larval habitat segregation between the molecular forms of the mosquito, *Anopheles gambiae* in a rice field area of Burkina Faso, West Africa. *Med Vet Entomol* 26(1):9–17. doi:10.1111/j.1365-2915.2011.00957.x.

Hamon J. 1963. Etude de l'âge physiologique des femelles d'anophèles dans les zones traitées au DDT, et non traitées, de la region de Bobo-Dioulasso, Haute-Volta. *Bull Wld Hlth Org* 28:83–109.

Hawley A.H. 1988. The biology of *Aedes albopictus*. *J Am Mosq Control Assoc* 4:2–39.

Hemingway J., Ranson H., Magill A., Kolaczinski J., Fornadel C., Gimnig J., Coetzee M., Simard F., Dabiré K.R., Kerah Hinzoumbe C., Pickett J., Schellenberg D., Gething P., Hoppé M., Hamon N. 2016. Averting a malaria disaster: Will insecticide resistance derail malaria control? *Lancet* 387(10029):1785–1788. doi:10.1016/S0140-6736(15)00417-1.

Hulme-Beaman A., Dobney K., Cucchi T., Searle J.B. 2016. An ecological and evolutionary framework for commensalism in anthropogenic environments. *Trends Ecol Evol* 31(8): 633–645.

Johnson M.T.J., Munshi-South J. 2017. Evolution of life in urban environments. *Science* 358:607.

Lyimo I.N., Ferguson H.M. 2009. Ecological and evolutionary determinants of host species choice in mosquito vectors. *Trends Parasitol* 25(4):189–196.

Martin L.J., Adams R.I., Bateman A. and the NESCent Working Group on the Evolutionary Biology of the Built Environment. 2015. Evolution of the indoor biome. *Trends Ecol Evol* 30:223–232. doi: 10.1016/j.tree.2015.02.001

Michalakis Y., Renaud F. 2009. Evolution in vector control. *Nature* 462:298–300.

Moyes C.L., Vontas J., Martins A.J., Ng L.C., Koou S.Y., Dusfour I., Raghavendra K., Pinto J., Corbel V., David J.P., Weetman D. 2017. Contemporary status of insecticide resistance in the major Aedes vectors of arboviruses infecting humans. *PLoS Negl Trop Dis* 11(7):e0005625. doi:10.1371/journal.pntd.0005625.

Neafsey D.E., Waterhouse R.M., Abai M.R., Aganezov S.S., Alekseyev M.A., Allen J.E., Amon J., Arcà B., Arensburger P., Artemov G., Assour L.A., Basseri H., Berlin A., Birren B.W., Blandin S.A., Brockman A.I., Burkot T.R., Burt A., Chan C.S., Chauve C., Chiu J.C., Christensen M., Costantini C., Davidson V.L., Deligianni E., Dottorini T., Dritsou V., Gabriel S.B., Guelbeogo W.M., Hall A.B., Han M.V., Hlaing T., Hughes D.S., Jenkins A.M., Jiang X., Jungreis I., Kakani E.G., Kamali M., Kemppainen P., Kennedy R.C., Kirmitzoglou I.K., Koekemoer L.L., Laban N., Langridge N., Lawniczak M.K., Lirakis M., Lobo N.F., Lowy E., MacCallum R.M., Mao C., Maslen G., Mbogo C., McCarthy J., Michel K., Mitchell S.N., Moore W., Murphy K.A., Naumenko A.N., Nolan T., Novoa E.M., O'Loughlin S., Oringanje C., Oshaghi M.A., Pakpour N., Papathanos P.A., Peery A.N., Povelones M., Prakash A., Price D.P., Rajaraman A., Reimer L.J., Rinker D.C., Rokas A., Russell T.L., Sagnon N., Sharakhova M.V., Shea T., Simão F.A., Simard F., Slotman M.A., Somboon P., Stegniy V., Struchiner C.J., Thomas G.W., Tojo M., Topalis P., Tubio J.M., Unger M.F., Vontas J., Walton C., Wilding C.S., Willis J.H., Wu Y.C., Yan G., Zdobnov E.M., Zhou X., Catteruccia F., Christophides G.K., Collins F.H., Cornman R.S., Crisanti A., Donnelly M.J., Emrich S.J., Fontaine M.C., Gelbart W., Hahn M.W., Hansen I.A., Howell P.I., Kafatos F.C., Kellis M., Lawson D., Louis C., Luckhart S., Muskavitch M.A., Ribeiro J.M., Riehle M.A., Sharakhov I.V., Tu Z., Zwiebel L.J., Besansky N.J. 2015. Mosquito genomics. Highly evolvable malaria vectors: The genomes of 16 anopheles mosquitoes. *Science* 347(6217):1258522. doi:10.1126/science.1258522.

Paupy C., Delatte H., Bagny L., Corbel V., Fontenille D. 2009. *Aedes albopictus*, an arbovirus vector: From darkness to the light. *Microbes & Infection / Institut Pasteur* 11:1177–1185.

Powell J.R., Tabachnick W.J. 2013. History of domestication and spread of *Aedes aegypti* – A review. *Mem Inst Oswaldo Cruz* 108(Suppl.1):11–17.

Reiter P. 2007. Oviposition, dispersal, and survival in *Aedes aegypti*: Implications for the efficacy of control strategies. *Vector Borne Zoonotic Dis* 7(2):261–273. doi:10.1089/vbz.2006.0630.

Roche B., Broutin H., Simard F., eds. 2018. *Ecology and Evolution of Infectious Diseases: Pathogen Control and Public Health Management in Low-Income Countries.* Oxford: Oxford University Press. 322p. doi:10.1093/oso/9780198789833.001.0001

Roiz D., Wilson A.L., Scott T.W., Fonseca D.M., Jourdain F., Müller P., Velayudhan R., Corbel V. 2019. Integrated *Aedes* management for the control of *Aedes*-borne disease. *PLoS Negl Trop Dis* 12(12):e0006845. doi:10.1371/journal.pntd.0006845

Rose N.H., Sylla M., Badolo A., Lutomiah J., Ayala D., Aribodor O.B., Ibe N., Akorli J., Otoo S., Mutebi J.P., Kriete A.L., Ewing E.G., Sang R., Gloria-Soria A., Powell J.R., Baker R.E., White B.J., Crawford J.E., McBride C.S. 2020. Climate and urbanization drive mosquito preference for humans. *Curr Biol* 30(18):3570–3579.e6. doi:10.1016/j. cub.2020.06.092.

Simard F., Ayala D., Kamdem G.C., Pombi M., Etouna J., Ose K., Fotsing J.M., Fontenille D., Besansky N.J., Costantini C. 2009. Ecological niche partitioning between *Anopheles gambiae* molecular forms in Cameroon: The ecological side of speciation. *BMC Ecol* 9:17.

Stearns S.C., Ackermann M., Doebeli M., Kaiser M. 2000. Experimental evolution of aging, growth, and reproduction in fruitflies. *Proc Natl Acad Sci U S A* 97:3309–3313.

World Health Organization. 2017. *Global Vector Control Response 2017–2030*. Geneva. http://www.who.int/vector-control/publications/global-controlresponse/en/.

17

MOSQUITO UTOPIAS AND DYSTOPIAS

A dispatch from the front lines

Indra Vythilingam

Utopia is a term to describe things that are perfect in all aspects whereas a dystopia is just the opposite; both share characteristics of science fiction and fantasy. But when considering mosquitoes, one should bear in mind that these creatures have lived for aeons on planet Earth and they too need to survive. As mentioned in earlier chapters there are about 3,500 species of mosquitoes but only a few hundreds of them are disease vectors. They carry either viruses or parasites that can infect humans and animals and which can lead to mortality if not treated. However, to a lay person, a mosquito is a mosquito, and is responsible for the misery it causes.

Control measures are instituted only towards mosquitoes that are vectors. This is especially true in tropical countries which are burdened with vector-borne diseases. The control measures are targeted to the behaviour of the mosquitoes and thus, only some non-vector mosquitoes and insects will be affected by these measures. The World Health Organization promotes elimination of diseases like filariasis and malaria (WHO 2017) and many countries have obtained elimination status. But this does not mean that the vectors have all been eliminated. Rather, we have achieved "anophelism without malaria": the requisite vectors are still there but without the pathogens they used to carry. And in the case of malaria as well as other vector-borne diseases, it is only the female mosquitoes feeding on blood that transmit the disease.

How do mosquitoes behave in the human community? What are the forces which determine whether the diseases carried by them will sweep through, leaving a trail of death and disaster; or entrench themselves for a long-drawn struggle; or invade but lightly and disappear? There is no simple answer to this complex situation. Vector-borne diseases in a community are social expressions of the biological relationship between the pathogens, their human hosts and the mosquitoes which bring all of them together. The different species of mosquitoes

DOI: 10.4324/9781003056034-17

responsible for these different diseases have developed their roles very well and each species has its own niche as described in the early chapters of this book. We know that *Ae. aegypti* and to some extent *Ae. albopictus* are responsible for the spread of many arboviral diseases such as dengue (Solomon 2006). Some species of *Anopheles* are responsible for the spread of malaria while *Culex quinqefasciatus* and species of *Mansonia* are responsible for the transmission of filariasis (Wharton 1960). Unfortunately, Southeast Asia has the greatest number of *Anopheles* species that are vectors of malaria (Hii and Rueda 2013).

Here I summarize the various control measures that have been instituted against the vector mosquitoes and the pros and cons of the new control measures to be instituted. It is very clear that countries plagued by vector-borne diseases are only targeting the vector mosquitoes. All other mosquitoes on this planet can survive.

Anopheles and malaria

Although there has been great progress in the reduction of malaria infections over the years, the number of malaria cases worldwide in 2018 was about 228 million, of which 93% occurred in the African region, followed by 3.4% in Southeast Asia (WHO 2019). Fortunately, there are reasonably effective drugs to control malaria and so some might raise the question why should one even try to kill the mosquitoes? An argument in point is that the threat of malaria is not shared equally across the population: pregnant women and children are most susceptible to the disease, with high risk of mortality if not treated early enough. It is therefore of crucial importance to control these vector mosquitoes to prevent the transmission of the parasites to humans.

Control of *Anopheles* larvae

The history of malaria control in Malaya must be attributed to Sir Malcolm Watson who started his work here in Klang in 1900 (Watson 1921, Singh et al. 1988). As a district surgeon he was seeing many malaria cases in a district hospital, as in 1901 when there was a huge epidemic rampant in that region. Watson was attracted to the idea of trying to prevent malaria rather than merely treating cases admitted to the hospital. He initiated a programme of clearing and drainage of the foothill swamps in and around the town. They used both the herringbone drains and the foothill contour drains which proved to be effective (Watson 1921). The number of malaria cases fell from more than 300 in 1901 to 50 in 1903.

At about the same time in Port Swettenham (near Klang), which was opened in 1901, about 68% of the labourers and government staff came down with malaria. The species that was responsible for malaria in the area was *An. sundaicus* which was breeding in brackish water. Thus, bunding (or diking), drainage and the exclusion of saltwater by building tide-gates were carried out. These measures proved to be successful in the port area (Figure 17.1). Subsoil drains were also built in other areas around Kuala Lumpur where *An. maculatus* was the vector (Singh et al. 1988). These mosquitoes breed in streams open to sunlight.

Anti-malaria oil was also applied to all breeding sites. This was discontinued when oil became expensive and the insecticide Abate 500E was introduced. However, over time when these drains with clean water became sullage drains as people settled in these areas, larviciding was stopped since *Anopheles* breed in clean water and not in sullage (or dirty) water. As Watson described his work controlling mosquitoes: "As we learn more, perhaps the time will come when we shall be able to say to one species of *Anopheles*, 'Come,' and to another, 'Go,' and shall be able to abolish malaria with great ease, perhaps at hardly an expense" ((Watson 1921: 292) (Figure 17.1).

Control of *Anopheles* mosquitoes

DDT has been used for control of malaria vectors with success as mentioned in several chapters of this book. The publication of Rachel Carson's *Silent Spring* caused a hue and cry against the use of DDT, especially for agricultural purposes. However, for malaria control it would still be allowed on a case-by-case basis (Mouchet 1994). In Malaysia, a pilot project was started in 1960 in the coastal area of Selangor to determine the efficacy of DDT to control malaria. There were 33 *Anopheles* species in the area and of these only five were known to be vectors (Moorhouse 1965). DDT was sprayed at 2gm/m^2 on the inside walls

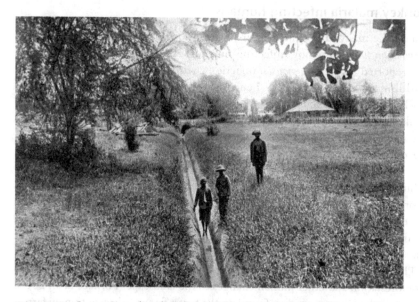

FIGURE 17.1 Inspecting a bunding near Klang. From Malcolm Watson 1921. The prevention of malaria in the Federated Malay States: a record of 20 years' progress. E.P. Dutton & Company.

of houses—referred to as indoor residual spraying (IRS). This was carried out because it was observed that the *Anopheles* mosquitoes, after entering the house, rest on the wall, bite a human and then rest on the wall again before flying out. Thus, *Anopheles* mosquitoes are able to absorb enough insecticide to kill themselves. The vectors were *An. campestris*, *An. letifer*, *An. maculatus*, *An. sundaicus* (now known as *An. epiroticus*) and *An. umbrosus*. The house-spraying apparently eradicated the *An. campestris* species but not the rest (Moorhouse 1965). This is mainly due to their different behaviour patterns.

With the introduction of DDT to malaria control and, of course, detection and treatment of human cases, malaria was considerably reduced in coastal areas but the results were less noticeable in the hilly areas of Malaysia. In the late 1980s it was observed that the *Anopheles* mosquitoes began entering houses to bite and then exit without resting on the walls. This was when insecticide-treated bed nets (ITNs) were tested and found to be useful. It has been reported that a large percentage of malaria has been reduced due to the use of ITNs (Fegan et al. 2007).

However, the problem now faced by the malaria programme is that the vectors are biting in the early part of the night and more commonly outdoors rather than indoors. Previously the peak biting times would be around 10.00–12.00 pm but now it is 7.00–8.00 pm. It should be noted that the control is targeted towards the vector; if other pest mosquitoes show similar behaviour, of course there is a possibility that they will be killed.

Monkey malaria infecting humans

Besides the main pathogens of human malaria, the simian malaria parasite of *Plasmodium knowlesi* is now infecting humans. All countries in Southeast Asia have reported cases of *P. knowlesi* infections, with the exception of Timor-Leste (Vythilingam et al. 2018). The Leucosphyrus group of *Anopheles* mosquitoes, which feeds on the long-tailed macaques, becomes infected by biting these monkeys and then transmitting the parasite to humans who they bite later. The first such case was reported in 1965 in Malaysia (Chin et al. 1965) and then a second case in the 1970s (Fong et al. 1971). After extensive research, it was postulated that simian malaria will remain in monkeys and will not be transmitted to humans (Warren et al. 1970). But then a large outbreak of *P. knowlesi* was reported in 2004 (Singh et al. 2004) to now become the predominant species affecting humans in Malaysia (Hussin et al. 2020). Moreover, a second simian malaria parasite, *P. cynomolgi*, is now being transmitted to humans in Southeast Asia (Ta et al. 2014, Singh et al. 2018, Grignard et al. 2019, Imwong et al. 2019).

The reason for the transmission of these two malaria parasites is perhaps due to deforestation and other human changes to the landscape (Fornace et al. 2019). Long-tailed macaques are now found on the forest fringe, adjacent to new farms, so that mosquitoes that were originally only forest-dwelling, have followed macaques to their new surroundings (Vythilingam et al. 2018). In the 1960s, mosquito species that were mainly biting macaques (Warren and Wharton 1963) are now biting both macaques and humans (Vythilingam et al. 2018). These mosquitoes are biting in the early part of the night and outdoors (Vythilingam et al. 2018), making control measures difficult to conduct since it is not possible to treat the macaques. Control of mosquitoes is especially difficult in the forest and forest fringes. This is how new diseases emerge all the time.

Aedes and arboviral diseases

Arboviruses transmitted by the *Aedes* mosquitoes (*Ae. aegypti* and *Ae. albopictus*) are mainly chikungunya, dengue and Zika. The history and natural history of each of these viruses have been well elaborated in various chapters of this book. Here I mainly add how other mosquitoes and insects can be affected by some indiscriminate methods used for controlling vector mosquitoes. For example, dengue became a problem in Southeast Asia in the early 1970s, but since there are no drugs to treat dengue, vector control became the hallmark for controlling this disease in the region.

House-to-house larval surveys

House-to-house larval surveys were conducted to compute the House Index and the Breteau Index, which are measures to determine the density of mosquitoes in an area. In most urban areas in the early 1970s and 1980s, water supply was a problem, so people used to store water, sometimes in open containers. As a result, the *Ae. aegypti* index was very high. With continuous house surveys and health education, the *Aedes* House Index in Malaysia has been reduced from 58.8% to 2.0% (Mudin 2015). Nonetheless, dengue cases have increased over the years. In Malaysia and in Singapore, the enactment of a new law, "The Destruction of Disease-Bearing Insects Act (DDBIA)," meant that people could be penalized if mosquitoes were found breeding in their homes (Ooi et al. 2006, Vythilingam and Wan-Yusoff 2017). People are now advised to apply the larvicide temephos (Abate 1 SG) to their storage water or else ensure that water containers are well covered to prevent mosquitoes from laying eggs there. In Vietnam, biological control with the crustacean, *Copepod mesocyclops*, has been used for feeding on the *Aedes* larvae (Nam et al. 2012).

Adult control

Fogging or ultra-low volume (ULV) insecticide spraying, is only carried out when dengue cases are reported, and this is done to kill infected adult mosquitoes to break the chain of transmission. All other mosquitoes and insects will be killed as well. Fogging is carried out at the house where the infection case occurred and in houses within 200 metres. However, during an epidemic, ULV spraying is conducted on a large scale since it can cover larger area. Studies have shown that ULV spraying is not very effective since the droplets only get carried as far as the living room of the house and thus mosquitoes hiding in closets and bedrooms will not be killed (Vythilingam and Wan-Yusoff 2017).

It was also found that there was no significant difference when ovitraps were set before fogging, during fogging and after fogging, as the first pupae emerged around day ten on all occasions (Chua et al. 2005). There was also no significant difference in the number of immature *Aedes* mosquitoes during the three fogging periods (Chua et al. 2005). It shows that the ULV spraying neither eliminated nor reduced the number of gravid *Aedes* mosquitoes. Forty-eight hours after ULV spraying, dead insects, spiders, and even small animals like frogs and snails were found in the ovitrap; in the garden, dead ants and spiders were also observed. Furthermore, one may assume that, following ULV treatment, the destruction of the natural predators of the mosquitoes could have contributed to the increase of immature mosquitoes (Chua et al. 2005). However, it is also known that *Ae. aegypti* are resistant to pyrethroids—the insecticides typically used in ULV (Leong et al. 2019)—especially in dengue epidemic areas. Other studies have also shown that space-spraying has not been effective in dengue epidemics (Esu et al. 2010). Since *Ae. aegypti* have been shown to be resistant to pyrethroids in most countries, mosquitoes are given an advantage if managers do not change insecticides.

Vectors of filariasis

Vectors of filariasis are varied. In Malaysia and the surrounding regions *Mansonia* mosquitoes are the main vector for Brugian filariasis. As a matter of fact, the first proof of transmission of a human disease by a mosquito was demonstrated by Patrick Manson in South China in 1878 (Mak 1983): Manson demonstrated that *Culex quinquefasciatus* was responsible for the transmission of *Wucheriria bancrofti* which had been discovered 15 years earlier. In India and other regions where *W. bancrofti* is predominant *Cx. quinquefasciatus* is the vector, whereas *Ae. Polynesinsis* is the vector in the Pacific islands. Some species of *Anopheles* are also vectors for filariasis. Thus, one can see that many different species of mosquitoes are involved in the transmission of filariasis. Unlike other vector-borne diseases, a single bite by an infected mosquito will not give rise to filariasis. A male and female microfilaria must be introduced before the person can be infected. In Malaysia, filariasis has been brought to very low levels. The control was based mainly on mass blood surveys and treatment of people rather than directed towards controlling mosquitoes.

Control of *Mansonia* mosquitoes

There are six species of *Mansonia* which have been incriminated as vectors: *Ma. annulata, Ma. annulifera, Ma. bonneae, Ma. dives, Ma. indiana* and *Ma. uniformis* (Wharton 1962). Early experiments in the laboratory showed that *Mansonia* were only moderately susceptible to DDT, dieldrin and benzene hexachloride (BHC). Semi-field trials in trap huts against three *Mansonia* species concluded that dieldrin was more effective than DDT and BHC. A pilot trial was conducted in an area along with mass treatment. There was a decrease in the microfilaria rate but no observable differences in the infection and transmission rates in the vectors (Wharton et al. 1958). This also could be due to animal reservoirs.

The physical removal of floating vegetation is one method of reducing the number of vectors since the immature stages are attached to the roots of plants. Large-scale drainage and irrigation schemes and developments like filling swamps have reduced vector populations. Along with drug administration it was possible to reduce the incidence of filariasis.

Culex and arboviral diseases

Various species of *Culex* mosquitoes are vectors of Japanese encephalitis (JE) and West Nile virus. West Nile virus occurs in North America, Africa, Europe, Middle East and West Asia. The *Culex* mosquitoes obtain the virus while feeding on birds and transmit it to humans. Human-to-human transmission does not take place in West Nile virus, nor in JE. JE is endemic in an area inhabited by about 1.9 billion people in Southeast Asia and Asia, being transmitted by many different species of *Culex* mosquitoes of which *Cx. tritaeniorhynchus* and *Cx. gelidus* are the main vectors (Vythilingam et al. 1997, Kabilan et al. 2004). Fortunately, a vaccine is available for JE. Although a number of JE isolates were found in various species of *Culex* mosquitoes in a study in Malaysia (Vythilingam et al. 1997), cases of JE are only sporadic and isolated transmissions occur occasionally.

Control of *Culex* vectors

To control the vectors of JE, it is recommended to carry out residual spraying of pig farms in endemic areas where the disease is a major problem. In other areas, houses surrounding the pig farms usually have screens on doors and windows to prevent the entry of mosquitoes. In rice-field areas where there is breeding of JE vectors, alternate wet and dry irrigation, or the use of fish or other natural products like *Azolla*, can be used to control the larvae (Keiser et al. 2005).

Culex quinquefasciatus is a cosmopolitan mosquito found in most parts of the world. It breeds in polluted water such as sewerage drains, cesspits, septic tanks, cesspools. This mosquito plays a major role in lymphatic filariasis; its control is difficult since it has developed insecticide resistance to all four classes of insecticides (Jones et al. 2012). Effective control of *Cx. quinquefaciatus* is best carried out by thoroughly cleaning the environment, as well as by source reduction and floating polystyrene beads into breeding sites (Jones et al. 2012).

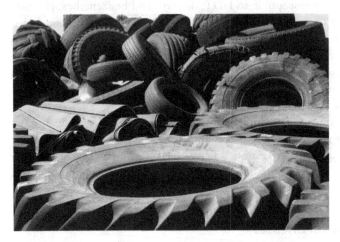

FIGURE 17.2 Discarded tyres near Perth, Australia (Creative Commons; photo by Alex
Dawson 2008).

Gene modification

Mosquitoes do not need passports to cross international borders. In an era in
which human agency has reached every corner of the globe and every aspect of
life on Earth, humans are responsible for the spreading of mosquitoes, especially
the *Aedes* genus whose eggs can withstand desiccation and are carried across
countries and oceans by water trapped in used tyres (Gubler 2012). Accordingly,
most of this genus and especially *Ae. albopictus* has established itself and will probably not be eliminated from the planet in the near future. Control measures are
only instituted if mosquitoes are found to be disease bearing (Figure 17.2).

One should also understand that it is not necessary for large numbers of mosquitoes to be present to cause a disease. For example, *Ae. aegypti* is easily dis-
turbed and thus can feed on multiple hosts to acquire a full blood meal (Scott et
al. 1993), meaning that if the mosquito is infected it can pass the pathogen on to
many people during a single blood meal (Platt et al. 1997). Singapore is a good
example, where the *Aedes* index is very low but where a large number of cases is
reported (Ooi et al. 2006).

Scientists have produced (and are producing) genetically modified (GM)
mosquitoes to help control the *Ae. aegypti* with mixed results. The UK biotech
company, Oxitec, has developed a mosquito inserted with a RIDL gene (release
of insects carrying a dominant lethal) that can only survive in water with tetracycline. The control strategy is to release the adult males into the wild so that
when they mate with the wild females, they will produce offspring that cannot
survive, since there is an absence of tetracycline (Massonnet-Bruneel et al. 2013).
In Brazil, following large releases of such a mosquito, there are now three different populations of the *Ae. aegypti* found in nature, with a significant transfer of
the tetracycline–dependent genome into the wild population. Eighteen months

after release of these GM mosquitoes, observations showed that the population which had been initially suppressed began to rebound, becoming as it was before release (Evans et al. 2019). The cautionary note is that these releases may end up promoting more robust populations of mosquitoes in the future, with ultimate effects on the ecosystem remaining unknown.

With the production of the GM mosquitoes, especially the *Anopheles*, one needs to understand that these mosquitoes are produced in laboratories either in the UK or in USA and they have to be shipped to and released in tropical countries where malaria occurs. The vectors for malaria are varied and many species are involved and the eggs cannot withstand desiccation. This would involve a huge sum of money for a developing country where malaria is occurring and specialized laboratories need to be set up for the production of the GM mosquitoes. Thus, such mosquitoes may only remain as a laboratory tool and are not realistic strategies for public health (Beisel and Boete 2013).

It is also a known fact that mosquitoes have developed resistance to insecticides by changing one or more of their genes (Hemingway et al. 2004) and that malaria parasites have developed resistance to drugs, including artemisinin (Ashley et al. 2014). It is therefore possible that in the long run these GM mosquitoes, which are refractory to the parasites, may one day become susceptible to them. At that point in time, malaria may rebound with a vengeance and the expertise to control the disease and vectors may not be available. We have lessons to learn from what has happened with the COVID-19 pandemic.

Most arthropods and insects are inhabited by *Wolbachia* bacteria (Moreira et al. 2009). However, *Wolbachia* is absent in *Ae. aegypti*. This observation led researchers to inoculate *Wolbachia* from drosophila into *Ae. aegypti*. Due to cytoplasmic incompatibility (CI), a male *Ae. aegypti* with *Wolbachia* that mates with the wild female will produce inviable progeny, meaning that release of male *Ae. aegypti* with *Wolbachia* can suppress this mosquito's population. In addition, a female *Ae. aegypti* with *Wolbachia* that mates with a wild male will produce all progeny with *Wolbachia*, which can be very advantageous for disease management since these bacteria are able to inhibit the ability of *Ae. aegypti* to carry dengue, chikungunya and Zika viruses (Moreira et al. 2009). As a result, the World Free Mosquito Programme felt it beneficial to release *Wolbachia*-infected *Ae. aegypti* in order to infect wild *Ae. aegypti* and make them incapable of spreading viral diseases. What will happen to this initiative in years to come? A recent study showed that *Ae. aegypti* infected with *Wolbachia* were still susceptible to chikungunya and Zika viruses at low levels and not entirely refractory as suggested in earlier studies (Tan et al. 2017). Studies also showed that *Wolbachia* blocked dengue virus in *Ae. aegypti* by 37.5% (Bian et al. 2010).

Community participation in vector control

It is not easy to eliminate mosquitoes from this planet. The common domestic *Ae. aegypti* was once nearly eliminated from the Americas in the 1930s but then rebounded after the programme was stopped (Dick et al. 2012). In theory it looks very simple to get rid of *Aedes* mosquitoes yet this species has been successful at colonizing new areas and causing more diseases despite human efforts to eradicate it. The typical top–down approach utilized by most governments was not very successful at removing breeding sites. Though successful for a short time, this eradication programme was not sustainable. Thus, it is now generally felt that a bottom-up approach will offer greater success at mosquito control. Community participation has been successful in Cuba, for example, where mosquito control has been more sustainable (Gubler and Clark 1996). Yet in Malaysia, even though community members have demonstrated good knowledge about dengue and its associated mosquitoes, they have shown little willingness to follow through with dengue control (Selvarajoo et al. 2020).

Even if a mosquito does not have the brain of a primate, it has been highly successful at living and sharing the planet with humans. Now researchers are producing GM mosquitoes and releasing them at large scale to outcompete wild mosquitoes. What researchers perhaps fail to appreciate is that GM mosquitoes will eventually die off, allowing wild mosquitoes to bounce back, possibly with a vengeance. Another irony is that we now tell community members that GM mosquitoes are our friends, so please do not kill them. What will happen in the future?

Environmental changes such as land-cover fluxes, deforestation and landscape modifications are also known to affect the distribution and density of mosquitoes. Such changes are the result of human processes. A changing climate can also promote a higher abundance of mosquitoes (Schaffner and Van Bortel 2013) and facilitate their development in a shorter time. It seems that the more humanity modifies the earth, the more that mosquitoes will thrive in our environment.

Conclusion

Since mosquito control is sometimes dependent on knowing the behaviour of the vectors, mosquitoes not exhibiting such behaviours may not be killed or eliminated. Mosquitoes also have the habit of changing their behaviour in order to escape being killed. When we speak of elimination of malaria or of filariasis, we are referring to eliminating the disease. But the species of mosquitoes responsible for transmitting these diseases will remain; thus the ecosystem will not be disrupted.

In the end, mosquitoes are part of the ecosystem and so will probably never be eliminated. Control measures only target the vector mosquitoes and will allow many other organisms to survive and provide food for still other organisms. The current trend in mosquito control is moving towards creating more mosquitoes, albeit ones that cannot transmit diseases. How far this strategy will succeed remains to be seen. Mosquitoes will not be wiped out from planet Earth. They are smarter than humans and will survive for years to come. To quote Andrew Spielman, "mosquitoes are well adapted to a very unstable, transient environment. They're the first organism in and the first out of a newly created body of water" (Spielman 2001). Mosquitoes are here to stay and there is a place for each species. Mosquitoes will thrive in the ecosystem as they have done for millions of years.

Bibliography

Ashley, E.A., M. Dhorda, R.M. Fairhurst, C. Amaratunga, P. Lim, S. Suon, S. Sreng, J.M. Anderson, S. Mao, B. Sam, and C. Sopha. 2014. Spread of artemisinin resistance in *Plasmodium falciparum* malaria. *New England Journal of Medicine* 371(5): 411–423.

Beisel, U., and C. Boëte. 2013. The flying public health tool: Genetically modified mosquitoes and malaria control. *Science as Culture* 22(1): 38–60.

Bian, G., Y. Xu, P. Lu, Y. Xie, and Z. Xi. 2010. The endosymbiotic bacterium *Wolbachia* induces resistance to dengue virus in *Aedes aegypti*. *PLoS Pathog* 6(4): e1000833.

Chin, W., P.G. Contacos, G.R. Coatney, and H.R. Kimball. 1965. A naturally acquired quotidian-type malaria in man transferable to monkeys. *Science* 149: 865.

Chua, K., I. Chua, I. Chua, and K. Chua. 2005. Effect of chemical fogging on immature *Aedes* mosquitoes in natural field conditions. *Singapore Medical Journal* 46: 639.

Dick, O.B., J.L. San Martín, R.H. Montoya, J. del Diego, B. Zambrano, and G.H. Dayan. 2012. The history of dengue outbreaks in the Americas. *American Journal of Tropical Medicine and Hygiene* 87: 584–593.

Esu, E., A. Lenhart, L. Smith, and O. Horstick. 2010. Effectiveness of peridomestic space spraying with insecticide on dengue transmission; systematic review. *Tropical Medicine & International Health* 15: 619–631.

Evans, B.R., P. Kotsakiozi, A.L. Costa-da-Silva, R.S. Ioshino, L. Garziera, M.C. Pedrosa, A. Malavasi, J.F. Virginio, M.L. Capurro, and J.R. Powell. 2019. Transgenic *Aedes aegypti* mosquitoes transfer genes into a natural population. *Scientific Reports* 9: 1–6.

Fegan, G.W., A.M. Noor, W.S. Akhwale, S. Cousens, and R.W. Snow. 2007. Effect of expanded insecticide-treated bednet coverage on child survival in rural Kenya: A longitudinal study. *Lancet* 370: 1035–1039.

Fong, Y.L., F.C. Cadigan, and G.R. Coatney. 1971. A presumptive case of naturally occurring *Plasmodium knowlesi* malaria in man in Malaysia. *Transactions of the Royal Society of Tropical Medicine and Hygiene* 65: 839.

Fornace, K.M., N. Alexander, T.R. Abidin, P.M. Brock, T.H. Chua, I. Vythilingam, H.M. Ferguson, B.O. Manin, M.L. Wong, and S.H. Ng. 2019. Local human movement patterns and land use impact exposure to zoonotic malaria in Malaysian Borneo. *eLife* 8: e47602.

Grignard, L., S. Shah, T.H. Chua, T. William, C.J. Drakeley, and K.M. Fornace. 2019. Natural human infections with *Plasmodium cynomolgi* and other malaria species in an elimination setting in Sabah, Malaysia. *The Journal of Infectious Diseases* 220: 1946–1949.

Gubler, D.J. 2001. Human arbovirus infections worldwide. *Annals of the New York Academy of Sciences* 951: 13–24.

Gubler, D.J. 2012. The economic burden of dengue. *American Journal of Tropical Medicine and Hygiene* 86: 743–744.

Gubler, D.J., and G.G. Clark. 1996. Community involvement in the control of *Aedes aegypti*. *Acta Tropica* 61: 169–179.

Hemingway J, Hawkes NJ, McCarroll L, Ranson H. 2004. The molecular basis of insecticide resistance in mosquitoes. *Insect Biochemistry and Molecular Biology* 34(7):653–665.

Hii, J., and L. Rueda. 2013. Malaria vectors in the Greater Mekong Subregion: Overview of malaria vectors and remaining challenges. *Southeast Asian Journal of Tropical Medicine and Public Health* 44(Supplement 1): 73–165.

Hussin, N., Y.A.L. Lim, P.P. Goh, T. William, J. Jelip, and R.N. Mudin. 2020. Updates on malaria incidence and profile in Malaysia from 2013 to 2017. *Malaria Journal* 19: 55.

Imwong, M., W. Madmanee, K. Suwannasin, C. Kunasol, T.J. Peto, R. Tripura, L. von Seidlein, C. Nguon, C. Davoeung, and N.P. Day. 2019. Asymptomatic natural human infections with the simian malaria parasites *Plasmodium cynomolgi* and *Plasmodium knowlesi*. *The Journal of Infectious Diseases* 219: 695–702.

Jones, C.M., C. Machin, K. Mohammed, S. Majambere, A.S. Ali, B.O. Khatib, J. Mcha, H. Ranson, and L.A. Kelly-Hope. 2012. Insecticide resistance in *Culex quinquefasciatus* from Zanzibar: Implications for vector control programmes. *Parasites & Vectors* 5: 78.

Kabilan, L., R. Rajendran, N. Arunachalam, S. Ramesh, S. Srinivasan, P.P. Samuel, and A. Dash. 2004. Japanese encephalitis in India: An overview. *Indian Journal of Pediatrics* 71: 609–615.

Keiser, J., M.F. Maltese, T.E. Erlanger, R. Bos, M. Tanner, B.H. Singer, and J. Utzinger. 2005. Effect of irrigated rice agriculture on Japanese encephalitis, including challenges and opportunities for integrated vector management. *Acta Tropica* 95: 40–57.

Leong, C.-S., I. Vythilingam, J.W.-K. Liew, M.-L. Wong, W.S. Wan-Yusoff, and Y.-L. Lau. 2019. Enzymatic and molecular characterization of insecticide resistance mechanisms in field populations of *Aedes aegypti* from Selangor, Malaysia. *Parasites & Vectors* 12: 236.

Mak, J. 1983. *Filariasis*. Kuala Lumpur: Institute for Medical Research, p. 108.

Massonnet-Bruneel, B., N. Corre-Catelin, R. Lacroix, R.S. Lees, K.P. Hoang, D. Nimmo, L. Alphey, and P. Reiter. 2013. Fitness of transgenic mosquito *Aedes aegypti* males carrying a dominant lethal genetic system. *PloS One* 8: e62711.

Moorhouse, D.E. 1965. Some entomological aspects of the malaria eradication pilot project in Malaya. *Journal of Medical Entomology* 2: 109–119.

Moreira, L.A., I. Iturbe-Ormaetxe, J.A. Jeffery, G. Lu, A.T. Pyke, L.M. Hedges, B.C. Rocha, S. Hall-Mendelin, A. Day, and M. Riegler. 2009. A *Wolbachia* symbiont in *Aedes aegypti* limits infection with dengue, chikungunya, and *Plasmodium*. *Cell* 139: 1268–1278.

Mouchet, J. 1994. DDT and public health. *Cahiers d'études et de recherches francophones / Santé* 4: 257–262.

Mudin, R.N. 2015. Dengue incidence and the prevention and control programme in Malaysia. *International Medical Journal Malaysia* 14: 5–9.

Nam, V.S., N.T. Yen, H.M. Duc, T.C. Tu, V.T. Thang, N.H. Le, L. Le Loan, V.T.Q. Huong, L.H.K. Khanh, and H.T.T. Trang. 2012. Community-based control of *Aedes aegypti* by using *Mesocyclops* in southern Vietnam. *American Journal of Tropical Medicine and Hygiene* 86: 850–859.

Ooi, E.-E., K.-T. Goh, and D.J. Gubler. 2006. Dengue prevention and 35 years of vector control in Singapore. *Emerging Infectious Diseases* 12: 887.

Platt, K.B., K.J. Linthicum, K. Myint, B.L. Innis, K. Lerdthusnee, and D.W. Vaughn. 1997. Impact of dengue virus infection on feeding behavior of *Aedes aegypti*. *American Journal of Tropical Medicine and Hygiene* 57: 119–125.

Schaffner F and Van Bortel AW. 2013. Public health significance of invasive mosquitoes in Europe. *Clinical Microbiology and Infection* 19: 685–692.

Scott, T.W., E. Chow, D. Strickman, P. Kittayapong, R.A. Wirtz, L.H. Lorenz, and J.D. Edman. 1993. Blood-feeding patterns of *Aedes aegypti* (Diptera: Culicidae) collected in a rural Thai village. *Journal of Medical Entomology* 30: 922–927.

Selvarajoo, S., J.W.K. Liew, W. Tan, X.Y. Lim, W.F. Refai, R.A. Zaki, N. Sethi, W.Y.W. Sulaiman, Y.A.L. Lim, and J. Vadivelu. 2020. Knowledge, attitude and practice on dengue prevention and dengue seroprevalence in a dengue hotspot in Malaysia: A cross-sectional study. *Scientific Reports* 10: 1–13.

Singh, B., K. Kadir, T. Hu, T. Raja, D. Mohamad, L. Lin, and K. Hii. 2018. Naturally acquired human infections with the simian malaria parasite, *Plasmodium cynomolgi*, in Sarawak, Malaysian Borneo. *International Journal of Infectious Diseases* 73: 68.

Singh, B., L.K. Sung, A. Matusop, A. Radhakrishnan, S.S.G. Shamsul, J. Cox-Singh, A. Thomas, and D.J. Conway. 2004. A large focus of naturally acquired *Plasmodium knowlesi* infections in human beings. *Lancet* 363: 1017–1024.

Singh, J., A.S. Tham, and WHO. 1988. *Case History on Malaria Vector Control Through the Application of Environmental Management in Malaysia*. Geneva: World Health Organization.

Solomon, T. 2006. Control of Japanese encephalitis-within our grasp? *New England Journal of Medicine* 355: 869.

Spielman, A. 2001. *Mosquito: A Natural History of Our Most Persistent and Deadly Foe*. New York: Hyperion.

Ta, T.H., S. Hisam, M. Lanza, A.I. Jiram, N. Ismail, and J.M. Rubio. 2014. First case of a naturally acquired human infection with *Plasmodium cynomolgi*. *Malaria Journal* 13: 1–7.

Tan, C.H., P.J. Wong, M.I. Li, H. Yang, L.C. Ng, and S.L. O'Neill. 2017. wMel limits zika and chikungunya virus infection in a Singapore Wolbachia-introgressed *Ae. aegypti* strain, wMel-Sg. *PLoS Neglected Tropical Diseases* 11: e0005496.

Vythilingam, I., K. Oda, S. Mahadevan, G. Abdullah, C.S. Thim, C.C. Hong, B. Vijayamalar, M. Sinniah, and A. Igarashi. 1997. Abundance, parity, and Japanese encephalitis virus infection of mosquitoes (Diptera: Culicidae) in Sepang District, Malaysia. *Journal of Medical Entomology* 34: 257–262.

Vythilingam, I., and W. Wan-Yusoff. 2017. Dengue vector control in Malaysia: Are we moving in the right direction. *Tropical Biomedicine* 34: 746–758.

Vythilingam, I., M. Wong, and W. Wan-Yussof. 2018. Current status of *Plasmodium knowlesi* vectors: A public health concern? *Parasitol* 145: 32–40.

Warren, M.W., W.H. Cheong, H.K. Fredericks, and G.R. Coatney. 1970. Cycles of jungle malaria in West Malaysia. *American Journal of Tropical Medicine and Hygiene* 19: 383.

Warren, M.W., and R.H. Wharton. 1963. The vectors of simian malaria: Identity, biology, and geographical distribution. *Journal of Parasitolology* 49: 892–904.

Watson, M. 1921. *The Prevention of Malaria in the Federated Malay States: A Record of Twenty Year's Progress*. New York: E.P. Dutton & Company.

Wharton, R. 1960. Studies on filariasis in Malaya: Field and laboratory investigations of the vectors of a rural strain of Wuchereria bancrofti. *Annals of Tropical Medicine and Parasitology* 54: 78–91.

Wharton, R., J. Edeson, T. Wilson, and J. Reid. 1958. Studies on filariasis in Malaya: Pilot experiments in the control of filariasis due to Wuchereria malayi in East Pahang. *Annals of Tropical Medicine & Parasitology* 52: 191–205.

Wharton, R.H. 1962. The biology of *Mansonia* mosquitoes in relation to transmission of filariasis in Malaya. *Bulletin of the Institute for Medical Research, Malaysia* 11: 1–114.

World Health Organization. 2017. *A Framework for Malaria Elimination*. Geneva: World Health Organization.

World Health Organization. 2019. *World Malaria Report 2019*. Reference Source.

AFTERWORD

Ashwani Kumar

Mosquitoes and their survival instincts fascinate. Yet, in matters of mosquitoes, one gets caught in a dilemma. Mosquitoes do both good and bad to humanity. One must consider whether nature could do without these blood seekers and disease agents? Not really—for not all mosquito species are disease vectors! Shall we or shall we not let them go? Have we not tried enough and failed? Have we learned our lessons yet or not? These are some of the questions that come to mind when considering the lessons of Mosquitopia.

Our knowledge about mosquitoes is not new. In ancient India, Susruta the author of Susruta Samhita in the second century AD described five kinds of mosquitoes (or "Mashakah") in Sanskrit, namely, Samudrah (marine or coastal mosquito), Parimandalah (very small mosquito), Hastimashakah (elephant mosquito), Krishnah (black mosquito) and Parawatiyah (hill/foothill mosquito). Rao (1984) mentions that from these divisions of mosquito taxa, knowledge about mosquitoes in India is at least 1,800 years old.

The destruction that mosquitoes cause!

Historically, mosquitoes were perceived as the agents of disruption and havoc of various human civilizations. Together with their pathogens and parasites, mosquitoes colluded in killing more people than all the wars fought on the earth. Even the mightiest of warriors, the likes of "Alexander the Great," fell to a bite of a mosquito laden with *Plasmodium*. Mosquitoes showed no mercy on the Vatican clergy either. In August 1590, Pope Sixtus V and, a month later, his successor Urban VII, died of malignant fever (Celli 1925). In a disastrous Vatican conclave of 1632, eight cardinals and 30 secretaries succumbed to the deadly *Plasmodium*. Mosquitoes were certainly not God-fearing.

Hate at first sight

The very sight of a mosquito annoys and irks. The immediate and voluntary response is to squash it before it syringes out the "red fluid" from the vein. Terrified humans have called mosquitoes "pesky bastards," "agents of doom," "flying syringes," "nasty and evil" and all else. Ranting frustration against a fellow species, however justified, is morally and ethically misplaced as we are informed by *Mosquitopia*. After all, it's simply the game of survival that species play in nature.

From sledge hammer to resurrection

From an evolutionary perspective, mosquitoes are far superior to humans. Mosquitoes display a remarkable instinct for survival through plasticity in their behaviour which is intimately attuned to their immediate environs. Perfecting life strategies seem to be their constant endeavour. It is in the greatest interest of humankind to preserve mosquitoes for the good they do by way of their ecosystem services in the food web and pollination of plants. They are the objects of scientific curiosity as one of nature's supreme manifestations of millions of years of evolution.

To start off this volume, Marcus Hall and Dan Tamir make a compelling case for a balanced approach while dealing with these wonderful creatures. The sledge hammer approach to eliminating mosquitoes has only led to their greater fitness, in their opinion. They conclude: In the end, rather than pushing an ultimatum that it must be us or them, can humans promote and practice a kind of "Mosquitopia" with these little humming creatures, humanity's most dangerous companions? Could we develop a relationship with this insect that will allow healthy cohabitation?

A manifestation of fascinating evolution

In Chapter 2, we have Hawkes and Hopkins's excellent descriptions of the mosquito's powerful sensors; its ability to match wingbeats as nuptial strategy; the variety of host-seeking cues; the advanced blood-sucking armature or proboscis; its blood-feeding strategies of piercing and locating the vein; the properties of its saliva that are angiogenic, inflammatory and anaesthetic; and its fecundity and breeding choices. Their indomitable survival instincts only raise one's inquisitiveness about the innumerable classical features of these amazing creatures and are a powerful reminder of how far mosquitoes have come in their evolutionary journey. By appearance, so beautiful are some of the mosquito species that they will give high-fashion models a run for their money! A look at the shiny and the multi-hued *Sabethes cyaneus* will leave no doubts in one's mind (Figure 18.1).

The discovery of an amber fossil of a mosquito in Canada resembling *Paleoculicis minutus* suggests that today's mosquito personifies a refined biological system by

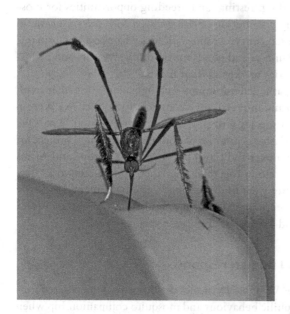

FIGURE 18.1 *Sabethes cyaneus*, mosquito (photo: Paul). Source: https://featuredcreature.
com/now-this-is-buzzworthy-species-of-mosquito-is-worlds-most-bea
utiful/

taking advantage of at least 79 million years of evolution. It then becomes obvious that a mere 300,000-year-old hominid, *Homo sapiens*, may be no match for
this sophisticated bio-machine that has been engineered, shaped and perfected
for millions of years.

Such different time scales suggest that human evolution is on a hopelessly slow
track when it comes to accumulating and transferring useful mutational changes
and genetic recombinations to future generations. Thus, it takes about 6,570
days (or 18 years) for humans to become biologically productive and start one
new generation. During the same time, with 40 days of maximum life, a typical mosquito would pass through some 164 generations. Even adjusting for the
several months spent in hibernating eggs (in inclement weather) and overlapping
generations, the mosquito's wheel of life turns much faster than that of humans
to provide these insects with much faster natural selection advantages.

An entangled destiny of mosquitoes and humans

Mosquitoes and humans are companions. Uli Beisel and Carsten Wergin
(Chapter 3) remind us that mosquito–human entanglements can be "infrastructuring environments." Loss of biodiversity, global warming, and heightening trade and travel provide new opportunities for sharing environments for
resources and habitats so that humans actively promote mosquito expansion with

their mobility and create feeding, resting, and breeding opportunities for mosquitoes. Citing the expanding distribution of *Aedes aegypti* and *Aedes albopictus* in Europe and Americas with used car tyres, and with lucky bamboo in Germany, they point out that "Just as humans and goods move, disease vectors and pathogens utilize global connectivities to expand their habitat."

Elaborating on human–pathogen–mosquito entanglements, together with global warming and accelerating inter-country connectivity, Beisel and Wergin predict that several mosquito species will find new ways to expand. The One Belt One Road (OBOR) initiative is just one ongoing infrastructural project for enhancing maritime trade and overland travel between Asia, Europe and Africa that will bring the world ever closer together. Vigilance of these networks may also provide insights into better ways for hindering vector movement, especially at the points of entry. The International Health Regulations division of WHO remind us that movement and expansion of invasive species is real.

The mosquito surge and human response

In Chapter 5, Urmi Engineer Willoughby argues that humans domesticated vectors by promoting anthropophilic behaviour and mosquito companionship when human settlers and slaves cultivated sugarcane in the Americas during the nineteenth century. Tenacious mosquito behaviour led to their evolutionary success, and their ability to pose an ongoing threat to humanity. Bill Gates calls them "the deadliest animal in the world" (Gates 2006).

Our early shot at a mosquito

Mosquito control campaigns in the last two centuries have been focused on water drainage and marsh reclamation resulting in a significant impact on vector populations and in reducing malaria burden (James Webb, Chapter 4). This was followed by the use of Paris Green, as in the project of eliminating *Anopheles arabiensis* from Northeast Brazil, and *Anopheles gambiae* from Egypt during one of the most meticulous anti-mosquito campaigns that led to the successful eradication of these two invasive malaria vectors. Buoyed by these successes led by Fred L. Soper, the Rockefeller Foundation sought to eradicate *Anopheles labranchiae* from the island of Sardinia in Italy with DDT as larvicide and adulticide. Although mosquito numbers were drastically reduced, thereby eliminating malaria, complete eradication of the vector proved elusive, with *An. labranchiae* returning to occupy its lost ground in later decades. Similar projects were carried out against *Aedes aegypti* in Brazil starting in 1947. Although highly successful in its initial years, *Aedes aegypti* numbers in South America would return by the 1960s. Moreover, the collateral damage of DDT was showing greater manifestations around the globe, leading to the destruction of non-target fauna. Rachel Carson's famous *Silent Spring* (1962), which painted a picture of a world without birdsong, evoked a strong response. Subsequent environmentalism and activism led to restricting DDT in agriculture and public health. Webb reminds us that only a few mosquito species are vectors, and that removing other species of mosquitoes and non-target organisms could prove perilous to humanity.

One sees that the battle of survival and superiority between humans and mosquitoes has been raging for centuries. And for the most part, mosquitoes have been holding the upper hand. One wonders who will have "the last laugh." Can humans achieve the Sisyphean task of exterminating mosquitoes even if they wished to? Could we or should we accept the inevitable and halt our fight for environmental, biological and mechanical reasons so that we can settle for something less than elimination of the invincible mosquito? Fred L. Soper's fight-to-finish strategy to William Gorgas' calibrated and selective approaches provide us with lessons to guide our future course as explained by Nancy L. Stepan (Chapter 6). The very thought of eradication appears to be misplaced and in a quagmire: the goal should remain that of reduction, not complete elimination, of vector populations.

The mosquito as art

What an inspiring and fascinating impression that artists Kerry Morrison and Helmut Lemke (Chapter 10) create in the minds of the wetland visitors and the readers from their mobile carrier, Wetlands on Wheels (WoW)! Viewing the world from the eyes of an artist adds another dimension to the nature of complexities. Fantasizing about mosquitoes to awaken human sensitivities through the medium of art brings together science and culture on the single canvas of life.

Mosquito and human rights

Do mosquitoes have rights as individuals and as species? Anna Wienhues (Chapter 13) questions the very morality of humans in killing an individual mosquito and also in trying to eliminate and eradicate mosquito species. It becomes apparent that the principle of hubris and risk applies to *Homo sapiens* in their quest to dominate all life forms on the planet in the sense of ownership. Wienhues points out that even if some mosquitoes act as vehicles for disease agents, they are, themselves, innocent victims. In defending their action for preventing infection and suffering, making a case for the extinction of an entire species is totally unjustified both morally and ethically, even though it may not be physically and biologically plausible. Also, can a few humans who venture to exterminate mosquitoes assume the moral and ethical responsibility of all humanity? Is moral, political, financial and informed consent crucial for such responsibility? Even if killing disease agents and vectors is justified as a matter of human rights, the talk of eradicating mosquitoes may be against a mosquito's natural rights.

Mosquito management

Management of pestiferous mosquitoes, and drainage of wetlands in the early twentieth century proved a practical and sustainable control strategy on Hayling Island, in South West England, and in the New Jersey marshlands. How mosquitoes harassed the guests of John F. Marshall, including Ronald Ross in 1922, is a telling story (Chapter 7, Peter Coates). The successes of the British Mosquito Control institute (BMCI) in draining the Hayling island marshlands in three years using tropical wisdom was an astonishing feat. During a subsequent visit to the same island in 1925, not a single bite was experienced by Ross and other guests. This points to the fact that today's highly chemical-dependent approach is short-term, never-ending and unsustainable. The integration of decades of gathered wisdom must shape the future of mosquito control. Suffice to mention that humans often live close to marshlands for food and livelihood, as emphasized by Ford, Gearey and Acott (Chapter 9).

In present times, William Takken (Chapter 8), advocates community engagement and implementing an integrated approach, that of combining environmental management (e.g. effective drainage) with housing improvements (mosquito-proofing and screening), biological control (with larvivorous fish and *Bacillus thruringiensis israelensis*), bio-rationale methods (insect growth regulators and attractive toxic sugar baits), chemical control (indoor residual spray and long-lasting insecticide nets) and behavioural control (repellents/attractants). All of these methods form the backbone of the Global Vector Control Response of the WHO which stresses operational research and global entomological capacity-building as a foundation for judicious interventions in a sustainable control strategy.

Alex Nading (Chapter 12) raises an interesting issue of ambivalence while dealing with mosquitoes. On the one hand, there is talk of extermination of mosquitoes, and on the other, the same insects are modified and propagated for human welfare. As an example of this ambivalence, *Wolbachia* is a gram-negative endosymbiont bacterium naturally present in about 60% of insect species and has the ability to check dengue, chikungunya, and Zika viruses. However, *Wolbachia* infection in *Aedes aegypti* (the vector of these viruses) is rare. This observation has convinced the World Mosquito Programme (WMP) to advocate the release of *Wolbachia*-infected *Aedes aegypti* from the laboratory for curbing these viruses. Interestingly, the mating of a *Wolbachia*-infected male *Aedes aegypti* with an uninfected wild female will cause cytoplasmic incompatibility, resulting in sterile eggs. Over a period of time, this mating process will eliminate the local wild *Aedes aegypti* population, thereby diminishing the associated vector-borne diseases.

Isabelle Dusfour and Sarah Cunard Chaney (Chapter 14) list various methods employed to control mosquitoes and feel that most such methods have reached the end of their chemical life since mosquitoes have become quite resistant to most insecticides. Biological control agent *Bacillus thuringiensis israelensis* has, by and large, proved itself to be safer and more effective than the larvicide temephos. Newer tools and techniques have become available such as releasing genetically modified insects with a dominant lethal gene (RIDL), sterile insect technique (SIT), insect incompatibilities with *Wolbachia*-modified mosquitoes (IIT) and gene drive. These methods are, however, at an early stage of experimentation as explained by Ramya Rajagopalan (Chapter 15). Paradoxically, many of the above techniques require mass production of mosquitoes in the laboratory for release in the field to control or replace wild populations. In the ongoing scrutiny of the safety and desirability of these latest control techniques, the authors conclude that it is more critical than ever to search for a sustainable and acceptable equilibrium that simultaneously preserves human health and protects the environment. One must aim to integrate the social aspects of mosquito-borne diseases with the ecological habits of the mosquitoes that transmit those diseases.

Indra Vythilingam (Chapter 17) highlights the worldwide campaign to eliminate malaria and filariasis with the support of the WHO. She professes how vectors and vector-borne diseases evolved and were addressed with different tools and strategies in Malaysia. Her most striking example shows how deforestation and human settlements led *Anopheles* to infect humans with *Plasmodium knowlesi*, a monkey malaria originating in local macaques. The author cautions against the use of genetically modified mosquitoes, citing the example of Oxitec *Aedes aegypti*. Eighteen months after the release of these GM mosquitoes, observations showed that the wild population which had initially been suppressed began to rebound to pre-release levels (Evans et al. 2019). The cautionary note here is that these releases may end up promoting more robust populations of mosquitoes in the future, with ultimate consequences for the ecosystem remaining unknown. It may also be an unrealistic or uneconomic strategy for many disease-endemic countries to set up sophisticated, GM-mosquito–producing laboratories, and then transport, monitor and evaluate GM- or *Wolbachia*-transinfected vector populations. Vythilingam underscores the paradox of convincing communities to carry out repeated releases of mosquitoes rather than preventing mosquito breeding in the first place.

An enigma of sorts!

From an anthropological perspective and the Brazilian narrations of Jean Segata (Chapter 11), one realizes the complexity of combining existing mosquito populations, patients ailing with yellow fever, and equivocal responses of authorities with yet another Aedes-borne outbreak that worsens incidence of dengue, chikungunya and Zika. As the face of disease changes its epidemiological dimensions, human perceptions and disease-detection technologies need to occupy the already crowded space for effective responses from municipalities, health workers, bureaucrats and political leaders. The mosquito, the scientists and their research and the healthcare institutions, alongside the human suffering, when combined with public health measures and job security of mosquito workers, all become nuts and bolts of the same inexorable machine: "the disease." The very movement of this machine depends on a disease continuum, its modulations and its dimensions in time and space. What an enigma of sorts!

The Mosquitome

Frederic Simard introduces (in Chapter 16) the intriguing concept of the "Mosquitome," which by his definition is the assemblage of mosquitoes that thrive where people live. He reminds us that human transformations of the natural environment are responsible for creating opportunities and habitat for mosquitoes, with the Mosquitome being composed of a handful of highly synanthropic mosquito species. This concept helps to separate mosquitoes into disease vectors living in the vicinity of human settlements from those that do not cause us harm—and indeed may carry out important roles in ecosystems. Here, elimination of mosquitoes should not be the goal; rather, the main strategy should focus on methods to reduce longevity and control mosquitoes of the Mosquitome so that they do not transmit their pathogens. Quoting Michalakis and Renaud (2009), Simard mentions that opportunities exist to disentangle vector fitness from pathogen transmission. *Beauvaria* and *Wolbachia* are considered good candidates for the late-life control of mosquitoes. In this way, mosquitoes can lay eggs but die before infecting humans with dangerous microbes. Local breeding containers and puddles must be drained; house-screening and insect-proofing will reinforce a methodology that targets the Mosquitome.

Mosquitopia

Mosquitopia is thus a treasure trove in the hands of explorers, nature lovers, entomologists and mosquito managers alike. It is an assemblage of deep insights into the world of mosquitoes, and is as much a philosophical expression of human appreciation of nature as it is a catalogue of the human successes and failures when dealing with mosquitoes. The volume sounds a wake-up call for the human race that stands at the crossroads of the old and the new, still searching for tools and methods to limit mosquitoes. *Mosquitopia* is a timely statement when global warming's effects are appearing more ominous in a world that is poised to further empower the old foe. Our wise authors implore us to raise human conscience and steer away from the aims of extermination and eradication and towards appreciating the moral and ethical rights of all life forms. Mosquitoes arrived several million years before *Homo sapiens* walked on this planet and will surely continue buzzing much after our species is gone. The sane approach? To "live and let live".

> A mosquito!
> Tiny and fascinating
> superbly adapted

amazingly powered
hated and victimized
facing extinction
returned emboldened
Better thee understand
my rights in thy space
A shared destiny
Better humans beware!

Bibliography

Balaji, Sivaraman, Seetharaman Jayachandran, and Solai Ramatchandirane Prabagaran. 2019. Evidence for the natural occurrence of *Wolbachia* in *Aedes aegypti* mosquitoes. *FEMS Microbiology Letters* 366(6):fnz055. doi: 10.1093/femsle/fnz055.

Celli, A. 1925. *Storia della malaria nell'agro romano*. Roma: Academia dei Lincei.

Evans, B.R., P. Kotsakiozi, A.L. Costa-da-Silva, R.S. Ioshino, L. Garziera, M.C. Pedrosa, A. Malavasi, J.F. Virginio, M.L. Capurro, and J.R. Powell. 2019. Transgenic *Aedes aegypti* mosquitoes transfer genes into a natural population. *Scientific Reports* 9: 1–6.

Gates, Bill. 2006. Mapping the end of malaria. In *GatesNotes*, October 10. https://www.gatesnotes.com/Health/Mapping-the-End-of-Malaria on 17.10.2020.

Michalakis, Y., and F. Renaud. 2009. Evolution in vector control. *Nature* 462: 298–300.

Rao, T.R. 1984. *The Anophelines of India*. New Delhi: Malaria Research Centre, 518.

INDEX

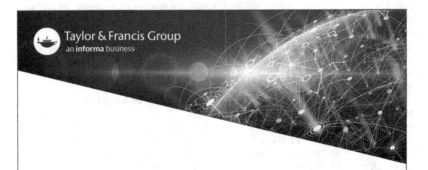

Printed in the United States
by Baker & Taylor Publisher Services